CHANGING PATTERNS
of INFECTIOUS
DISEASE

CHANGING PATTERNS of INFECTIOUS DISEASE

LOIS M. BERGQUIST, Ph.D.

Professor of Microbiology,
Los Angeles Valley College,
Van Nuys, California

and

Consulting Microbiologist,
Saint Joseph Medical Center,
Burbank, California

Lea & Febiger   *Philadelphia   1984*

Lea & Febiger
600 Washington Square
Philadelphia, Pa. 19106-4198
U.S.A.
(215) 922-1330

Library of Congress Cataloging in Publication Data

Bergquist, Lois M.
  Changing patterns of infectious disease.

  Bibliography: p.
  Includes index.
  1. Communicable diseases—Diagnosis. 2. Micro-
organisms, Pathogenic—Identification. I. Title.
[DNLM: 1. Communicable diseases—Microbiology. WC 100
B499c]
RC112.B37   1984   616.9′0475   84-3957
ISBN 0-8121-0940-6

Printed in the United States of America

Print Number: 4   3   2   1

To Scott Barrett Paul

PREFACE

Life is unfair. No sooner do you get one problem solved than another one, often worse, rises up to take its place.

—John F. Kennedy

Despite the large number of texts available on infectious disease and clinical microbiology, few books present both clinical and laboratory diagnostic criteria for diseases caused by classic pathogens. Even fewer books examine the changing patterns of infectious disease associated with alterations in microorganisms, with opportunistic modes of transmission, with the practice of modern medicine, and with certain lifestyles. Yet infectious disease specialists and clinical microbiologists must work closely in the diagnosis and management of both long-recognized infectious diseases and those which are emerging in the latter twentieth century as significant causes of morbidity and mortality.

Changing Patterns of Infectious Disease examines the changing patterns of some classic infectious diseases, of lesser known opportunistic infections, of some newly described disease entities induced by antimicrobial or chemotherapeutic agents, and of some clinical syndromes that possibly occur as sequelae of viral or bacterial infections. An introductory chapter explores both the progress that has been made in controlling infectious disease and the remaining and emerging problems that can be attributed to microbial agents. Each of the following 19 chapters discusses a specific infectious disease or clinical syndrome and contains sections on clinical diagnostic criteria, etiology, predisposing factors, epidemiology, laboratory diagnosis, and prognosis. Each of the 19 chapters includes 2 to 5 case reports that have been selected to demonstrate the clinical spectrum, course, and management of the particular disease. A final chapter is devoted to the examination of perspectives for the future of infectious disease.

A broader understanding of host-parasite relationships in infectious disease may one day lead to the eradication or diminution of some of the most vexing of the disease-producing agents. The changing patterns of infectious disease present a constant challenge to all of us serving those who are victimized by microbial mischief.

The scope and content of the book were largely influenced by my experience as a consulting microbiologist at Saint Joseph Medical Center in Burbank, California. No book represents a single effort, however, and I am indebted to numerous individuals who supplied material or suggestions. Those deserving acknowledgment include Ian M. Baird, Riverside Methodist Hospital, Columbus, Ohio; George H.

Cannon, L.D.S. Hospital, Salt Lake City; F.H. Chan, Children's Hospital of Eastern Ontario, Ottawa; William L. Current, Auburn University, Auburn, Alabama; Richard L. Guerrant, University of Virginia, Charlottesville; Robert W. Horne, John Innes Institute, Norwich, England; Thomas B. Hugh, Saint Vincent's Medical Center, Sydney, Australia; Steven L. Johnson, Centers for Disease Control, Atlanta; Raymond L. Kaplan, Rush-Presbyterian-St. Luke's Medical Center, Chicago; Carol A. Kauffman, Veterans Administration Medical Center, Ann Arbor, Michigan; Gary L. Lattimer, Williamsport General Hospital, Williamsport, Pennsylvania; A. Julio Martinez, Presbyterian University Hospital, Pittsburgh; James S. Nelson, Washington University School of Medicine, St. Louis; Steven R. Peikin, Jefferson Medical College, Philadelphia; Michael Radetsky, The Children's Hospital, Denver; John W. Rippon, The University of Chicago, Chicago; Ronald L. Searcy, St. Louis; Hans Sepp, Toronto East General Hospital, Toronto; Y. Shapira, Hadassah University Hospital, Hadassah, Israel; Sister Naomi Hurd, Saint Joseph Medical Center, Burbank, California; John P. Utz, Georgetown University Hospital, Washington, D.C.; David H. Walker, University of North Carolina, Chapel Hill; William R. Weisburger, Maryland Medical Laboratory, Baltimore; and Alice S. Weissfeld, Cedars-Sinai Medical Center, Los Angeles.

Those deserving of special recognition for their help include my colleague, Leslie P. Boston, Los Angeles Valley College, Van Nuys, for library research, for editorial assistance, and for reading proof; Ellen M. Swartzenburg for preparing final manuscript material; and staff members of Lea & Febiger for their additional assistance and expertise.

Van Nuys, California   Lois M. Bergquist

CONTENTS

CHAPTER 1 INFECTIOUS DISEASE: PROGRESS AND PROBLEMS

Remarkable progress has been made in controlling infectious disease since Edward Jenner introduced a smallpox vaccine in 1796. By far the most dramatic victory has been the elimination of smallpox by a worldwide immunization program. The decline in morbidity and mortality from diphtheria, pertussis, poliomyelitis, rubella, measles, and mumps can likewise be attributed to the availability of vaccines.

Since Alexander Fleming's serendipitous discovery that penicillin, a product of a common mold, could inhibit bacterial growth, an increasing number of natural and synthetic antimicrobial agents has become available for treating infections. The antimicrobial agents are credited with saving millions of lives each year and with reducing some of the serious complications that sometimes follow the infections.

The availability of potent insecticides has made it possible to break life cycles of parasites transmitted by arthropods or insects. With the use of DDT and other powerful insecticides, malaria is no longer a problem in most temperate regions.[1] Unfortunately, eradication methods have been less successful in other parts of the world where the potential for transmission appears to be close to the original level.[2] Schistosomiasis is reported to be largely under control in the People's Republic of China owing to the effective use of molluscicides and environmental sanitation methods.[3]

Other control measures have concentrated on purification of water supplies and prevention of transmission of infectious diseases by emphasizing personal hygiene. Yet, infectious disease still ranks fourth as a cause of death in the United States. It remains the major cause of death in most undeveloped countries.

Some countries have national organizations that require reporting of particular infectious diseases. Other independent organizations gather information on infectious diseases from hospital records and death certificates. In many instances, statistics do not reflect the actual incidence of a disease because standard diagnostic criteria have not been applied. In addition, most opportunistic infections are not reportable. Yet they comprise an increasing percentage of the total number of cases of infectious disease.

It is, nevertheless, still possible to examine the changing patterns of infectious disease caused by the emergence of new or altered pathogens and opportunistic organisms. The emergence or survival of twentieth century pathogens or opportunistic organisms can be attributed to (1) alterations in microorganisms, (2) opportunistic modes of transmission, (3) the practices of modern medicine, and (4) certain lifestyles of the twentieth century.

ALTERATIONS IN MICROORGANISMS

Microorganisms are constantly undergoing changes that enable them to cope with increasingly hostile environments. The development of mechanisms that permit survival of the most adaptable microorganisms is more rapid than the development of defense mechanisms that allow their hosts to combat microbial invaders. The adaptive process involves finding and exploiting weaknesses in defenses of the host.

Treponema pallidum, the cause of syphilis, is but one example in which a microorganism adapted to a changing environment.[4] With the movement of people from warm climates to cooler climates came the necessity for covering the body with more clothes. The spirochete, which formerly caused skin lesions, adapted to colonization on the warm, moist environment of the genitalia. Prior to that time, syphilis was probably relatively benign, but a mutation of the organism is believed to have occurred near the end of the fifteenth century, AD. That mutant causes the serious venereal disease known today.

Alterations in Antigenic Identity

The antigenic changes of influenza viruses that permit the almost annual emergence of virulent strains of influenza viruses A or B are well known.[5] The history of influenza viruses indicates that pandemics of influenza have been caused by viruses possessing new antigenic determinants. Influenza viruses contain a segmented genome of at least seven fragments of single-stranded RNA. The segmented genome appears to favor production of recombinant variants in mixed infections. The phenomenon is known as *antigenic shift.*

A more subtle variation in influenza A virus is believed to be related to mutation and a process of immunologic selection. The mutant virus particles possess a growth advantage in the presence of preformed specific antibody. The phenomenon is called *antigenic drift.*

As new strains of influenza viruses emerge, preceding strains tend either to disappear or become sequestered for long periods of time. Only rarely do they reappear as significant causes of influenza. The fear that a pig influenza virus Hsw INI, a virus closely related to the strain involved in the pandemic of 1918 to 1919, would spread in epidemic proportions when it briefly surfaced in the United States in 1976 did not materalize.

Emergence of Drug-Resistant Strains

After a few years of widespread use of antimicrobial agents, it became apparent that some strains of microorganisms could survive in the hostile environment of drugs while susceptible strains were killed. As a result of the selective pressure associated with the use of penicillin G, more than 80% of isolates of Staphylococcus aureus were resistant to that drug by 1960. The indiscriminate or persistent use of any antimicrobial agent can provide a survival advantage to a variety of microorganisms.

Drug resistance can be associated with the chromosome or plasmids of bacteria. The most common type of drug resistance is due to chromosomal mutations occurring in a single step or in multiple steps. A single point mutation can interfere with the binding of a drug with a receptor protein, but additional mutations can promote actual destruction of a drug.[6] Mutations that produce resistance occur as rare and random events in a bacterial population, but can only reach a position of dominance in the presence of a particular antimicrobial agent.

Resistance can also be conferred on a once drug-susceptible strain of a bacterium by transfer of R-plasmids that contain genes carrying resistance factors for one or more drugs. It is well documented that nonpathogenic coliforms can transfer plasmids for multiple drug resistance by a process of conjugation in the alimentary tract.[7]

Public health authorities have been concerned about the emergence of strains of Neisseria gonorrhoeae that produce β-lactamase (penicillinase) as an inducible enzyme in the presence of penicillin.[8] The β-lactamase of Neisseria gonorrhoeae is associated with an R-plasmid that is similar to a plasmid of Haemophilus influenzae or H. parainfluenzae. The enzyme degrades penicillin and cyclosporin by cleaving bonds that separate side chains from the molecules.[9]

Development of Multiple-Host Pathogens

In many instances, at least one vertebrate and one invertebrate host are required to complete the life cycle of a microorganism. A classic example is supplied by human malarian parasites, in which the sexual cycle (sporogony) takes place in the Anopheles mosquito and the asexual cycle (schizogony) takes place in the human. This appears to be an example of host-range extension. A variety of vertebrates, all of which were once arboreal, were probably the original parasite-hosts. The survival capacity of malarian parasites in an invertebrate host required development of new immune mechanisms to resist defenses of the host and development of new enzyme systems to assimilate nutrients.[10] The adaptation has been so highly specific that the species of Plasmodium affecting the human does not cause malaria in other vertebrates and develops only in anopheline mosquitoes.

There are many other examples of extensions to two-host systems. In some instances, arthropod hosts have become immune to actual disease and act merely as mechanical vectors or vehicles of transportation from one vertebrate host to another. An example of a mechanical vector is the wood tick, Dermacentor andersoni, which transmits the rickettsial agent of Rocky Mountain spotted fever.

It is often necessary to study records of infectious disease over several centuries to trace the development of two-host or multiple-host systems. The enteric bacteria causing salmonelloses are classic examples of multiple-host pathogens. Many domestic and wild animals, including dogs, birds, cats, turtles, cattle, horses, and sheep, harbor the organisms, but domestic fowl constitute the largest single reservoir of salmonellae. An exception to the salmonellae as multiple-host pathogens is the bacterium, Salmonella typhi, which causes disease only in humans. The newly recognized human cryptosporidiosis, gastrointestinal yersiniosis, and Campylobacter infections appear to be current examples of extension of previously recognized animal pathogens to the human host.[11-13] Since human dependence on animals and the human love affair with pets is likely to continue, other heretofore host-specific pathogens will predictably adapt to the human host.

OPPORTUNISTIC MODES OF TRANSMISSION

The incidence of infectious disease is dependent on the opportunities afforded for transmission of etiologic agents from their natural reservoirs. Infectious disease may be spread indirectly, by contact with contaminated food, water, air, dressings, instruments, body discharges, and other fomites or directly, by contact with an infected individual or animal, or with carriers of infectious agents. Some infectious agents are transmitted by biting insects or arthropods. Greater human mobility, industrialization, crowding of individuals in large cities made possible by rapid methods of transportation, certain practices of modern medicine, and even lifestyles of the twentieth century have provided unique ways for human hosts to accommodate microorganisms.

Human Mobility

The opening of intercontinental trade routes in previous centuries was responsible for the dissemination of pathogenic microorganisms from regions of endemicity to highly susceptible populations. The form of plague known as the Black Death destroyed at least a quarter of the population of Europe during the fourteenth century when

Yersinia pestis was transmitted by rodents of Burma and of Yunnan province in China to rodents of Europe.[14] Additional infectious diseases were spread by migrations of people along the trade routes.

The exact role of twentieth century modes of transportation in the transmission of infectious disease cannot be completely assessed; however, one example gives us at least a hint of the magnitude of the effect. In 1963, as many as 10,000 people were believed to have ingested water that contained Salmonella typhi, the cause of typhoid fever, at a ski resort in Switzerland.[15] Several weeks later, more than 430 cases of typhoid fever in 6 countries were traced to the contaminated drinking water.

Although cruise ships cannot be considered a form of rapid transportation for passengers or microorganisms, sometimes cruises do provide a unique setting for disseminating pathogens. Most outbreaks of infectious disease aboard cruise ships have been linked to a common food source or food handler. Since passengers are often from widely separated geographic areas, the microorganisms that disembark with their hosts can spread to places far from their source.

Wars have provided additional opportunities for the transportation of microorganisms. The spread of leprosy from the Middle East to Europe in the sixth century was accelerated by the Crusades. More recently, the movement of large numbers of troops by aircraft from Southeast Asia to the Pacific Islands during World War II contributed to the introduction of dengue in the South Pacific.

Other, undisclosed opportunities probably exist for microorganisms to travel from endemic areas to countries with susceptible individuals. The sometimes frightening thought is the unparalleled speed with which the microorganisms can travel in or on their human hosts. It means constant surveillance on the part of microbial sleuths everywhere.

Industrialization and Urbanization

Industrialization and urbanization during the last two centuries have led to high-density populations in large cities throughout the world. High-density populations facilitate the spread of respiratory diseases. Respiratory pathogens are disseminated by coughing, sneezing, and speaking. Other pathogens are shed by body secretions and skin lesions into the air.

The quartering of large work forces in the limited space of urban areas presents special problems. Aerosols containing microorganisms can fall as far as 3 or 4 feet away from the person discharging mucus or saliva into the air. Although most aerosols fall to the ground and dry, the dried material can become airborne again with the slightest change in air currents. The humid atmosphere of air-conditioned buildings, auditoriums, hospitals, and homes favors the survival of some microorganisms.

A consequence of industrialization and urbanization has been an alarming increase in air pollutants. Many of the chemicals released by mobile or stationary sources are health hazards. Some pollutants are known to induce cancer. Other pollutants contribute to particulate matter suspended in the air and provide ideal shelters and vehicles of transportation for microorganisms.

PRACTICES OF MODERN MEDICINE

The cure-oriented intervention techniques of modern medicine, which permit the liberal use of antimicrobial and chemotherapeutic agents, the increasing number of manipulative procedures, and the replacement of vital organs, are not without risk to patients.

More than 100 antimicrobial and chemotherapeutic agents are in use today. Side effects associated with their use include vertigo, deafness, depression of bone marrow, gastrointestinal disturbances, allergic reactions, and superimposed infections. Individuals with impaired host defenses, such as those occurring in cancer, diabetes, severe burns, collagen diseases, and neurologic disorders, or after an organ transplant, are particularly susceptible to superimposed infections.

One newly recognized example of a superimposed infection is antibiotic-associated colitis caused by Clostridium difficile.[16] The colitis can be induced by most antimicrobial agents except parenteral aminoglycosides and vancomycin. The lack of competition of indigenous organisms is presumed to permit colonization and proliferation of the anaerobe. A cytopathic toxin is believed to be responsible for the inflammatory response.

The association of the serious and often fatal Reye syndrome with aspirin following a viral infection has been a curious phenomenon.[17] Some researchers suspect that a synergistic relationship between a virus and the medication may be responsible for promoting the characteristic liver dysfunction. The true cause remains an enigma.

The goal in any organ transplant is to prevent rejection of the graft. Corticosteroids have been used extensively as immunosuppressive agents in organ-transplant recipients.[18] Hormone-induced immunosuppression is not specific, however, and individuals receiving corticosteroids are prime candidates for potentially lethal infections.

Infections associated with manipulative techniques arise in three major areas: (1) in the diagnosis and treatment of obstructive respiratory disease; (2) in the prolonged use of indwelling catheters; and (3) in the administration of anesthetics.[19] Most of the infections are caused by gram-negative bacteria. If aerosol particles are 6 μm or less and contain bacteria from contaminated nebulizers or IPPB machines, they gain access to respiratory bronchioles, alveolar ducts, or alveolar sacs.

It is well known that urethral catheters permit bacteria to gain access to the bladder, kidney, and prostate gland. Although Escherichia coli is the most common cause of urinary tract infections in a general population, hospital patients with indwelling catheters often develop infections caused by drug-resistant strains of Proteus, Pseudomonas, or Enterobacter.

Rebreathing bags, suction tubes, face masks, and endotracheal tubes are all possible reservoirs for microorganisms. Microorganisms that sometimes contaminate hoses of anesthesia equipment include Candida, Staphylococcus, Neisseria, Branhamella, and Pseudomonas species.[20] Pseudomonas species represent a greater threat than the others, which can be found normally in the upper respiratory tract.

LIFESTYLES OF THE TWENTIETH CENTURY

Times of economic prosperity and scientific advancement have long been associated with greater sexual freedom. The present sexual revolution began in the late 1950s when the postwar economy was healthy once again and when the launching of Sputnik started the space race. Greater sexual promiscuity resulted in an increase in cases of reportable and nonreportable sexually transmitted diseases (STDs). The number of cases of gonorrhea doubled in the United States from 1969 to 1980. Not only did the incidence of gonorrhea and syphilis rise, but a variant of herpes simplex virus 1 (HSV-1), herpes simplex virus 2 (HSV-2), emerged as the major cause of herpes genitalia.[21] Although herpes simplex 1 usually causes most oral, ocular, and brain infections, either HSV-1 or HSV-2 can cause lesions on a variety of body sites. The herpesviruses can remain latent, and tend to surface again and again to produce the sometimes painful lesions. It is estimated that at least 20 million Americans are victims of herpes genitalia.

Infectious mononucleosis, sometimes called glandular fever, is a disease of teenagers and adults associated with the Epstein-Barr virus (EBV) in economically privileged countries. In less affluent societies, 90 to 95% of children may acquire EBV antibodies by the time they are 6 years old.[22] Conversely, 60 to 70% of the teenagers and young adults in Europe and the United States are susceptible to EBV. The virus is shed in the saliva of infected individuals and spread by the extensive salivary exchange that takes place during kissing. EBV also seems to be associated with a type of lymphoma and a form of nasopharyngeal carcinoma.

The two major problems of promiscuous heterosexual intercourse have traditionally been conception and transmission of STDs. The development of contraceptives has minimized conception and made sex a frequent and an increasingly acceptable form of recreation.

Homosexuality has a unique role in the transmission of the classic STDs and of other infectious diseases not known previously to be spread by sexual activity. Not only do homosexuals have a greater number of sexual partners than do heterosexuals, but the practices common to homosexual activity provide greater opportunities to transmit microorganisms. Anal intercourse, in particular, may afford a special opportunistic mode of transmission. Shigella species, hepatitis B virus (HBV), human cytomegalovirus (HCV), and, apparently, the agent of acquired immune deficiency syndrome (AIDS) can be transmitted sexually in that manner.

Although homosexuals remain the largest "at risk" group for developing AIDS, spread to heterosexual populations is predictable. AIDS is especially frightening because it provides the opportunity for microorganisms that have previously established a compatible host-parasite relationship to emerge as pathogens, causing death in at least 40% of the cases.

SUMMARY

The full impact of alterations in microorganisms, opportunistic modes of transmission, practices of modern medicine, and certain lifestyles of the twentieth century can only be surmised. Those forces which are continuous and simultaneous, but not always symbiotic, have led to changing patterns of infectious disease. With the disappearance of the classic pathogens, some newly recognized lethal and potentially lethal infectious diseases have emerged. Some of the microbial agents of the newly recognized diseases may have been living in harmony with their human hosts while humans were battling the ravages of serious infectious diseases that are now under control. Other microbial agents of newly recognized infectious diseases represent distinct alterations in microorganisms that permit them to survive despite rigorous attempts to eliminate them. Some humans are victimized only when their immune mechanisms are compromised or overwhelmed.

It is important that health care personnel everywhere be willing to maintain constant vigilance by examining diagnostic criteria, etiologic agents, epidemiology, pertinent laboratory procedures, and prognosis of newly recognized or remaining infectious diseases or those syndromes occurring as complications of infections.

REFERENCES

1. Wyler, D.J.: Malaria—resurgence, resistance and research. N. Engl. J. Med., *308*:875, 1983.
2. Bruce-Chwatt, J.J.: Man against malaria: conquest or defeat. Trans. R. Trop. Med. Hyg., *73*:605, 1979.
3. Grove, D.I.: Schistosomes, snails and man. *In* Changing Disease Patterns and

Human Behavior. Edited by N.F. Stanley and R.A. Joske. New York, Academic Press, 1980.

4. Hackett, C.J.: On the origin of the human treponematoses. Bull. WHO, *29*:7, 1963.
5. Webster, R.G., and Laver, W.G.: Antigenic variation of influenza viruses. *In* The Influenza Viruses and Influenza. Edited by E.D. Kilbourne. New York, Academic Press, 1975.
6. Pratt, W.B.: Chemotherapy of Infection. New York, Oxford University Press, 1977.
7. Watanabe, T., and Fukasawa, T.: Episome-mediated transfer of drug resistance in Enterobacteriaceae, transfer of resistance factors by conjugation. J. Bacteriol., *81*:669, 1961.
8. Centers for Disease Control: Penicillinase-producing Neisseria gonorrhoeae. Morbid. Mortal. Weekly Rept., *32*:181, 1983.
9. Citric, N., and Pollock, M.R.: The biochemistry and function of β-lactamase (penicillinase). Adv. Enzymol., *28*:237, 1966.
10. Busvine, J.R.: The evolution and mutual adaptation of insects, microorganisms and man. *In* Changing Disease Patterns and Human Behavior. Edited by N.F. Stanley and R.A. Joske. New York, Academic Press, 1980.
11. Centers for Disease Control: Human cryptosporidiosis—Alabama. Morbid. Mortal. Weekly Rept., *31*:252, 1982.
12. Asakawa, Y., et al.: Two community outbreaks of human infection with Yersinia enterocolitica. J. Hyg. (Lond.), *71*:715, 1973.
13. Pearson, A.D., et al.: Campylobacter-associated diarrhoeae in Southampton. Br. Med. J., *2*:955, 1977.
14. Lechevalier, H.A., and Solotorovsky, M.: Three Centuries of Microbiology. New York, McGraw-Hill, 1965.
15. Bernard, R.P.: The Zermatt typhoid outbreak in 1963. J. Hyg. Camb., *63*:537, 1965.
16. George, W.L., Rolfe, R.D., and Finegold, S.M.: Clostridium difficile and its cytotoxin in feces of patients with antimicrobial-agent-associated diarrhea and miscellaneous conditions. J. Clin. Microbiol., *15*:1049, 1982.
17. Centers for Disease Control: Surgeon general's advisory on the use of salicylates and Reye syndrome. Morbid. Mortal. Weekly Rept., *31*:289, 1982.
18. Fauci, A.S., Dale, D.C., and Balow, J.E.: Glucocorticoid therapy: Mechanism of action and clinical consideration. Ann. Intern. Med., *84*:304, 1976.
19. Knight, V.: Instruments and infection. Hosp. Pract., *2*:82, 1967.
20. Bergquist, L.M.: Microbiology for the Hospital Environment. New York: Harper & Row, 1981.
21. Hutfield, D.C.: History of herpes genitalia. Br. J. Vener. Dis., *42*:263, 1966.
22. Evans, A.S., and Niederman, J.C.: Epstein-Barr virus. *In* Viral Infections of Humans, Epidemiology, and Control. New York, Plenum, 1976.

CHAPTER 2 AMEBIC MENINGOENCEPHALITIS

Amebic meningoencephalitis is a rare but usually fatal infection caused by free-living amebas. The term primary amebic meningoencephalitis (PAM) was coined by Butt in 1964 for two cases of the fatal cerebral infection that occurred in Florida.[1] Similar infections were described a year later in four Australian children and also in an elderly drug addict.[2,3] Although originally it was thought that this meningoencephalitis was caused by the free-living ameba known as Acanthamoeba, in retrospect, it appears that another free-living ameba belonging to the genus Naegleria may have been the etiologic agent.

It has now been established that the disease associated with Acanthamoeba causes a granulomatous amebic encephalitis (GAE) that lasts from 1 week to several months.[4-6] PAM is a more rapidly fulminating disease which terminates in death 5 to 7 days after the onset of symptoms.[7] At least 130 cases of PAM and more than 100 cases of GAE have occurred since they were first described. Unfortunately, most have been diagnosed only after examination of autopsy material.

The initial symptoms of PAM are not unique to that form of meningoencephalitis, but a history of swimming in freshwater lakes, ponds, or backwater bays is universal in children and young adults in whom the disease has occurred.[8,9] The typical course of amebic meningoencephalitis is headache, fever, malaise, lethargy, nuchal rigidity, a positive Kernig's sign, disorientation, and ataxia, followed by a comatose state.

Although meninogencephalitis has been the most frequent infection, it now appears that the protozoan can promote a wide spectrum of opportunistic infections in individuals with underlying disease or immune deficiencies and no history of swimming in stagnant water.[9-12] At least 10 cases of keratitis caused by Acanthamoeba have been reported in the past decade.[13] All but 1 individual had serious complications that required enucleation, keratoplasty, or corneal graft. The course of opportunistic infection is affected adversely by a delay in diagnosis and treatment. The devastating consequences of amebic meningoencephalitis or opportunistic acanthamoebiasis indicate an increased need for a complete history of the patient, particularly as it pertains to swimming in landlocked water, underlying disease, or drug use.[14]

ETIOLOGY

A single species of Naegleria, N. fowleri, is known to be a human pathogen. Several species of Acanthamoeba, including A. culbertsoni, A. castellanii, A. polyphaga, and A. astronyxis, are known to cause human disease.[9] In a fatal case of meningocencephalitis occurring in a diabetic woman, the identification of the responsible free-living ameba could not be confirmed as Naegleria or Acanthamoeba.[15] It is probable that several free-living amebas can invade human tissue with serious consequences. None of the soil amebas, when provided opportunistic circumstances, can be eliminated as causes of infection.

Damage to the spinal cord and brain is attributed to the ability of the amebas to disseminate, proliferate, and destroy tissue in a relatively short period. The nutritious milieu supplied by the cerebrospinal fluid promotes the rapid proliferation of the parasites, and the flow of cerebrospinal fluid permits the amebas to move into the subarachnoid space or lining of the ventricles with ease (Fig. 2–1). An acute inflammatory or granulomatous response follows invasion of the cerebrum and cerebellum by hundreds of amebas.[10] Although differences in virulence among soil amebas have been demonstrated, much remains to be learned about the factors determining the virulence of particular strains in human hosts.

PREDISPOSING FACTORS

Development of amebic meningoencephalitis in children or young adults appears to follow exposure to large quantities of the soil amebas, Naegleria or Acanthamoeba, in contaminated water. An unusually large number of cases seems to be associated with diving or swimming under water.[1,15] In a few cases of amebic meningoencephalitis in adults, no history of contact with landlocked water could be established.[16] Predisposing factors in adults include diabetes, neoplasms, alcoholism, radiation therapy, and a history of immunosuppressive, antimicrobial, or chemotherapeutic drugs. Trauma resulting from a foreign object or blowing dust was the most common predisposing factor in 10 reported cases of keratitis caused by Acanthamoeba.[13] The significance of underlying disease and immune deficiencies in the development of acanthamoebiasis has not been studied in depth, but past experience with other opportunistic infections would indicate that either or both provide a host with unique susceptibility to otherwise saprophytic microorganisms.

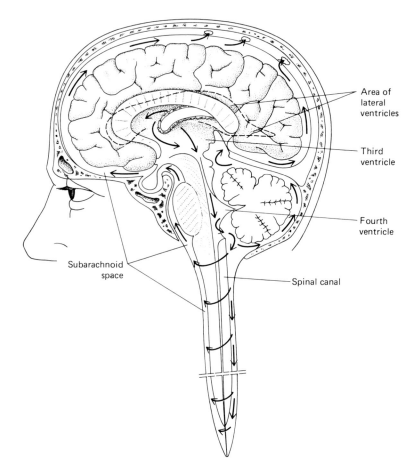

Figure 2–1. Postulated pathways of soil amebas moving into cerebrospinal fluid. (From Bergquist, L.M.: Microbiology for the Hospital Environment. New York, Harper & Row, 1981.)

EPIDEMIOLOGY

Although the reported cases of amebic meningoencephalitis are limited to parts of Australia, England, the United States, Africa, and Czechoslovakia, it is likely that the disease occurs but is not recognized in many parts of the world. The distribution of soil amebas Naegleria and Acanthamoeba is known to be widespread. The trophozoites of Naegleria are believed to enter the nasal passages when people swim in water contaminated with the amebas. The cysts may be inhaled during blowing dust storms and undergo excystation into trophozoites before invading the nasal mucosa.[13] Subsequently, the trophozoites penetrate the cribriform plate and migrate to the cortical areas, where they multiply. It is postulated that Acanthamoeba species may enter through the skin, the eye, the genitourinary tract, or the respiratory tract.[17] Involvement of the central nervous system follows metastatic spread from a primary focus. Following excystation, the trophozoites invade the intestinal mucosa. No person-to-person transmission has been demonstrated.

LABORATORY DIAGNOSIS

Primary amebic meningoencephalitis cannot always be distinguished from other types of meningoencephalitis by standard laboratory tests. Examination of cerebrospinal fluid may be of limited value because, at least early in the disease, amebas may not be present in the CSF. Cultural and serologic techniques or demonstration of the parasites in tissue sections of autopsy specimens may be required to confirm a diagnosis of naegleriasis or acanthamoebiasis.

Microscopic Examination

Centrifuged specimens of cerebrospinal fluid are best examined under diminished light of a brightfield microscope or a phase-contrast microscope. The motile amebas are readily distinguishable from any surrounding blood cells. Trophozoites of Naegleria fowleri measure 10 to 35 μm and demonstrate motility by lobopodia.[18] A single nucleus with a prominent karyosome is readily observable (Fig. 2–2). Smooth-walled cysts, measuring 7 to 15 μm in diameter, occur in soil and frequently contaminate stagnant water.

Acanthamoeba trophozoites are somewhat larger than those of Naegleria, measuring 15 to 45 μm, with a single prominent nucleus and pulsating vacuoles (Fig. 2–3). The trophozoites move by means of

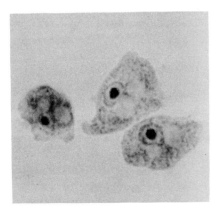

Figure 2–2. Trophozoite of Naegleria fowleri showing prominent karyosome and lobopodia on a trichrome stain. (From Visvesvara, G.S.: Free-living pathogenic amoebae. *In* Manual of Clinical Microbiology, 3rd Ed. Edited by E.H. Lennette. Washington, D.C., American Society for Microbiology, 1980.)

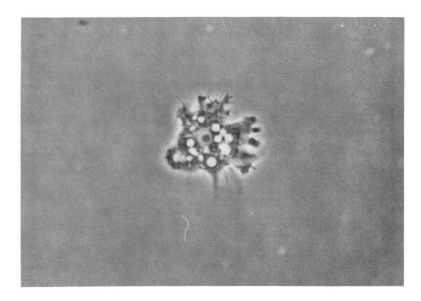

Figure 2–3. Trophozoite of Acanthamoeba culbertsoni showing prominent kar-yosome and acanthopodia by phase-contrast microscopy. (From Visvesvara, G.S.: Free-living pathogenic amoebae. *In* Manual of Clinical Microbiology, 3rd Ed. Edited by E.H. Lennette. Washington, D.C., American Society for Microbiology, 1980.)

fine tapering projections known as acanthopodia. The cysts are dou-ble-walled and measure 10 to 25 mμ. Naegleria can be differentiated from Acanthamoeba by demonstration of the biflagellate stage. In a drop of centrifuged cerebrospinal fluid containing Naegleria placed in 1.0 ml of sterile distilled water and incubated at 37°C for 2 or 3 hours, approximately 30 to 50% of the amebas will convert to pear-shaped biflagellated organisms.

An alternate method of demonstrating enflagellation is to place a drop of the mixture of cerebrospinal fluid and distilled water on a cover slip. A mixture of petroleum jelly and paraffin in equal pro-portions applied to the edges of the cover slip allows an inverted hanging drop slide to be positioned and sealed over the drop. Enflag-ellation of Naegleria occurs after incubation of the upright slide in a moist chamber for 2 or 3 hours at 37°C. Both tube and slide prepa-rations can be checked for the biflagellates as time permits.

Permanent stained smears are easily prepared by placing a drop of centrifuged cerebrospinal fluid or incubated mixture on a clean glass slide and incubating it in a moist chamber for 10 minutes. The amebas will adhere to the surface of the slide and can be fixed by placing a few drops of Schaudinn's fixative, heated to 37°C, on the slide and allowing it to react for 1 minute. After processing in a Coplin jar containing Schaudinn's fixative for 1 hour at room temperature, trichrome or iron-hematoxylin stain may be applied.

Postmortem examination of brain or other tissue sections stained with hematoxylin-eosin may be required to diagnose amebic meningoencephalitis. The olfactory lobes are primarily involved in naegleriasis, but are usually spared in acanthamoebiasis. Hemorrhagic necrosis is found in both PAM and GAE, but lesions of GAE are usually granulomatous rather than characteristic of the acute inflammatory response associated with PAM (Fig. 2–4). Opportunistic acanthamoebiasis may promote an acute inflammatory response more typical of PAM (Fig. 2–5). Trophozoites are usually abundant, especially around blood vessels.

Cultural Techniques

Naegleria fowleri or Acanthamoeba species grow well on prewarmed 1.5% nonnutrient agar plates, prepared with Page's ameba saline and precoated with a saline suspension of Escherichia coli or Aerobacter aerogenes. Excystment is stimulated by the presence of gram-negative bacilli.[19] Two or three drops of centrifuged cerebrospinal fluid, or tissue triturated in Page's ameba saline, placed in the center of the plates is a sufficient inoculum. The amebas can often be demonstrated after a day of incubation at 37°C, but plates should

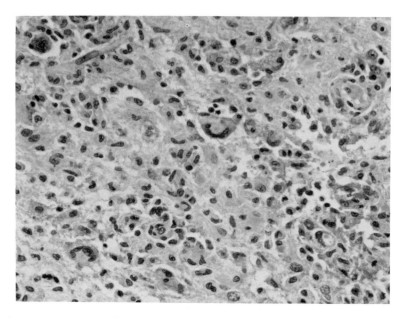

Figure 2–4. Histopathology of granulomatous amebic encephalitis (GAE) with multinucleated giant cells. (From Martinez, A.J.: Is Acanthamoeba an opportunistic infection? Neurology, 30:567, 1980.)

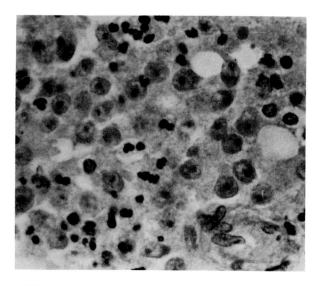

Figure 2–5. Histopathology of acute inflammatory response and trophozoites in opportunistic acanthamoebiasis. (From Grunnet, M.L., Cannon, G.H., and Kushner, J.P.: Fulminant amebic meningoencephalitis due to Acanthamoeba. Neurology, *31*:174, 1981.)

be kept for at least 7 days. Movement of amebas can be observed under the low-power objective of a brightfield microscope. Encystation frequently occurs on the second or third day of incubation. Both trophozoites and cysts may be present after 4 or 5 days. The pathogenic soil amebas are thermophilic and will grow at 43 to 46°C.

Pure cultures of amebas may be obtained by suspending some growth from an agar plate in Page's ameba saline, centrifuging, and using the sediment to inoculate an antibiotic-containing proteose peptone-yeast extract glucose medium for Acanthamoeba or Nelson's medium enriched with 0.2% heat-inactivated fetal calf serum for Naegleri.[20,21] Penicillin in a concentration of 400 U/ml and streptomycin in a concentration of 400 μg are sufficient to destroy bacterial contaminates. Several mammalian cells, including those of chicken fibroblasts, support the growth of Naegleria and Acanthamoeba. Cytopathic effects (CPE) are similar to those produced by viruses.[18] The CPE are not specific enough to identify the particular ameba responsible for an infection, but cell cultures may be useful in isolating the protozoa if few amebas are present.

Serologic Tests

It is doubtful that patients with naegleriasis have sufficient time to mount a demonstrable antibody reponse to the invasion of the soil amebas. The sometimes longer course of acanthamoebiasis may make serologic studies a bit more feasible. A rising complement-fixing (CF) antibody titer was demonstrated in a patient whose serum was obtained three times during the course of brain disease caused by Acanthamoeba.[22] Indirect immunofluorescence may have some value in confirming the presence of soil amebas in brain sections or spinal fluid. The lack of commercially available standardized antigens or antibodies, however, limits the value of serologic tests in the diagnosis of amebic meningoencephalitis.

Animal Pathogenicity Studies

Mice are susceptible to pathogenic soil amebas. Intranasal inoculation causes mice to die within 5 to 7 days. Amebas in brains of mice can be demonstrated by microscopic examination of brain sections or by cultural techniques.

PROGNOSIS

Primary amebic meningoencephalitis is usually fatal, although a few instances of survival have been described in the literature. In 1971, a patient from Queensland, Australia is reported to have recovered from meningoencephalitis caused by Naegleria fowleri, which was isolated from cerebrospinal fluid.[23] Recovery from a documented case of PAM caused by Naegleria in the United States occurred in California in 1978.[24] Survival in the first instance was attributed to intensive parenteral intrathecal and ventricular treatment with amphotericin B. Survival in the second case was attributed to aggressive treatment with amphotericin B, supplemented by therapeutic doses of miconazole and rifampin. Unfortunately, similar drug regimens have not affected the fatal course of the disease in other patients.

CASE REPORTS

Case 1

A previously healthy 14-year-old boy was admitted to a central Florida hospital on July 4, 1978. During the preceding 3 weeks, he had been swimming (primarily underwater) and diving in a freshwater lake. On July 2 he complained of increasingly severe frontal and bitemporal headache. He then developed a low-grade fever (38.1°C) and malaise and was treated with diazepam (Valium; Roche Laboratories, Nutley, New Jersey) and analgesic. On admission the patient was lethargic and disoriented and had mild nuchal rigidity, an oral temperature of 40°C, nystagmus, and a disconjugate gaze. Treatment with 3 g of penicillin G IV every 4 hours and 500 mg of chloramphenicol every 6 hours was begun. Shortly thereafter, examination of a wet preparation of cerebrospinal fluid (CSF) showed motile amoebae, which were subsequently identified as N. fowleri by Dr. F. M.

Wellings (Epidemiology Research Center, Tampa, Florida) on the basis of flagellate formation, the indirect fluorescent antibody test (IFAT), and mouse pathogenicity studies.

Amphotericin B was administered IV (10 mg once daily) and intrathecally (0.05 mg once daily). Despite this therapy and measures to decrease intracranial pressure, the patient's condition deteriorated from agitation to total unresponsiveness within 18 hours. On the second hospital day, he developed anisocoria and evidence of neurogenic pulmonary edema, which was treated with positive pressure ventilation. Therapy with miconazole administered IV (200 mg/day) and intrathecally (20 mg/day) was begun on day 2. There was no neurologic improvement, and the patient died on day 5.

Postmortem examination of the brain showed the typical neuropathologic changes observed in PAM. The other organs were normal, with the exception of the lungs, which showed severe passive congestion without inflammation or the presence of organisms.*

Case 2

A 57-year-old woman first became ill in the spring of 1976 with autoimmune hemolytic anemia, manifested by a positive direct Coombs test, increased bilirubin, and decreased serum haptoglobin concentration. Prednisone therapy produced a partial hematologic response, and she was referred to us in September, 1976. She had a malar rash and swollen knees. Evaluation confirmed the Coombs-positive hemolytic anemia, with an anti-I cold agglutinin, abnormal liver function tests, a circulating nonspecific anticoagulant, positive antinuclear antibody test, cold agglutinin titer of 1:256, and subnormal levels of the third and fourth levels of complement. A diagnosis of systemic lupus erythematosus was made and therapy with prednisone continued. In addition, she received azathioprine and cyclophosphamide at times during the next 21 months.

The hemolytic anemia was partially corrected, but because of marked side effects of the chronic steroid therapy, gradual splenic enlargement, and thrombocytopenia, splenectomy was performed on July 20, 1978. She was discharged on July 27, taking 10 mg prednisone daily. On August 9 she developed a fever which persisted until she was readmitted on August 13.

On admission, she was disoriented and exhibited mild left facial weakness, but there were no other neurologic abnormalities. A 3- to 4-cm subcutaneous mass was noted in the left lower quadrant. There was no nuchal rigidity. Her temperature was 39.5°C. The hematocrit was 45.6%, platelets $118-10^9$ per liter, and the white blood count

*From Stevens, A.R., et al.: J. Infect. Dis. *143*:193–199, 1981. © 1981 by the University of Chicago.[15]

7.9–10^9 per liter, with a differential count of 6 bands, 86 neutrophils, 7 lymphocytes, 1 monocyte, and 3 nucleated red blood cells. Urinalysis showed 1+ protein, 8 to 10 white blood cells per high-power field, and numerous gram-negative rods. A urine culture grew greater than 10^5 colonies of Escherichia coli per cubic millimeter, but three sets of blood cultures were negative. Chest x-ray showed diffuse interstitial pulmonary infiltrates, and blood gases revealed a Po_2 of 59 mm Hg, Pco_2 of 19 mm Hg, and pH of 7.50.

Cerebrospinal fluid (CSF) pressure was 80 mm H_2O. There were 85 RBC per cubic millimeter. The protein content was 59 mg per deciliter, the glucose content 30 mg per deciliter (simultaneous serum glucose 117 mg per deciliter), and CSF bacterial cultures were negative. Computerized tomography (CT) revealed decreased density in the right parietal area. She was treated with intravenous methylprednisolone, piperacillin, and amikacin.

On the second hospital day, CSF findings were 80 mm H_2O pressure, 350 RBC per cubic millimeter and 7 WBC per cubic millimeter (75% neutrophils), protein 112 mg per deciliter, and glucose 84 mg per deciliter (simultaneous serum glucose 218 mg per deciliter). Bilateral Babinski signs were noted. On the third day, CT showed a huge area of decreased density in the right frontal parietal and temporal lobe with a shift of the midline. After developing signs of transtentorial herniation, she died on the third day of hospitalization.

At autopsy, the brain showed severe asymmetric edema with transtentorial herniation. The surfaces of the right temporal, parietal, and frontal lobes were hemorrhagic and necrotic. Hemorrhagic necrosis involved the major portion of the right cerebral hemisphere, and smaller areas of hemorrhagic necrosis were seen in the left cerebral hemisphere, lower pons, left cerebellar hemisphere, and vermis.

Microscopic examination of the brain revealed extensive fibrinoid necrosis of medium and small arteries, with thrombosis of many vessels and an extensive perivascular and tissue infiltrate composed primarily of neutrophils. No giant cells were seen. Amebic trophozoites were seen within the inflammatory infiltrate. The amebae measured 20 μm in diameter, with a single eccentric nucleus. Double-walled cysts were rare. Electronmicroscopy of the trophozoites revealed an organism with a round, eccentric nucleus, prominent round nucleolus, round mitochondria, and empty cytoplasmic vacuoles. Indirect immunofluorescent studies were performed by Dr. Eddy Willaert, Veterans Administration Hospital, Gainesville, Florida, by the method of Stamm. Antisera against Acanthamoeba were produced in rabbits and made species-specific by adsorption. Deparaffinized routine histologic sections were then incubated with dilutions of the antisera. A second incubation with fluorescein-conjugated anti-immunoglobulin allowed visualization of the immune complexes bound to the amebae.

Antisera to four species of Acanthamoeba were tested, and A. castellanii was identified as the etiologic agent by indirect immunofluorescent studies.

Amebic trophozoites were also found in the lungs and skin. Grossly, the lungs were firm, with several small (0.5 cm) pale parenchymal nodules. Microscopically, focal acute bronchopneumonia was seen, with areas of granulomatous pneumonitis containing giant cells. No vasculitis was present. Amebic trophozoites were seen within the alveolar exudate, and one was seen in an alveolar multinucleated giant cell. Stains for fungi and bacteria were negative. In the 3 × 4-cm subcutaneous nodule from the left lower quadrant of the abdomen there was no overlying ulceration, and microscopic sections showed fat necrosis, acute and chronic inflammation, and scattered amebic trophozoites. No vasculitis or giant cells were seen in the skin. No amebae or granulomas were found in other tissues.*

Case 3

An 8-month-old female Hausa infant was admitted to the hospital on January 29, 1977, with a 2-day history of fever, vomiting, and convulsions, as described by the mother. The infant was taken during this period to a nearby clinic, where she was given an injection of chloroquine, as malaria is one of the most common diseases in these parts. There was no improvement in her condition; it was, in fact, deteriorating, and hence the infant was brought to the hospital.

On admission, the infant was febrile and already in an unconscious, flaccid state, with no neck stiffness and moderate dehydration. A provisional diagnosis of gastroenteritis was made. Blood was drawn for determinations of electrolytes and glucose, culture, and investigation for malarial parasites. None of these contributed to the diagnosis. The patient was given intravenous fluids, but her condition did not improve. She became dyspneic and had convulsions; hence, a lumbar puncture was done. The cerebrospinal fluid was blood-tinged and opalescent. Pressure was not recorded. The total cell count was 1.288/µl, of which 87% were neutrophils and 13% lymphocytes; erythrocytes, 900/µl; protein, 200 mg/dl; glucose 21.6 mg/dl; chlorides, 106 mEq/L. Cerebrospinal fluid was negative for bacteria by Gram- and Ziehl-Neelsen-stained smears, and the culture was subsequently sterile. The cerebrospinal fluid was also negative for antigens of Meningococcus, Pneumococcus, Haemophilus, and Staphylococcus.

The infant was treated as for pyogenic meningitis, pending a definitive diagnosis, but her condition did not respond to the treatment. The opinion of the bacteriologist was sought regarding the possibility

---

*From Grunnet, M.L., Cannon, G.H., and Kushner, J.P.: Neurology, *31*:174–177, 1981.[25]

of other microorganisms. A possibility of Torulopsis or soil ameba infection was suggested, taking into consideration the harmattan, a period of the year during which the whole atmosphere of the city is dusty, and one breathes air containing fine dust. The incidence of meningitis also increases during this period. Lumbar puncture was therefore repeated, revealing xanthochromia and increased pus cells, predominantly neutrophils. Examination of a wet mount with India ink did not reveal Cryptococcus; however, examination of a wet mount of the centrifuged sample of cerebrospinal fluid revealed elongated phagocytic forms that were first thought to be phagocytic neutrophils. However, when 0.5% eosin solution was allowed to pass under the coverslip, the elongated phagocytic forms became rounded but did not take the color of eosin, whereas the polymorphonuclear cells were readily stained with eosin. The cerebrospinal fluid was inoculated onto Sabouraud dextrose agar for fungal culture, which was subsequently negative, and onto nonnutrient agar for free-living amebas with Escherichia coli as food. After 24 hours incubation at 37°C, the nonnutrient agar plate was examined under low power for the growth of free-living amebas. A fairly luxurious growth of the amebas was seen. A scraping of the growth was then put into 2 drops of distilled water in a cavity slide and incubated in a simple moist chamber (Petri dish with wet filter paper) at 37°C for flagellation. The flagellates were observed after 2 hours, moving freely in the distilled water. The possibility of Naegleria species was suggested, with advice to start treatment with amphotericin B, pending further identification of the species. In the meantime, nasal swabs were also taken for culture of free-living amebas. This also yielded a pure culture of amebas that subsequently proved to be Naegleria.

Amphotericin B was given for a period of 7 days, 1.500 units daily, intravenously. On the second day of treatment, there was a considerable improvement in the level of consciousness of the infant. She was responding to stimuli; some muscle tone had been regained, and she was no longer flaccid. Feeble attempts to nurse were noticed. There was no improvement beyond this stage. The child by now had a normal temperature; twitching and convulsions were not seen. At this stage, amphotericin B was stopped, because it was thought that no further treatment was necessary, in view of the clinical improvement in the patient's condition and the toxicity of the drug.

On the third day after discontinuation of treatment, fever developed again, and the infant succumbed to it on February 16, 1977. Unfortunately, necropsy could not be carried out, as the parents refused permission.*

---

*From Lawande, R.V., John, I., Dobbs, R.H., and Egler, L.J.: Am. J. Clin. Pathol., *71*:591–594, 1979.[26]

Case 4

A 47-year-old, black, diabetic woman was admitted to Riverside Hospital, Newport News, Virginia, on 17 May 1974, complaining of "weakness, loss of appetite, and diabetes." Two weeks previously she had been hospitalized elsewhere for "jerking of her extremities, shaking all over, and decreased vision;" she had been discharged on Diabinese, an oral hypoglycemic agent. No recent history of nausea, vomiting, diarrhea, dyspnea or trauma had been documented. The family lived in a rural area of Smithfield, Virginia, and used well water. Their house was without heat or electricity.

Examination at the time of admission showed an emaciated, uncooperative, chronically ill woman with a temperature of 38.3°C, blood pressure, 128/70, and pulse, 100 per min. Her eyes were deviated to the right; she was unable to move them to the left; and her neck was stiff. No abnormalities of the pupils were detected; no nystagmus was present; and the fundi were normal. Her tongue was believed deviated leftward, but no spacial asymmetry was noted. Her deep tendon reflexes were equal and active. The results of the remainder of her examination were not remarkable.

Admission laboratory work showed a blood leukocyte count of 8200 with 74% neutrophils, 5% band forms, 12% lymphocytes, 8% monocytes, and 1% basophils. Her hemoglobin was 14.2 g/dl; hematocrit, 43.9%, and platelets normal. A serum Na was 132; K, 5.8; Cl, 88; and CO_2, 10 mEq/L. The blood urea nitrogen was 48; serum creatinine, 1.9; and blood glucose, 510 mg/dl. A PCO_2 of arterial blood was 17 mm Hg; blood pH, 7.36; and serum acetone, 160 mg/dl. The serum bilirubin, alkaline phosphatase, creatine phosphokinase, glutamic oxaloacetic transaminase, calcium, and uric acid levels were all normal. A serum total protein was 7.4 with an albumin of 3.4 g/dl. A urinalysis showed a specific gravity of 1.029, was positive for ketones, had a pH 5.0, and contained 3 to 4 leukocytes per high-powered field. Cerebrospinal fluid was clear, but contained 110 cells per mm^3 (5 neutrophils and 105 lymphocytes), 84 mg/dl protein, and 240 mg/dl sugar. India ink, Gram's stain, and stains for acid-fast bacilli were negative; studies for amoebae were not done.

Results of chest roentgenogram and intravenous pyelograms were normal; however, calcifications over the pancreas were visible. An electrocardiogram showed sinus tachycardia with poor R-wave progression. The electroencephalogram exhibited a low-amplitude delta activity during the entire recording and was interpreted as subacute or acute cortical dysfunction of a generalized nature. There was no shift of structures as determined by echo sound. A radioisotope scan of the brain showed minimal increased activity over the right parietal area. A routine skull roentgenogram was not remarkable nor was an epidurogram. A retrograde right brachial arteriogram was interpreted as compatible with hydrocephalus and a mass in the right anterior parietal and posterior frontal cortex as associated with a spreading of surface branches of the right middle cerebral artery.

The patient received parenteral insulin, and although ketosis was eliminated, her blood sugars ranged between 250 and 420 mg/dl. Her serum Na remained low, and she was believed to have an inappropriate secretion of antidiuretic hormone. A 5-U tuberculin PPD skin test was positive, and she was started on isoniazid, streptomycin, and ethambutol.

By the second hospital day she was thought to have developed a left homonymous hemianopsia and left facial and palatal palsies. Her deep-tendon knee reflexes were 3 + on the left and 2 + on the right. She remained uncooperative but appeared to understand simple commands and could verbalize.

By the third hospital day she became increasingly dyspneic, was unable to handle her secretions, and she was intubated and supported artificially with ventilation. At this time she also received Decadron parenterally.

By the fifth hospital day she was essentially unresponsive, with a left hemiparesis and persistent deviation of her eyes to the right. Her Na was 125; K, 4.2; Cl, 85; and CO_2, 21 mEq/L. Her blood urea nitrogen was 17 and glucose, 295 mg/dl. The P_{CO_2} of arterial blood was 31 mm Hg, and the pH was 7.43.

On the sixth hospital day she developed decorticate posturing, her neck became 4 + stiff, Babinski's was present bilaterally, and a left lateral nystagmus was noted.

She died on the seventh hospital day.*

SUMMARY

Primary amebic meningoencephalitis (PAM) and granulomatous amebic meningoencephalitis (GAE) are rare but serious infections caused by ubiquitous free-living soil amebas. Although most cases of amebic meningoencephalitis in humans have been associated with Naegleria fowleri, several species of Acanthamoeba and at least one unidentified free-living ameba have been reponsible for human disease. The course of the infection varies with the etiologic agent, but PAM is usually fatal. Naegleria are believed to gain entrance through intranasal instillation of contaminated fresh water, but primary foci for Acanthamoeba may be the skin, the eye, the genitourinary tract, or the respiratory tract. The association of Acanthamoeba with keratitis in the last decade in immunocompromised hosts suggests that

---

*From Duma, R.J., Helwig, W.B., and Martinez, A.J.: Ann. Intern. Med., *88*:468–473, 1978.[16]

the protozoan has the potential for causing opportunistic as well as primary infections.

REFERENCES

1. Butt, C.G.: Primary amebic meningoencephalitis. Presented at the joint annual meeting of the American Society of Clinical Pathologists and College of American Pathologists. Bal Harbour, Florida. October 16–24, 1964.
2. Fowler, M., and Carter, R.F.: Acute pyogenic meningitis probably due to Acanthamoeba sp.: a preliminary report. Br. Med. J., *2*:740, 1965.
3. Patras, D., and Andujar, J.J.: Meningoencephalitis due to Hartmanella (Acanthamoeba). Presented at scientific assembly of the American Society of Clinical Pathologists, Chicago, Illinois. October 15–23, 1965.
4. Duma, R.J.: Primary amoebic meningoencephalitis. Crit. Rev. Clin. Lab. Sci., *3*:163, 1972.
5. Martinez, J.A., et al.: Meningoencephalitis due to Acanthamoeba sp.: pathogenesis and clinico-pathological study. Acta. Neuropathol., *37*:183, 1977.
6. Visvesvara, G.S., et al.: Isolation of two strains of Acanthamoeba castellanii from human tissue and their pathogenicity and isoenzyme profiles. J. Clin. Microbiol., *18*:1405, 1983.
7. Carter, R.F.: Primary amoebic meningo-encephalitis. An appraisal of present knowledge. Trans. R. Soc. Trop. Med. Hyg., *66*:193, 1972.
8. Willaert, E.: Primary amoebic meningoencephalitis. A selected bibliography and tabular survey of cases. Ann. Soc. Belg. Med. Trop., *54*:429, 1974.
9. Griffin, J.L.: Pathogenic free-living amoebae. *In* Parasitic Protozoa. Vol. 2. Edited by J. Kreier. New York, Academic Press, 1979.
10. Červa, L.: Amebic meningoencephalitis. *In* Medical Microbiology and Infectious Disease. Edited by A.I. Braude. Philadelphia, W.B. Saunders, 1981.
11. Nagington, J., et al.: Amoebic infections of the eye. Lancet, *2*:1537, 1974.
12. Jones, D.B., Visvesvara, G.S., and Robinson, N.M.: Acanthamoeba polyphaga keratitis and Acanthamoeba uveitis associated with fatal meningoencephalitis. Trans. Ophthalmol. Soc. U.K., *95*:221, 1975.
13. Ma, P., Eddy, W., Juechter, K.B., and Stevens, A.R.: A case of keratitis due to Acanthamoeba in New York, New York, and features of 10 cases. J. Infect. Dis., *143*:662, 1981.
14. Martinez, A.J.: Is Acanthamoeba encephalitis an opportunistic infection? Neurology, *30*:567, 1980.
15. Stevens, A.R., et al.: Primary amoebic meningoencephalitis: A report of two cases and antibiotic and immunologic studies. J. Infect. Dis., *143*:193, 1981.
16. Duma, R.J., Helwig, W.B., and Martinez, A.J.: Meningoencephalitis and brain abscess due to a free-living amoeba. Ann. Intern. Med., *88*:468, 1978.
17. Martinez, A.J., et al.: Meningoencephalitis due to Acanthamoeba sp. Acta Neuropathol., *37*:183, 1977.
18. Visvesvara, G.S.: Free-living pathogenic amoeba. *In* Manual of Clinical Microbiology, 3rd Ed. Edited by E.H. Lennette. Washington, D.C., American Society for Microbiology, 1980.
19. Singh, B.N.: Inter-relationship between micropredators and bacteria in soil. Presented at Forty-seventh Session, Indian Science Congress Association. Calcutta, India, July 20, 1960.
20. Visvesvara, G.S., and Balamuth, W.: Comparative studies on related free-living and pathogenic amebae with special reference to Acanthoamoeba. J. Protozool., *22*:245, 1975.
21. Visvesvara, G.S., and Healy, G.R.: Comparative antigenic analysis of pathogenic and free-living Naegleria species by the gel diffusion and immunoelectrophoresis techniques. Infect. Immunol., *11*:95, 1975.
22. Kenney, M.: The micro-Kolmer complement fixation test in routine screening for soil amoeba infection. Health Lab. Sci., *8*:5, 1971.
23. Anderson, K., and Jamieson, A.: Primary amoebic meningoencephalitis. Lancet, *1*:902, 1972.

24. Center for Disease Control: Primary amebic meningoencephalitis. Morbid. Mortal. Weekly Rept., *27*:343, 1978.
25. Grunnet, M.L., Cannon, G.H., and Kushner, J.P.: Fulminant amebic meningoencephalitis due to Acanthamoeba. Neurology, *31*:174, 1981.
26. Lawande, R.V., John, I., Dobbs, R.H., and Egler, L.J.: A case of primary amebic meningoencephalitis in Zaria, Nigeria. Am. J. Clin. Pathol., *71*:591, 1979.

CHAPTER 3 ANTIBIOTIC-ASSOCIATED COLITIS

Antibiotic-associated pseudomembranous colitis is a serious intestinal disease usually precipitated by antimicrobial therapy.[1,2] The inflammatory process can be induced by most antimicrobial agents except parenteral aminoglycosides and vancomycin. Clindamycin was implicated as the initiating therapeutic agent in 1974.[3,4] Penicillins, cephalosporins, tetracycline, cephamycins, lincomycin, moxalactam, erythromycin, chloramphenicol, and trimethoprim-sulfamethoxazole, however, have all been associated with antibiotic-associated colitis.[5,6] The stool specimens of patients in whom the clindamycin-associated colitis occurred in 1974 were later found to contain Clostridium difficile. The stool filtrates produced a cytopathic effect in tissue cultures. This was consistent with the observed effects of clindamycin in hamsters.[7]

Pseudomenbranous colitis has also been reported following chemotherapy for cancer.[7] Because therapeutic regimens in cancer patients often consist of more than one drug, the specific effects of any one chemotherapeutic agent are less well defined than those of antimicrobial agents. Clearly, any interference in normal intestinal flora can induce colitis. At least one case of pseudomembranous colitis associated with intestinal colonization in the absence of recent antibiotic therapy or chemotherapy has been reported.[8]

ETIOLOGY

The role of Clostridium difficile as a major cause of antibiotic-associated colitis is well established.[1,5,6,9] C. difficile is a large anaerobic gram-positive bacillus that produces elongated subterminal spores. The bacterium is a part of the indigenous flora of the colon and urogenital tract of some healthy humans.[11-14] Administration of antimicrobial agents is believed to permit C. difficile to flourish in the intestine while more susceptible indigenous organisms are destroyed. In simultaneous and deferred test procedures, growth of the intestinal organisms Streptococcus, Bifidobacterium, and Lactobacillus was inhibited by C. difficile.[10] C. difficile also interfered with the growth of the intestinal organisms Bacteroides, Peptococcus, and Peptostreptococcus. The significance of the in vitro tests to possible in vivo mechanisms in antibiotic-associated colitis remains speculative.

C. difficile was first isolated from stool specimens of healthy infants ranging in age from 2 weeks to 1 year.[15,16] The cytotoxic effect of C. difficile is produced by an exotoxin called toxin B. An immunologically distinct enterotoxin, designated as toxin A, has been isolated from cultures of C. difficile. Sloughing of intestinal epithelial tissue, hemorrhaging, and deposition of polymorphonuclear cells in characteristic plaques are hallmarks of antibiotic-associated colitis.

PREDISPOSING FACTORS

Administration of antibiotics or chemotherapeutic agents predisposes some individuals to pseudomembranous colitis. Underlying neoplastic disease may also favor growth of C. difficile. In one study, 40% of the patients on an oncology ward were colonized with the anaerobe.[9] It cannot be completely ascertained whether C. difficile is of endogenous or exogenous origin in antibiotic-associated colitis. Epidemiologic studies have demonstrated that C. difficile-induced colitis can be a nosocomial infection.

EPIDEMIOLOGY

Carrier rates up to 3% or higher have been reported for C. difficile.[2,10] The carrier rates are higher in infants, although the reason C. difficile can be isolated with greater frequency from asymptomatic infants is unclear. It has been proposed that neonates may have passively acquired immunity or undeveloped binding sites for the toxin or the organism. No documented cases of person-to-person transmission have been reported, but C. difficile can be isolated from the environment of patients with antibiotic-associated diarrheal syndromes.[13,17]

C. difficile has been isolated from the hands of health care professionals attending colitis patients and from fecal-contaminated toilet seats, hoppers, sinks, scales, floors, mops, and bed clothing. Cross infection has been suspected of being a factor in three outbreaks of antibiotic-associated colitis in the United States and in one outbreak in England.[3,4,18–20] As awareness of antibiotic-associated colitis increases, it is hoped that more can be learned about the epidemiology of the disease.

LABORATORY DIAGNOSIS

A clinical diagnosis of antibiotic-associated colitis is dependent on a history of antibiotic therapy and diarrhea. Stools may be liquid or soft in consistency and as frequent as five per day. Radiographic, sigmoidoscopic, or colonoscopic techniques may be used to demonstrate lesions in the colon (Fig. 3–1). C. difficile and toxin B have

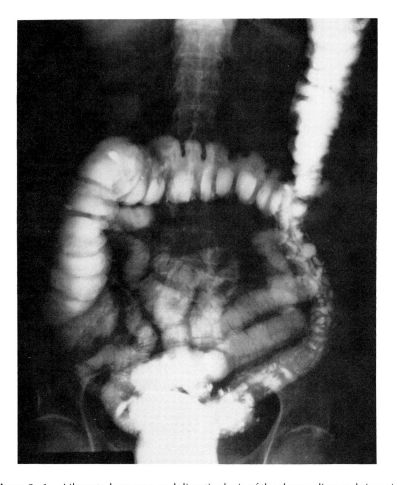

Figure 3–1.   Ulcerated mucosa and diverticulosis of the descending and sigmoid colon revealed by barium enema in a patient with pseudomembranous colitis. (Reprinted by permission of the publisher from Peikin, S.R., Galdibini, J., and Bartlett, J.G.: Role of Clostridium difficile in a case of nonantibiotic-associated pseudomembranous colitis. Gastroenterol., 79:948–951, 1980. Copyright 1980 by the American Gastroenterological Association.)

been isolated from stools of asymptomatic patients. Therefore, its presence alone without documentation of a pseudomembrane or plaques is not diagnostic for antibiotic-associated colitis.

Microscopic Examination

When pseudomembranous colitis is suspected, a Gram stain of a smear prepared from stool is indicated. In antibiotic-induced colitis caused by C. difficile, large numbers of polymorphonuclear white blood cells are usually present. Sometimes, gram-positive bacilli, with or without subterminal spores, can be seen.

Cultural Techniques

Prereduced cycloserine-cefoxitin-fructose-egg yolk agar (CCFEYA) is recommended as a highly efficient selective and differential plating medium.[21] Plates can be incubated for 48 to 72 hours at 37°C in a GasPak jar or in an anaerobic chamber. Colonies of C. difficile are slightly raised, moist, and white, with filamentous edges; they change the color of the medium from orange to yellow. The colonies fluoresce yellow in ultraviolet light.[22]

Biochemical Characterization

C. difficile ferments fructose, but does not degrade lecithin. If appropriate, additional biochemical tests and gas chromatography of volatile organic acids can be performed by the procedures recommended by the Virginia Polytechnic Institute and State University Anaerobe Laboratory in Blacksburg, Virginia (Fig. 3–2).[23] C. difficile is motile, produces gelatinase, but does not produce lipase, indole, or esculin. In addition to fructose, the organism ferments glucose, mannitol, and mannose.

Cytotoxic Assay

The toxin of C. difficile can be recovered by inoculating prereduced anaerobically sterilized chopped meat with a stool specimen.[21] After incubation at 37°C for 48 to 72 hours, broth is centrifuged for 20 minutes at 2000 rpm. The supernatant is filtered, using a 0.45 μm pore-size membrane filter. Tubes or flasks of human fibroblasts WI-38 (Microbiological Associates, Bethesda, Maryland) are inoculated with 0.1 ml aliquots of filtrate. Other 0.1 ml aliquots of filtrate are mixed with equal volumes of antitoxin of Clostridium sordellii (Food and Drug Administration Bureau of Biologics, Rockville, Maryland) and allowed to stand at room temperature for 1 hour before inoculating cell cultures. Tissue cultures can be maintained with Medium 199 (Flow Laboratories, Inglewood, California), penicillin (100 U/ml), streptomycin (100 μg/ml), and 2% fetal bovine serum. All cultures should be examined after 4 hours and held for at least 48 hours. Cytopathic effect (CPE) of C. difficile toxin consists of increased refractility, rounding of cells, or partial destruction of the monolayer of tissue cells. The degree of CPE is scored on a 0 to 4 scale used for cell cultures of viruses.[23]

$$
\begin{aligned}
0 \quad &= \text{no CPE} \\
\pm \quad &= \text{suggestion of beginning CPE} \\
1+ \quad &= 25\% \text{ or less cells affected} \\
2+ \quad &= 25 \text{ to } 50\% \text{ cells affected} \\
3+ \quad &= 50 \text{ to } 75\% \text{ cells affected} \\
4+ \quad &= 75 \text{ to } 100\% \text{ cells affected or sloughed from glass}
\end{aligned}
$$

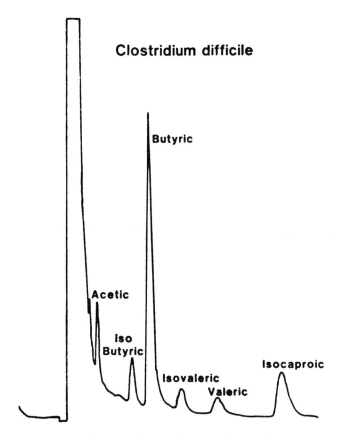

Figure 3–2. Pattern of volatile fatty acid peaks obtained from the fermentation of glucose by Clostridium difficile detected by gas liquid chromatography. (From Rosenblatt, J.E.: Anaerobic bacteria. III. Identification of anaerobic bacteria. *In* Laboratory Procedures in Clinical Microbiology. Edited by J.A. Washington. New York, Springer-Verlag, 1981.)

The CPE of the toxin is neutralized by C. sordellii or C. difficile antitoxin.

If fecal specimens are used for toxin detection, stool should be diluted 1:10 with sterile 0.85% saline and filtered through a 0.45-μm pore-size membrane filter. If tests cannot be performed immediately, diluted and filtered fecal specimens may be stored at $-70°C$. A reference or public health laboratory should be consulted if methodology or trained personnel are not available in a hospital setting.

An enzyme immunoassay (EIA), using rabbit and goat antisera to C. difficile, an alkaline phosphatase-labeled antibody to goat IgG, and p-nitrophenol phosphate, appears to be a sensitive and rapid assay for C. difficile antigen.[24]

PROGNOSIS

Diarrhea may be mild to severe in antibiotic-associated colitis and may last 4 to 6 weeks after discontinuation of antibiotics. C. difficile is susceptible to vancomycin, but, unfortunately, relapses occur in approximately 20% of cases treated with vancomycin. Studies in hamsters indicate that recurrences may result from spore survival in the colon or from environmental contamination.[2,25,26]

Severe complications, including toxic megacolon, colonic perforation, and hypoproteinemia, appear to be rare in antibiotic-associated colitis. It is possible that more than one toxin is elaborated by C. difficile in vivo or that there are strain differences that account for varying degrees of severity. It is also possible that as yet unidentified host factors participate in the disease process.

CASE REPORTS

Case 1

On August 30, 1980, a 64-year-old woman was admitted for high fever and somnolence. She had had cavitary lung tuberculosis in 1946 and had had a subfebrile state for the 4 months before admission.

Laboratory data were (with upper limits of normal in parentheses): serum bilirubin 13 μmol/L(21), SGOT 28(20), SGPT 10(17), γ-glutamyl transpeptidase 49(28), alkaline phosphatase 38(30) (IU/L). Chest x-ray showed diffuse micronodulary opacities a few days after the beginning of treatment only. Liver biopsy disclosed granulomatous hepatitis, and a suspicion of miliary tuberculosis was later confirmed by the growth of Mycobacterium tuberculosis.

Chemotherapy with rifampicin 600 mg, isoniazid 500 mg, ethambutol 1600 mg daily (patient's weight 70 kg) was started in September. The patient was afebrile for the first 10 days of treatment.

On October 10, she became slightly febrile and from October 15 onwards she complained of diffuse abdominal pain. Her stool frequency was 5 to 6 times daily and she was febrile up to 39°C. Pseudomembranous colitis (PMC) was diagnosed by rectoscopy, biopsy, and isolation of C. difficile in stool cultures. She was given 2 g vancomycin daily by mouth. 2 days later, agranulocytosis developed and she died in acute heart failure on October 19. Necropsy revealed miliary tuberculosis of lung, liver, spleen, and bone marrow and confirmed extensive pseudomembranous rectocolitis.

In this woman without pre-existing liver disease, PMC developed after 26 days of uninterrupted rifampicin treatment, a short period in the light of O'Connor's hamster studies of PMC due to rifampicin-resistant C. difficile after 6 months of treatment. The delays in the other cases were 9 months and a few weeks. Liver dysfunction in our patient was slight and there was no cholestasis; thus the PMC could not be explained by one of the two hypotheses described above. Decreased resistance associated with diffuse miliary tuberculosis may nevertheless have favoured infection with C. difficile.*

Case 2

A 26-year-old man with embryonal cell carcinoma of the testicle underwent orchiectomy and retroperitoneal lymph node dissection and received local x-ray treatment (4400 rads). A lung metastasis was surgically resected, and 4 months later the patient was given chemotherapy that consisted of cisplatin, bleomycin sulfate, and vinblastine sulfate. Three days later the patient developed abdominal cramping and mild diarrhea, which were treated successfully with nasogastric aspiration and IV fluids. Four weeks after this episode, a second course of chemotherapy was given with reduced doses, and the patient developed severe diarrhea, which started promptly after reinstitution of chemotherapy and lasted for 8 to 10 days; chemotherapy was continued for 14 days.

Pseudomembranous colitis was shown by sigmoidoscopy. Clostridium difficile was cultured from 2 stool specimens, and the toxin assay was positive. Treatment with oral vancomycin for 10 days cleared the organism.

Over a 6-month interval, 3 additional episodes of severe colitis occurred. All episodes were caused by toxigenic C. difficile and responded to treatment with oral vancomycin. A stool culture taken between treatment cycles was negative when the patient was asymptomatic. Each episode of colitis occurred with the readministration of cancer chemotherapy, even when the doses were further reduced. Antibiotics were given only once.

Pseudomembranous colitis usually follows the administration of antibiotics, but cases without this antecedent have been described. Suppression of the normal bowel flora by drugs used for cancer chemotherapy may be one mechanism by which pseudomembranous colitis due to toxigenic C. difficile occurs as a complication of cancer chemotherapy.†

Case 3

A 57-year-old woman was admitted to the Massachusetts General Hospital because of chronic diarrhea. She was in apparent good health until 2 months before admission, when she noted the onset of diarrhea associated with mild crampy abdominal pain. Over the following 2-month period, she developed anorexia and lost 10 lbs. She complained

---

*From Klaui, H., and Leuenberger, P.: Lancet, 2:1294, 1981.[27]
†From Fainstein, V., Bodey, G.P., and Fekety, R.: J. Infect. Dis. *143*:865, 1981. © 1981 by the University of Chicago.[7]

of chills and excessive sweating. Detailed questioning of the patient and her family physician, as well as a search of her medicine cabinet, failed to disclose evidence of antimicrobial agent use.

Physical examination revealed a blood pressure of 120/80 mm Hg, a heart rate of 110 beats/min, 16 respiration per minute, and a temperature of 100.2°F per rectum. The results of examination of the head, neck, chest, heart, and breasts were within normal limits. The abdomen was soft and nontender with normal bowel sounds. There was no palpable organs or masses. There were no rectal masses, and the stool was guaiac negative. There was mild pedal edema. The neurologic examination was physiologic. Laboratory data included a hematocrit of 31% and a white blood cell count of 7400 cells/mm³ with 14% polys, 64% band forms, 10% lymphocytes, 9% monocytes, and 3% eosinophils. The erythrocyte sedimentation rate was 136 mm/hour. Urinalysis was significant for 2+ protein, 10 to 20 white cells, 20 to 50 red cells, and occasional red cell casts. The CH50, C'3, C4, and Raji cell assay were within normal limits.

Percutaneous kidney biopsy showed membranoproliferative glomerulonephritis. The azotemia and active urine sediment resolved spontaneously without therapy. Evaluation of her diarrhea revealed a negative routine stool culture for Salmonella and Shigella, stool for ova and parasites, and qualitative stool fat. Occasional polymorphonuclear leukocytes were seen on Wright stain of the stool. Sigmoidoscopy to 18 cm was normal. Barium enema showed diverticulosis with ulcerated mucosa of the descending and sigmoid colon. Colonoscopy to 40 cm revealed multiple white-based superficial ulcers with mild erythema and granularity in the intervening mucosa. No gross pseudomembrane was seen. Biopsy at the edge of an ulcer yielded the diagnosis of pseudomembranous colitis. Tissue culture assay of stool using WI-38 cells showed a cytopathic toxin that was neutralized by C. sordellii antitoxin. Serial 10-fold dilutions of the specimen indicated the cytotoxin titer was 1:100. Culture of the stool on a selective medium incorporating cycloserine and cefoxitin yielded C. difficile in a concentration of $10^{2.3}$/g wet weight. The isolate was grown in chopped meat glucose broth culture for 5 days; all free supernatant applied to tissue cultures produced cytopathic changes that were neutralized by C. sordellii antitoxin, indicating in vitro production of cytotoxin that was similar or identical to the cytotoxin noted in the stool specimen.

The patient was given vancomycin 500 mg orally every 6 hours for 1 week. She defervesced, and the differential white count normalized with only modest improvement in her diarrhea. Twenty-four hours after starting vancomycin the stool was negative for cytotoxicity. However, 1 week after finishing the course of vancomycin her diarrhea worsened, and the stool again contained a cytopathic toxin that was again neutralized by C. sordellii antitoxin. She received a second course of vancomycin, had moderate improvement in her diarrhea, and was discharged.

One week later the patient was admitted because of a colonic perforation. At laparotomy, a walled-off diverticular perforation of the sigmoid colon was encountered. Good pulses were felt in the vessels supplying the colon. The colon appeared inflamed, especially in the sigmoid and cecal regions, and a diverting ileostomy was performed. The stool was negative for cytotoxicity. The patient developed sepsis and low cardiac output postoperatively. A total colectomy was then performed in order to remove the presumed source of sepsis. The colon contained large areas of mucosal ulceration. There were linear and irregular areas of denuded mucosa with intervening patches of edematous but otherwise unremarkable mucosa. Microscopically, the ulcerations were morphologically nonspecific, but were consistent with a "late" stage of pseudomembranous colitis. Some of the ulcers were nearly transmural, and there was no evidence of reepithelialization over any of the ulcers. The patient continued to do poorly, and died on the second postoperative day.*

SUMMARY

Antibiotic-associated colitis is induced primarily by the administration of antimicrobial agents and is caused by toxigenic strains of Clostridium difficile, an organism that is sometimes indigenous to the colon. The disease is usually benign and may be self-limiting in some individuals. In other individuals, serious complications can occur. Although C. difficile is susceptible to vancomycin, recurrences have been reported in approximately one out of five cases.

The presence of distinct plaques on the intestinal wall and demonstration of a cytotoxin are necessary to confirm a diagnosis of antibiotic-associated colitis. The cytotoxin is distinct from the enterotoxin causing the in vivo lesions in individuals with pseudomembranous colitis. An enzyme immunoassay (EIA) technique holds promise as a rapid and sensitive means for detecting antigens of C. difficile.

REFERENCES

1. Bartlett, J.G., et al.: Antibiotic-associated pseudomembranous colitis due to toxin-producing clostridia. N. Engl. J. Med., *298*:531, 1978.
2. George, W.L., Rolfe, R.D., Mulligan, M.E., and Finegold, S.M.: Infectious diseases 1979—antimicrobial agent-induced colitis: an update. J. Infect. Dis., *140*:266, 1979.

---

*Reprinted by permission of the publisher from Peikin, S.R., Galdibini, J., and Bartlett, J.G.: Gastroenterol. *79*:948–951, 1980. Copyright 1980 by the American Gastroenterological Association.[8]

3. Ramirez-Ronda, C.H.: Incidence of clindamycin-associated colitis. Ann. Intern. Med., *81*:860, 1974.
4. Tedesco, F.J., Barton, R.W., and Alpers, D.H.: Clindamycin-associated colitis: a prospective study. Ann. Intern. Med., *81*:429, 1974.
5. George, W.L., Rolfe, R.D., and Finegold, S.M.: Clostridium difficile and its cytotoxin in feces of patients with antimicrobial-agent-associated diarrhea and miscellaneous conditions. J. Clin. Microbiol., *15*:1049, 1982.
6. Gilligan, P.H., McCarthy, L.R., and Genta, V.M.: Relative frequency of Clostridium difficile in patients with diarrheal disease. J. Clin. Microbiol., *14*:26, 1981.
7. Fainstein, V., Bodey, G.P., and Fekety, R.: Relapsing pseudomembranous colitis associated with cancer chemotherapy. J. Infect. Dis., *143*:865, 1981.
8. Peikin, S.R., Galdibini, J., and Bartlett, J.G.: Role of Clostridium difficile in a case of nonantibiotic-associated pseudomembranous colitis. Gastroenterol., *79*:948, 1980.
9. Bartlett, J.G., Chang, T.W., Taylor, N.S., and Onderdonk, A.B.: Colitis induced by Clostridium difficile. Rev. Infect. Dis., *1*:370, 1979.
10. Rolfe, R.D., Helebian, S., and Finegold, S.M.: Bacterial interference between Clostridium difficile and normal fecal flora. J. Infect. Dis., *143*:470, 1981.
11. Bartlett, J.G., Onderdonk, A.B., Cisneros, R.L., and Kasper, D.L.: Clindamycin-associated colitis due to a toxin-producing species of Clostridium in hamsters. J. Infect. Dis., *136*:701, 1977.
12. Bartlett, J.G., Taylor, N.S., Chang, T.W., and Dzink, J.A.: Clinical and laboratory observations in Clostridium difficile colitis. Am. J. Clin. Nutr., *33*:2521, 1980.
13. Kim, K.H., et al.: Isolation of Clostridium difficile from the environment and contacts of patients with antibiotic-associated colitis. J. Infect. Dis., *143*:42, 1981.
14. Hafiz, S., McEntegart, M.G., Morton, R.S., and Waitkins, S.A.: Clostridium difficile in the urogenital tract of males and females. Lancet, *1*:420, 1975.
15. Hall, I.C. and O'Toole, E.: Intestinal flora in new-born infants with a description of a new pathogenic anaerobe, Bacillus difficilis. Am. J. Dis. Child., *49*:390, 1935.
16. Snyder, M.L.: The normal fecal flora of infants between two weeks and one year of age. I. Serial studies. J. Infect. Dis., *66*:1, 1940.
17. Mulligan, M.E., Rolfe, R.D., Finegold, S.M., and George, W.L.: Contamination of a hospital environment with Clostridium difficile. Curr. Microbiol., *3*:173, 1979.
18. Kabins, S.A., and Spira, T.J.: Outbreak of clindamycin-associated colitis. Ann. Intern. Med., *83*:830, 1975.
19. Kappas, A., et al.: Diagnosis of pseudomembranous colitis. Br. Med. J., *1*:675, 1978.
20. Keighley, M.R.B., et al.: Randomized controlled trial of vancomycin for pseudomembranous colitis and postoperative diarrhea. Br. Med. J., *2*:1667, 1978.
21. George, W.L., Sutter, V.L., Citron, D., and Finegold, S.M.: Selective and differential medium for isolation of Clostridium difficile. J. Clin. Microbiol., *9*:214, 1979.
22. Rosenblatt, J.E.: Anaerobic bacteria. III. Identification of anaerobic bacteria. *In* Laboratory Procedures in Clinical Microbiology. Edited by J.A. Washington. New York, Springer-Verlag, 1981.
23. Smith, R.F.: Viruses. II. Processing of specimens and cultures. *In* Laboratory Procedures in Clinical Microbiology. Edited by J.A. Washington. New York, Springer-Verlag, 1981.
24. Yolken, R.H., et al.: Enzyme immunoassay for the detection of Clostridium difficile antigen. J. Infect. Dis., *144*:378, 1981.
25. Fekety, R., et al.: Antibiotic-associated colitis: Effects of antibiotics on Clostridium difficile and the disease in hamsters. Rev. Infect. Dis., *1*:386, 1979.
26. Tosnival, R., Silva, J., Jr., Fekety, R., and Kim, K-H.: Studies on the epidemiology of colitis due to Clostridium difficile in hamsters. J. Infect. Dis., *143*:51, 1981.
27. Klaui, H., and Leuenberger, P.: Pseudomembranous colitis due to rifampicin. Lancet, *2*:1294, 1981.

CHAPTER 4 ASPERGILLOSIS

Aspergillosis is a noncommunicable complex group of infectious diseases caused by a dimorphic fungus belonging to the genus Aspergillus. Rudolf Virchow, the eminent pathologist, is believed to have reported one of the first cases of aspergillosis over 125 years ago.[1] Renon's classic monograph in 1897 describing six cases of human aspergillosis did much to stimulate interest in the disease in France.[2]

Today, the disease is recognized as being worldwide in distribution. Aspergillosis may manifest itself in a variety of clinical forms, but it is primarily an opportunistic infection of the lung. If dissemination occurs, aspergillosis usually has a rapidly fulminating course, which results in death.

The increasing use of immunosuppressive drugs and organ transplants has widened the range of host susceptibility in recent years. It is doubtful that accurate statistics exist for the actual incidence of aspergillosis, because multiple opportunistic infections sometimes occur in immunocompromised hosts. In addition, the ubiquitous nature of the organisms causing aspergillosis make them frequent laboratory contaminants. In some instances, an unequivocal diagnosis of aspergillosis is difficult to establish.

The infections caused by Aspergillus species may be divided into five major types of disease. Three forms of pulmonary aspergillosis are recognized: allergic aspergillosis, primary aspergilloma, and invasive pulmonary aspergillosis. In addition, a noninvasive localized form of aspergillosis and Aspergillus infections of nosocomial origin have been described. The clinical manifestations of the disease are generally related to the species of Aspergillus involved. Certain toxic metabolites, known as aflatoxins, produced by some Aspergillus species have long been suspected of having a role in human liver disease, but a definitive association between the fungal products and disease has yet to be proven.

ALLERGIC ASPERGILLOSIS

Allergic bronchopulmonary aspergillosis (ABPA) causes symptoms indistinguishable from those of asthma caused by pollen, animal danders, or ordinary house dust.[3-5] Awareness is increasing that ABPA

36

can occur as a complication of atopic asthma. The asthma tends to be episodic, occurring with the appearance of fleeting pulmonary infiltrates.

Complete accord on additional criteria for establishing a diagnosis of ABPA has not been reached. Several groups of investigators accept six of the following seven diagnostic criteria.[5,6]

1. Wheezing
2. Episodic pulmonary filtrates
3. Isolation of Aspergillus from sputum
4. Precipitating antibodies for Aspergillus fumigatus
5. A markedly elevated IgE
6. Eosinophilia
7. Positive skin tests for Aspergillus fumigatus

In addition to these criteria, proximal bronchiectasis has been reported in ABPA. It may be difficult to distinguish ABPA from steroid-dependent asthma.[6]

PRIMARY ASPERGILLOMA

Aspergilloma or "fungus ball" is a chronic infection that occurs when Aspergillus grows in a pre-existing cavity of the lung. A compact mass of mycelium and debris of cellular origin combine to form the "fungus ball" within the cavity. The ball typically measures 1.0 to 5.0 cm in diameter. No invasion of surrounding tissue occurs. Tomography or radiography reveals the presence of a crescent-shaped air space surrounding the cavity (Fig. 4–1). Pulmonary aspergillomas develop slowly and usually produce mild symptoms. If hemoptysis occurs, the loss of blood may be profuse and life-threatening.[7]

INVASIVE PULMONARY ASPERGILLOSIS

Invasive pulmonary aspergillosis is most often a complication of chronic lung disease and only rarely is found in previously healthy individuals.[8] The fungi invade lung tissue and may disseminate to points distant from the primary site of infection. The disease is characterized by granulomatous lesions that extend into the lung parenchyma.[1] A single lesion may resolve itself to form a "coin lesion," but multiple lesions are associated with the production of cavitation and necrosis. Symptoms include a productive cough, low-grade fever, weight loss, and toxemia.[1] Dissemination of Aspergillosis is particularly common in immunocompromised hosts and in patients receiving support for respiratory, renal, or hepatic failure.[9,10]

NONINVASIVE ASPERGILLOSIS

Aspergillus has been implicated in a number of noninvasive diseases of varying severity. The fungus can colonize the external auditory

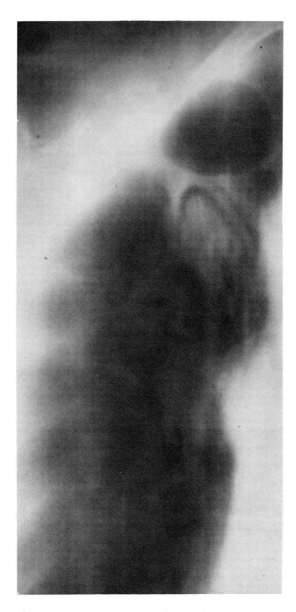

Figure 4–1.　Chest tomogram showing a fungus ball (aspergilloma) in an old cavity just below a larger bulla in the right upper lobe of a lung. The meniscus of air can be seen above the ball and below the superior wall of the cavity. (From Utz, J.P.: Aspergillosis. *In* Infectious Diseases, 3rd Ed. Edited by P.D. Hoeprich. Hagerstown, Maryland, Harper & Row, 1983.)

canal. If a plug containing a mycelium, cerumen, and debris occludes the canal, pruritus, irritation, and impairment of hearing can occur. Damage to the tympanic membrane is rare, and the infection responds well to antifungal therapy. Aspergillus can also cause keratitis, orbital cellulitis, sinusitis, and infections of a variety of other organs.[11-14]

NOSOCOMIAL ASPERGILLOSIS

Several factors contribute to nosocomial aspergillosis. Hospital patients, by the nature of underlying disease or immunosuppressive therapy, are particularly susceptible to a number of opportunistic microorganisms. A variety of Aspergillus species can be isolated from air and horizontal surfaces in the hospital environment.[15] In one instance, retrospective evaluation found that a clustering of nosocomial infections appeared to be related to recent nearby road construction and the presence of Aspergillus in window air conditioners.[16] Unfortunately, nosocomial aspergillosis is often fatal, and diagnosis is made only on autopsy.[17]

AFLATOXIN POISONING

Aflatoxins are heat-stable metabolites, which when ingested, cause severe poisoning and liver damage in animals and possibly in humans. The toxins have been isolated from contaminated grains, corn, and peanuts. Some Aspergillus and Penicillium species are prolific producers of aflatoxins. At least eight aflatoxins—B_1, B_2, B_{2a}, G_1, G_2, G_{2a}, M_1, and Q_1—have been described. Aflatoxin B_1, the most potent aflatoxin, produces hepatocarcinoma in laboratory animals.[18]

The role of aflatoxins in human cancer remains speculative. It is not known whether ingestion of low levels of the toxin over a period of time can produce liver disease, but epidemiologic evidence suggests that aflatoxin B_1 may cause endemic hepatocarcinoma in Africa and South Asia.[19] Some attempts have been made to associate aflatoxins with Reye syndrome, but a direct cause and effect relationship has not been demonstrated.[20,21]

ETIOLOGY

Aspergilli are ubiquitous in nature and particularly abundant on decaying vegetation. Several Aspergillus species have been associated with aspergillosis, but Aspergillus fumigatus is the most aggressive pathogen and the cause of most invasive pulmonary aspergilloses. A. flavus and A. oryzae have been isolated from sputum in pulmonary disease.[1] A. niger is more frequently implicated in noninvasive aspergillosis. It is the most common cause of "fungus ball" in the United States. A. fumigatus and A. niger are the most common causes of ocular aspergillosis, but both A. oryzae and A. flavus have been isolated from oculomycoses.[11,22]

All species of Aspergillus are considered potentially allergenic. In many instances, the fungi are not recovered from clinical specimens, and the only evidence of invasion is the presence of branching hyphae in tissue sections obtained on autopsy. Identification, therefore, is not always extended to the species level. It is likely that several saprophytic species can colonize the immunocompromised host.

PREDISPOSING FACTORS

A history of underlying chronic asthma is a significant risk factor in allergic bronchopulmonary aspergillosis (ABPA). The allergic response in many cases of atopic asthma is initiated by a variety of substances, including the spores of fungi. ABPA is reported in some parts of the world to be a common complication in children with cystic fibrosis.[23,24] Underlying disease and immunosuppression, resulting from prolonged use of antibiotics, steroids, or drugs, are known to predispose individuals to invasive aspergillosis. In a study of 98 patients with confirmed aspergillosis, nearly 90% of the individuals had neoplasms.[9] The use of immunosuppressive drugs in transplant recipients makes those persons prime candidates for several opportunists, including Aspergillus species.[25] Patients on support systems for respiratory, renal, or hepatic failure are also uniquely susceptible to aspergillosis.[26] Hemodialysis has been shown to diminish the ability of an individual to respond to various antigens.[27]

An increasing number of reports indicate that the immunocompromised state is not a prerequisite for invasive pulmonary or disseminated aspergillosis;[28–30] however, in vitro tests of lymphocyte function might reveal defects undetected by the clinical status of the affected patients or by conventional laboratory tests. Studies in mice suggest that immunity to invasive aspergillosis in that animal is multifactorial, but largely T-cell dependent.[31]

Consumption of large quantities of grains, nuts, corn, or rice may predispose some individuals to aflatoxin poisoning. The climate in the southeastern states of the United States favors growth of fungi in stored crops.[21] Thirty-five percent of corn samples from that part of the country were found to contain 6 to 348 μg of aflatoxin per kg in a survey conducted by the United States Department of Agriculture.[18] More studies are needed to assess dosages of aflatoxin required to cause hepatic dysfunction.

EPIDEMIOLOGY

The most common means of transmission of aspergillosis is by inhalation of spores of the fungi, but the portal of entry can also be the skin or the gastrointestinal tract. Nosocomial aspergillosis has been related to contaminated window air conditioners, road construction, hospital ventilation systems, and fireproofing material in ceilings.[16,32–34] At least one case of death from aspergillosis occurred following infection at the site of insertion of a Hickman catheter.[35] There is no evidence of person-to-person transmission.

LABORATORY DIAGNOSIS

A prerequisite for a diagnosis of aspergillosis is isolation of Aspergillus species or demonstration of characteristic hyphae in tissue sections or clinical specimens. Unfortunately, disseminated aspergillosis is too often discovered on examination of autopsy material. The value of serologic tests for the diagnosis of aspergillosis is somewhat controversial.[36,37]

Microscopic Examination

Sputum, earwax, skin or nail scrapings, material from lesions, biopsy specimens, or material obtained on autopsy may be used to demonstrate the presence of the branching hyphae of Aspergillus species. It may be necessary to treat sputum with 10% potassium hydroxide (KOH) to digest extraneous material. A warm 20% solution of KOH clears earwax. A pepsin solution (6 g pepsin in 600 ml of water and 10 ml concentrated HCl) will free hyphae from minute tissue samples if incubation is carried out at 37°C for 24 to 48 hours.[38] Mounting of fresh or formalin-fixed specimens directly in a solution of 40% KOH and Parker Blue-Black Quink is a rapid and efficient method for staining hyphae of Aspergillus in wet mounts.[39] In biopsy material, only short fragments of hyphae can be seen when sections are stained with hematoxylin-and-eosin, Gridley, periodic acid-Schiff (PAS), or Gomori methenamine silver nitrate (GMSN) techniques (Fig. 4–2).

Cultural Techniques

Aspergillus fumigatus grows readily at 37°C on Sabouraud's dextrose agar or Czapek-Dox medium containing chloramphenicol (0.05 mg per ml), but other species grow more readily at 25°C. All Aspergillus species are inhibited by cyclohexamide.[40] Certain species of Aspergillus grow better in the presence of the high osmotic pressure afforded by Czapek-Dox agar.

It is customary to set up duplicate plates, bottles, or tubes for incubation at 37°C and at room temperature. Material from lesions or solid tissue needs to be washed in physiologic saline containing penicillin and streptomycin to eliminate contamination by bacteria.[38] Pieces of tissue 1 to 2 mm in diameter can be used as inocula. It is preferable to use screw-capped bottles or tubes for reasons of safety if the presence of more virulent fungi has not been ruled out. All cultures should be maintained for a minimum of 3 weeks. Aspergillus organisms are usually rapid growers, and it is preferable to examine

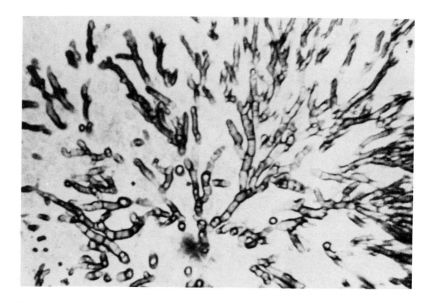

Figure 4–2. Short fragments of hyphae of Aspergillus fumigatus in lung tissue. (From Hazen, E.L., Gordon, M.A., and Reed, F.C.: Laboratory Identification of Pathogenic Fungi Simplified, 3rd Ed. Springfield, Illinois, Charles C Thomas, 1970.)

Table 4–1. Cultural characteristics of three common Aspergillus species grown on Czapek-Dox medium.

	A. fumigatus	A. niger	A. flavus
Surface colony color	blue-green	brown or black	yellow-green
Reverse colony color	brown	yellow	red-brown
Growth at 45°C	+	–	–

Adapted from Austwick, P.K., and Longbottom, J.L.: Medically important fungi. *In* Manual of Clinical Microbiology, 3rd Ed. Edited by E.H. Lennette. Washington, D.C., American Society for Microbiology, 1980.

young cultures in which morphologic and cultural characteristics are more apt to be typical. Cultures should be opened only in microbiologic safety hoods. Small amounts of material from centers of colonies can be mounted in a drop of lactophenol cotton blue for microscopic examination. Important identifying characteristics include colony color, rate of growth, and microscopic morphology. Morphologic and cultural characteristics for 3 common Aspergillus species are listed in Tables 4–1 and 4–2. The significance of the isolation of species other than A. fumigatus from a single specimen must be assessed carefully since the fungi are such common laboratory contaminants.

Table 4–2. Morphologic characteristics of three common Aspergillus species grown on Czapek-Dox medium.

	A. fumigatus	A. niger	A. flavus
Shape of mature vesicle	flask-shaped	spherical	spherical or subspherical
Rows of sterigmata	1	2	1–2
Maximum vesicle diameter (μm)	30	100	65
Maximum conidiophore length	300 μm	6 mm	2 mm
Conidia (μm)	2.5–3.5	5.5–8.0	3.5–4.5

Adapted from Austwick, P.K., and Longbottom, J.L.: Medically important fungi. *In* Manual of Clinical Microbiology, 3rd Ed. Edited by E.H. Lennette. Washington, D.C., American Society for Microbiology, 1980.

Serologic Tests

Serologic tests can be of some value in establishing a diagnosis of aspergillosis if certain limitations are recognized. The Ouchterlony comparative double diffusion (CDD) and immunoelectro-osmophoresis (IEOP) have been used extensively for the detection of precipitating antibodies against Aspergillus antigens;[41,42] however, precipitating antibodies to Aspergillus antigens have not been demonstrated in all instances of aspergillosis.[43] Other, less time-consuming methods for detection of antibodies have been introduced over the years, but a rapid enzyme-linked immunosorbent assay (ELISA) for A. fumigatus appears to be applicable for demonstrating IgG antibodies.[44]

Negative results on the available serologic tests do not rule out aspergillosis. Immunocompromised hosts are often incapable of mounting a response that produces detectable antibodies. An alternative procedure would be to detect Aspergillus antigen in the host. Antiserum designed to detect Aspergillus antigenemia has been produced in rabbits;[45] however, the applicability of the antiserum for the diagnosis of human aspergillosis will require further studies.

Aflatoxin Detection

Aflatoxin B_1 can be quantitated in serum and urine with methodology now available. High-pressure liquid chromatography has been used successfully to quantitate aflatoxin B_1 in serum.[46] The limit of detection approximates 0.5 ng of aflatoxin B_1. A radioimmunoassay (RIA) is sensitive enough to be used to demonstrate aflatoxin B_1 in urine samples.[21] The method detects aflatoxin B_1 concentrations as low as 20 pg. No extensive surveys have been conducted to determine the prevalence of aflatoxin in sera or urine. In one limited, but controlled, study of children with Reye syndrome and control subjects, aflatoxin was detected in the serum or urine of 23% of the participants.[21] None of the children in control groups was ill despite the presence of the toxin. The significance of finding aflatoxin in apparently healthy individuals is not known.

PROGNOSIS

Prognosis in aspergillosis is dependent on the seriousness of any accompanying underlying disease or immunosuppression. Allergic bronchopulmonary aspergillosis (ABPA) is disabling and can be fatal. Noninvasive aspergillosis is not usually serious. Infections of the external ear are often self-limiting. Aspergilloma or "fungus ball" is frequently benign, but surgical intervention may be necessary.

Invasive aspergillosis involving the lung or other organs is always serious and usually fatal. The course is related to the severity of immune deficiency. Invasive aspergillosis has a rapidly fulminating course in patients with underlying malignancy.[47]

The severity and course of nosocomial aspergillosis is probably related to numbers of inhaled spores.[16] More aggressive attempts in monitoring the environment of high-risk patients and in screening for Aspergillus in nasal swabs could permit application of appropriate antifungal therapy and prevent overt disease.

Reports of human intoxication attributed to aflatoxins have been relatively rare, but in animals, aflatoxins are known to cause hemorrhage, hepatic dysfunction, and hepatic tumors with grave prognoses.[48] It is probable that the long-term effect of ingesting aflatoxin B_1 may be associated with neoplastic transformation of liver cells, but the mere presence of aflatoxin is not definitive evidence of a cause-effect relationship.

CASE REPORTS

Case 1

This white girl was well until she was 5½ years old when a tonsillectomy and adenoidectomy were performed. Six to 9 months afterwards, a cough began and became progressively worse over the next 4 years. Episodes of wheezing first occurred during upper respiratory infections and later became more spontaneous. The illness was diagnosed as asthma when she was 9 years old.

She was first brought to the Out-Patient Department of the Long Island Jewish Medical Center when she was 11 years old, in June 1965, with the complaint of recurrent coughs and frequent rhinitis. Anti-allergic therapy consisting of desensitization to house dust, molds, and ragweed was started. The episodes of wheezing persisted throughout this course of desensitization. In the initial tests for allergens, she showed a moderate reaction to house dust, feathers, penicillin, and Hormodendrum, and a marked reaction to Alternaria and

Aspergillus. Her asthmatic attacks were treated with drugs and antihistamines; no steroid therapy was given.

At age 12½, when assessed in the Adolescent Clinic, she was thin and small and sexually immature. Her weight was only 77 lb (15 percentile); her height 58½ inches (25 percentile). Her first menstrual period was attended by considerable anxiety. Because of recurrent and almost continuous wheezing, it was agreed to treat her with steroids. These were first utilized in October (aged 13½) for acute episodes of asthma. Additional medication at this time included antibiotics for respiratory infections, tranquilizers, antihistamines and adrenalin, all when indicated. At home she used inhalations of Isuprel (an anti-asthmatic preparation) when her condition warranted it. During January 1968, she had almost constant wheezing and required intensive medication. In May 1968, when ill with fever, a chest x-ray revealed an infiltrate in the left upper lobe and tomograms showed 3 separate opaque nodular lesions in the left upper lobe. She was hospitalized and given 3 g of intramuscular cephaloridine per day for 1 week. She had no anemia or leukocytosis. Urinalysis was negative. Sputum cultures were negative for pathogens. Skin tests with histoplasmin, coccidioidin, blastomycin, and tuberculin were negative, the latter with PPD of intermediate strength. Because the radiographic nodular lesions in the lingular segmental region persisted, a bronchoscopy and a bronchogram were performed on June 3, 1968. No evidence of bronchiectasis was found, though nodular infiltration in the left lung field remained unchanged. A left scalene node biopsy did not show any lesions.

On June 4, 1968, a left thoracotomy was undertaken to explore the involved upper left lobe. Three solid lesions were excised by segmental resection; these proved to be abscesses from which Aspergillus fumigatus were grown. Precipitation studies of the child's serum then proved positive for Aspergillus fumigatus antigens (precipitation tests were performed by Dr. I. Abrams, Nassau County Hospital for Pulmonary Diseases, Plainview, New York). The patient was now given iodide treatment consisting of an intravenous dose of 1 g every other day for 4 days and then orally as potassium iodide 300 mg 3 times daily for 6 weeks. Asthmatic attacks continued for the next 4 months. She developed a fever and a chest roentgenogram revealed a nodular infiltrate of the right upper lobe along with hilar adenopathy. The question of recurrence of aspergillosis in the opposite lung was considered. She was followed with serial roentgenograms until April 1969, when a large area of consolidation in the right mid-lung field associated with hilar and mediastinal adenopathy became evident. The left lung remained entirely clear. Bronchoscopy showed some redness of the mucous membrane of the right upper lobe bronchus, but no other abnormality. Smears and bronchial washings from the right side grew Aspergillus fumigatus.

The patient was then given amphotericin B intravenously, starting with 0.25 mg per kg for 3 days and increasing this to 1 mg per kg per day for 4 weeks and then 3 times a week for the next 4 months. The pulmonary infiltrate appeared to decrease under this regimen. In addition, amphotericin B was given by aerosol inhalation 3 times a week over a 6 week period; 1 mg in 10 ml distilled water was used. The total dose of amphotericin B was 2.5 g over a 4 month period. Nausea and wheezing occurred. When a rising BUN was found, this treatment was stopped (August 1969).

In September 1969, hemoptysis developed. A chest roentgenogram showed a fibrotic scar in the right upper lung and a bronchogram revealed bronchiectasis in this area. A right thoracotomy with resection of the anterior segment of the upper lobe of the right lung was then done. The resected specimen contained a bronchiectatic abscess from which Staphylococcus aureus and Aspergillus niger were grown. The patient was given amphotericin B intravenously after the operation and 3 times weekly for the next month (50 mg per dose). She would react to these latter doses of medication with severe wheezing episodes; and therefore, the drug was stopped. Since then, she has had several minimal episodes of hemoptysis and some recurrence of evening temperatures. All sputum cultures have now been negative for Aspergilli, and the roentgenograms of the chest have shown no evidence of active disease over an 18-month period.*

Case 2

A 59-year-old woman with a previous history of acute granulocytic leukemia, diagnosed 14 months prior to admission, was admitted for chemotherapy of a relapse. Outpatient treatment had consisted of maintenance chemotherapy, including cytosine arabinoside and 6-thioguanine. She had no complaints other than mild headache. Physical examination disclosed moderate obesity, but was otherwise unremarkable. She was afebrile.

Laboratory data on admission included the following: hemoglobin, 9.0 g/dl; leukocyte count, 4000/mm^3, with 18% segmented neutrophils, 4% band forms, 34% lymphocytes, 3% monocytes, and 41% blast-like cells. Smears of the bone marrow aspirate disclosed hypercellularity with replacement of the marrow elements by leukemic blast cells. Cerebrospinal fluid showed no evidence of CNS leukemia or infection. Chest roentgenogram was normal.

Reinduction chemotherapy was begun with intravenous infusions

---

*From Berger, I., Phillips, W.L., and Shenker, I.R.: Clin. Pediatr., *11*:178–182, 1972.[49]

of doxorubicin and cytosine arabinoside. Her headache resolved spontaneously on the first day.

In order to establish venous access for IV infusions and frequent blood samples, a silicone rubber catheter, as described by Hickman, et al., was placed via the right cephalic vein, into the superior vena cava. A subcutaneous tunnel was constructed such that the catheter entry site was at the level of the right nipple. Eleven days after insertion of the catheter, she developed temperature to 40°C associated with cellulitis around the cephalic vein cut-down site. The infection occurred 3 days after completion of chemotherapy when the leukocyte count was 500/mm^3 with approximately 100 segmented neutrophils per cubic millimeter. Blood cultures were obtained, but material at the site of infection was unobtainable for culture. Chest roentgenogram was normal. Broad spectrum antimicrobial therapy was started.

Fever continued along with progression of the cellulitis. Granulocyte transfusions were added on the twenty-second hospital day. The wound was opened, and on the following day, black necrotic tissue with a "moldy" appearance was noted. Cultures revealed Aspergillus species and biopsy showed invasive hyphae. No leukemic cells were noted. Amphotericin B was started. Three days later she began complaining of right arm weakness. Examination disclosed slight weakness of the extensors of the wrist and interossei muscles with paralysis of the biceps, brachioradialis, deltoid, and triceps muscles. Muscle stretch reflexes of the right arm were absent, and the sensory exam was normal except for a small area of anesthesia over the lateral right shoulder. Nerve stimulation studies and motor latencies revealed no response in the deltoid, biceps, and triceps muscles. A gallium-67 scan revealed intense uptake of gallium in the right shoulder area. Tomograms with gallium suggested the possibility of infection in the humeral head. Exploration and debridement of the wound was undertaken and revealed an abscess, which dissected over the chest wall posterior to the pectoralis major muscle. The neurovascular structures were involved with the purulent infection. Biopsy of the humeral head did not reveal bony involvement. Repeat biopsy and culture of the area grew Aspergillus species and Staphylococcus epidermidis. A second microscopic examination of a biopsy specimen again disclosed invading hyphal elements, morphologically consistent with Aspergillus species. Over the next week, her bone marrow recovered, the fever subsided, but arm weakness and purulent drainage continued. Nine days following surgical debridement, she sustained a major hemorrhage from one of the shoulder vessels. Resuscitation was unsuccessful, and the patient died.*

*From Krol, T.C. and O'Keefe, P.: Cancer *50*:1214–1217, 1982. © by the American Cancer Society.[35]

Case 3

A 54-year-old man was admitted to another hospital on March 19, 1979, with a 4-day history of fever, chills, and myalgias. No hematuria or dark urine was observed.

He had a history of diabetes mellitus, but used no medications of any kind and denied recent change in urinary frequency, nocturia, or thirst. There was no weight loss or anorexia. There was also a history of substantial alcohol intake since losing his job 4 months before admission. He had had measles and mumps in childhood. This was his first hospital admission.

Physically, he was well developed and nourished. He appeared to be in a toxic condition, although alert and oriented. He was febrile (temperature 38.9°C). Pulse rate was 130 beats per minute and regular; respirations were 24/min. He was icteric and had generalized muscle tenderness. No rash or adenopathy was noted. He had normal bowel sounds. Heart sounds were normal, with no murmurs or rub. Neurologic findings were unremarkable. The clinical impression on admission was that he had a urinary tract infection with sepsis.

Sputum and blood cultures were obtained; a Foley catheter insertion yielded only 15 ml of bloody urine that was culture negative. Laboratory studies showed metabolic acidosis, hyperkalemia, azotemia, and elevated transaminase levels with hyperbilirubinemia. A renal scan demonstrated bilaterally diminished perfusion, and a renal ultrasound examination showed normal-sized kidneys with no obstruction.

He was treated with ion-exchange resin enemas, glucose, insulin, and antibiotics and was transferred to Thomas Jefferson University Hospital, Philadelphia, on day 2.

On admission, he was febrile (temperature, 40°C) and appeared toxic, confused, and tremulous, with a BP of 182/90 mm Hg and a respiratory rate of 40/min. No asterixis was noted. He had no rash or adenopathy and was icteric. His abdomen was distended with periumbilical and right upper quadrant tenderness and normal bowel sounds. There were no palpable masses or organomegaly. Rectal examination disclosed a moderately enlarged prostate with dark-brown stools that were positive for blood. Neurologically, he had no focal signs or meningism, and his fundi were unremarkable.

About 1 hour after admission, his BP was 110/80 mm Hg, and he was diaphoretic and lethargic. He was treated with intravenous albumin and saline infusions, which raised his BP. His admission studies showed azotemia with metabolic acidosis, hyperkalemia, and a prolonged prothrombin time. Sputum, urine, CSF, and blood cultures were obtained. Spinal fluid was chemically and cytologically unremarkable. He was treated with fluid restriction, glucose and insulin, polystyrene sodium sulfonate (Kayexelate), and sodium bicarbonate, and parenteral aminoglycoside and cephalosporin therapy was begun. He was also given vitamin K_1, thiamine, and multivitamins. An abdominal obstruction series was nondiagnostic and a nasogastric tube was placed. Specifically, the chest roentgenogram showed increased interstitial markings but no discrete infiltrates.

Hemodialysis was started the next morning. A heavy-metal screen was negative. Severe thrombocytopenia was noted, and his prothrombin time remained slightly prolonged. A bone marrow aspirate demonstrated adequate megakaryocytes and was unremarkable.

As the nasogastric drainage was positive for blood, he was given platelet transfusions and fresh-frozen plasma. High-dose methylprednisolone was administered. Aqueous penicillin G sodium therapy was started as the diagnosis of leptospirosis was considered.

Two days after admission, he was stuporous. He remained febrile and anuric. Abdominal distention was still present, with moderate tenderness. Three days after admission, he remained in poor condition, semicomatose, and febrile. A gingival biopsy specimen was unremarkable. The next day, he had a respiratory arrest and was intubated. A chest roentgenogram now also showed a right lower lobe infiltrate consistent with aspiration or other infection. He was deeply comatose. Hemodialysis on a daily basis and antibiotic therapy were continued, as were corticosteroid administration (methylprednisolone, 40 mg every 12 hours) and calcium infusions. Creatine phosphokinase level was greatly elevated, as was aldolase level. Six days after admission, he was hypotensive, requiring dopamine. An EEG demonstrated no activity. He died 1 day later. A sputum culture done yielded Aspergillus fumigatus on the day of death.*

SUMMARY

Aspergillosis is a complex group of diseases caused by dimorphic fungi belonging to the genus Aspergillus. Localized ear infections are rarely serious, and surgery is often curative for aspergillomas. Aspergillus fumigatus is the most common cause of the usually fatal form of invasive pulmonary disease. Underlying neoplastic disease and immunosuppression predispose individuals to aspergillosis, but invasive aspergillosis may also occur in apparently healthy individuals. A diagnosis of aspergillosis is complicated by the ubiquitous nature of the fungus in the environment. Aspergillus species may be transient residents of the nose and are frequent laboratory contaminants. No person-to-person transmission of aspergillosis is known to occur. More aggressive monitoring of the environment, use of radiographic or

---

*From DiSilva, H., Burke, J.F., and Cho, S.Y.: JAMA, *248*:1495–1497, 1982. Copyright 1982, American Medical Association.[30]

tomographic techniques, and repeated attempts to culture Aspergillus species may be needed to diagnose the potentially lethal infection.

REFERENCES

1. Emmons, C.W., Binford, C.H., Utz, J.P., and Kwon-Chung, K.J.: Medical Mycology, 3rd Ed. Philadelphia, Lea & Febiger, 1977, p. 285.
2. Renon, L.: Étude sur l'Aspergillose Chez les Animaux et Chez l'Homme. Paris, Masson et Cie, 1897.
3. Goodman, N.L.: Aspergillosis. Clin. Microbiol. Newsl., *4*:9, 1982.
4. Chetty, A., Monon, R.K., and Malviya, A.N.: Allergic bronchopulmonary aspergillosis in children. Indian J. Pediatr., *49*:203, 1982.
5. Wang, J.L.F., et al.: Allergic bronchopulmonary aspergillosis in pediatric practice. J. Pediatr., *94*:376, 1979.
6. Henry, R.L., Mellis, C.M., Simpson, S.J., and South, R.T.: Allergic bronchopulmonary aspergillosis in cystic fibrosis. Aust. Paediatr. J., *18*:110, 1982.
7. Sarosi, G.A.: Aspergillosis. *In* Medical Microbiology and Infectious Disease. Edited by A.I. Braude. Philadelphia, W.B. Saunders, 1981.
8. Brown, E., et al.: Invasive pulmonary aspergillosis in an apparently non-immunocompromised host. Am. J. Med., *69*:624, 1980.
9. Young, R.C., et al.: Aspergillosis—the spectrum of the disease in 98 patients. Medicine, *49*:147, 1970.
10. Park, G.R., et al.: Disseminated aspergillosis occurring in patients with respiratory, renal, and hepatic failure. Lancet, *2*:179, 1982.
11. Teoh, G.H., Yow, C.S., and Soo-Hoo, T.S.: Fungal keratitis—A case report of Aspergillus infection of the cornea. Singapore Med. J., *23*:42, 1982.
12. Green, W.R., Fout, R.L., and Zimmerman, L.E.: Aspergillosis of the orbit. Report of ten cases and review of the literature. Arch. Ophthalmol., *82*:302, 1982.
13. Kulkarni, R., et al.: Multiple splenic aspergillomas in a patient with acute lymphoblastic leukemia. Am. J. Ped. Hematol. Oncol., *4*:141, 1982.
14. Utz, J.: Aspergillosis. *In* Infectious Diseases, 3rd Ed. Edited by P.D. Hoeprich. New York, Harper & Row, 1983.
15. Gage, A.A., Dean, D.C., Schimert, G., and Minsley, N.: Aspergillus infection after cardiac surgery. Arch. Surg., *101*:384, 1970.
16. Lentino, J.R., et al.: Nosocomial aspergillosis. A retrospective review of airborne disease secondary to road construction and contaminated air conditioners. Am. J. Epidemiol., *116*:430, 1982.
17. Fuchs, P.C.: Epidemiology of Hospital-Associated Infections. Chicago, American Society of Clinical Pathologists, 1979, p. 113.
18. Stoloff, L.: Aflatoxin—an overview. *In* Mycotoxins in Human and Animal Health. Edited by J.V. Rodricks, C.W. Hesseltine, and M.A. Mehlman. Park Forest South, Illinois, Pathotox Publishers, 1977.
19. Shank, R.C.: Mycotoxicoses in man: dietary and epidemiological conditions. *In* Mycotoxic Fungi, Mycotoxins, and Mycotoxicoses. Vol. 3. Edited by L.G. Morehouse. New York, Marcel Dekker, 1978.
20. Ryan, N.J., et al.: Aflatoxin B_1: Its role in the etiology of Reye's syndrome. Pediatrics, *64*:71, 1979.
21. Nelson, D.B., et al.: Aflatoxin and Reye's syndrome: A case control study. Pediatrics, *66*:865, 1980.
22. Stenon, S., Brookner, A., and Rosenthal, S.: Bilateral endogenous necrotizing scleritis due to Aspergillus oryzae. Ann. Ophthalmol., *14*:67, 1982.
23. Nelson, L.A., Calleraine, M.L., and Schwartz, R.H.: Aspergillosis and atopy in cystic fibrosis. Am. Rev. Respir. Dis., *120*:863, 1979.
24. Brueton, M.J., Ormerod, L.P., Shah, K.J., and Anderson, C.M.: Allergic bronchopulmonary aspergillosis complicating cystic fibrosis in childhood. Arch. Dis. Child., *55*:348, 1980.
25. Evans, D.B.: Invasive fungal infections in transplant patients. Hosp. Update, *7*:701, 1981.

26. Bailey, R.G., Woolf, H., Cullens, H., and Williams, R.: Metabolic inhibition of polymorphonuclear leucocytes in fulminant hepatic failure. Lancet, *1*:1162, 1976.
27. Touraine, J.L., et al.: T lymphocytes and serum inhibitors of cell mediated immunity in renal insufficiency. Nephron, *14*:195, 1975.
28. Ahmand, M., Weinstein, A.J., Hughes, J.A., and Cosgrove, D.E.: Granulomatous mediastinitis due to Aspergillus flavus in a non-immunosuppressed patient. Am. J. Med., *71*:903, 1981.
29. Cooper, J.A.D., Weinbaum, D.L., Aldrick, T.K., and Mandel, G.L.: Invasive aspergillosis of the lung and pericardium in a non-immunocompromised 33-year-old man. Am. J. Med., *71*:903, 1981.
30. D'Silva, H., Burke, J.F., and Cho, S.Y.: Disseminated aspergillosis in a presumably immunocompetent host. JAMA, *248*:1495, 1982.
31. Williams, D.M., Weiner, M.H., and Drutz, D.J.: Immunologic studies of disseminated infection with Aspergillus fumigatus in the nude mouse. J. Infect. Dis., *143*:726, 1981.
32. Arnow, P.M., et al.: Pulmonary aspergillosis during hospital renovation. Am. Rev. Respir. Dis., *118*:49, 1978.
33. Burton, J.R., et al.: Aspergillosis in four renal transplant recipients. Ann. Intern. Med., *77*:383, 1972.
34. Aisner, J., et al.: Aspergillus infections in cancer patients: association with fireproofing materials in a new hospital. JAMA, *235*:411, 1976.
35. Krol, T.C., and O'Keefe, P.: Brachial plexus neuritis and fatal hemorrhage following Aspergillus infection of a Hickman catheter. Cancer, *50*:1214, 1982.
36. Bardana, E.J., Jr.: Measurement of humoral antibodies to Aspergillus. Ann. N.Y. Acad. Sci., *221*:64, 1974.
37. Young, R.C., and Bennett, J.E.: Invasive aspergillosis, absence of detectable antibody response. Am. Rev. Respir. Dis., *104*:910, 1971.
38. Austwick, P.K.C., and Longbottom, J.L.: Medically important Aspergillus species. *In* Manual of Clinical Microbiology, 3rd Ed. Edited by E.H. Lennette. Washington, D.C., American Society for Microbiology, 1980.
39. Balogh, N.: Diagnostik Pilzkrankheiten bei Tieren mit modifizierte Parker Blue-Black Superchrome Tintensärbung. D.T.W., *71*:327, 1974.
40. Campbell, M.C., and Stewart, J.L.: The Medical Mycology Handbook. New York, John Wiley & Sons, 1980.
41. Pepys, J., and Turner-Warwick, M.: The lung in allergic diseases. *In* Clinical Aspects of Immunology. Edited by P.G.H. Gell, R.A. Coombs, and P.J. Lachmann. Oxford, Blackwell Scientific Publications, 1975.
42. Longbottom, J.R., and Pepys, J.: Diagnosis of fungal diseases. *In* Clinical Aspects of Immunology. Edited by P.G.H. Gell, R.A. Coombs, and P.J. Lachmann. Oxford, Blackwell Scientific Publications, 1975.
43. Drouhet, E., Camey, L., and Segretain, G.: Valeur de l'immuno-precipitation et de l'immunofluorescence indirecte dans les aspergilloses bronchopulmonaires. Ann. Inst. Pasteur, *123*:379, 1972.
44. Richardson, M.D., Stubbins, J.M., and Warnock, D.W.: Rapid enzyme-linked immunosorbent assay (ELISA) for Aspergillus fumigatus antibodies. J. Clin. Pathol., *35*:1134, 1982.
45. Lehman, P.F., and Reiss, E.: Invasive aspergillosis: Antiserum for circulating antigen produced after immunization with serum from infected rabbits. Infect. Immun., *20*:570, 1978.
46. Unger, P.D., Mehendale, H.M., and Hayes, A.W.: Hepatic update and disposition of aflatoxin B_1 in isolated perfused rat liver. Toxicol. Appl. Pharmacol., *4*:523, 1977.
47. Bodey, G.P.: Fungal infections complicating acute leukemia. J. Chron. Dis., *19*:667, 1966.
48. Enomoto, M.: Fungal toxins. *In* Medical Microbiology and Infectious Diseases. Edited by A.I. Braude. Philadelphia, W.B. Saunders, 1981.
49. Berger, I., Phillips, W.L., and Shenker, I.R.: Pulmonary aspergillosis in childhood—a case report and discussion. Clin. Pediatr., *11*:178, 1972.

CHAPTER 5 CAMPYLOBACTER INFECTIONS

Although Campylobacter enteritis has been described as a new disease, it has been known as a cause of infectious abortion in cattle and sheep and as a form of enteritis in calves and pigs for more than 60 years.[1] The Greek term, campylobacter, means a curved rod. The name was proposed by Sebald and Veron in 1963 as a generic name for a group of microaerophilic curved rods that differed from typical vibrios.[2] During the last 10 years, Campylobacter enteritis has emerged as a significant diarrheal disease in humans.[3-7] Bacteremia, salpingitis, endocarditis, meningitis, abscesses, pustules, arthritis, pericarditis, peritonitis, cholecystitis, phlebitis, septic abortions, central nervous system infections, mycotic aortic aneurysms, Reiter syndrome, erythema nodosum, colitis, and urinary tract infections have been associated with Campylobacter organisms.[8-13]

Classic features of Campylobacter enteritis include fever, abdominal pain, and diarrhea. The ileum and the jejunum are the primary sites affected, but the large bowel can be involved.[1,14] The acute inflammatory colitis observed on histologic sections is indistinguishable from that of amebiasis, salmonellosis, shigellosis, ulcerative colitis, and Crohn disease.[6] Blood may be found in the stool 2 to 4 days after onset.[15] Vomiting and dehydration are not common, but malaise, headache, musculoskeletal pain, rigors, and delirium have been reported.[14]

The severity of symptoms in Campylobacter enteritis is variable, but the duration of morbidity is usually limited to 1 week or less. If untreated, a period of asymptomatic excretion of vibrios may last as long as 6 to 8 weeks.

It is likely that most cases of acute inflammatory joint disease as a sequela of Campylobacter infection go unrecognized. Yet, the arthritic complication has been estimated to occur in 2 to 10% of cases in pediatric patients.[16-18] Reactive arthritis following Campylobacter enteritis in adults appears to be rare. Involvement of 1 or more joints and isolation of the etiologic agent from stool or evidence from antibody titers against C. jejuni are the criteria needed to establish a diagnosis of reactive arthritis associated with Campylobacter enteritis.[19] The symptoms of Campylobacter-reactive arthritis are clinically indistinguishable from postinfective arthritis following Salmonella, Shigella, or Yersinia enteritis.[20–22]

Extraintestinal Campylobacter infections tend to be opportunistic infections, occurring most frequently in patients with malignancies, diabetes, or cardiovascular disease. Febrile episodes may be prolonged or relapsing, such as those observed in malaria or brucellosis.[14] Age and status of underlying disease are factors in the severity of symptoms.

Perinatal infections constitute the most serious Campylobacter-associated diseases. Most cases occurring in neonates are fatal. Campylobacter infections are common and provide another example of an extension of host-range by microorganisms.

ETIOLOGY

Campylobacter fetus and C. jejuni have been implicated in human disease. Enteritis is usually caused by C. jejuni, but at least one case of gastroenteritis associated with C. fetus was reported in an otherwise healthy man.[23] Extraintestinal infections are more commonly caused by C. fetus subsp. intestinalis. The campylobacters are microaerophilic, gram-negative, curved rods that demonstrate pleomorphic forms consisting of spiral, gull-winged, or S shapes (Fig. 5–1). The vibrios exhibit typical darting motility when viewed by darkfield or

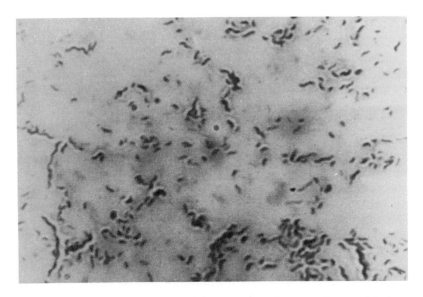

Figure 5–1. Gram stain of Campylobacter jejuni showing pleomorphic forms. (From Kaplan, R.L.: Campylobacter. *In* Manual of Clinical Microbiology, 3rd Ed. Edited by E.H. Lennette. Washington, D.C., American Society for Microbiology, 1980.)

phase-contrast microscopy. The organisms do not ferment or oxidize carbohydrates, but can be differentiated by temperature requirements, hippurate hydrolysis, and nalidixic acid susceptibility. C. fetus appears to be widely distributed among animals, including cattle, sheep, pigs, turkeys, chickens, and dogs.[1,24]

PREDISPOSING FACTORS

The presence of underlying disease, contact with farm animals, and deficient immune status of neonates or older individuals appear to be risk factors in the development of Campylobacter infections. More than half of the reported cases of reactive arthritis in pediatric patients following Campylobacter enteritis have been associated with HLA-B27.[19] Infections caused by C. fetus subsp. intestinalis have been associated with alcoholism.[25–27] Since isolation of the etiologic agent in human campylobacteriosis is now feasible for most laboratories, other predisposing factors may become apparent in the future.

EPIDEMIOLOGY

Campylobacter jejuni is a cosmopolitan pathogen found in both temperate and tropical regions. The bacterium has been isolated from the intestines of a wide variety of wild and domestic animals.[28–31] C. jejuni can persist in carcasses of chickens and turkeys processed for marketing.[24,32] The presence of the vibrios in domestic birds may be related to their high body temperatures.

Although chilling of carcasses in cold water is a uniform procedure in poultry-processing plants, the United States Department of Agriculture does not require chlorination of the chilled water. Processing without chlorination probably permits survival of larger numbers of organisms. Appropriate cooking of all poultry is an important measure in the prevention of human campylobacteriosis. Bacteria indigenous to poultry are usually destroyed by heating to an internal temperature of 145°F (62.8°C) in traditional ovens. Microwave ovens may require higher internal temperatures to kill the same organisms because of the shorter cooking time. It appears that eating undercooked barbecued chicken may have been the source of Campylobacter in an outbreak of enteritis in Iowa in 1979.[33]

Dogs, raw milk, and contaminated water have been implicated as sources of human campylobacteriosis. A waterborne outbreak of Campylobacter gastroenteritis, which is believed to have affected 2000 persons, occurred in the town of Bennington, Vermont in 1978.[34] All age groups and both sexes were affected equally. Person-to-person transmission of C. jejuni has been reported in some family and community outbreaks.[35–37]

C. jejuni has been isolated from healthy children in South Africa and in Bangladesh.[38,39] Colonization with C. jejuni may not necessarily be associated with disease in developing countries.

The carrier state has been difficult to establish definitively in developing countries. Since the organism is ubiquitous in nature, exposure is bound to be frequent. One study of children in South Africa reported that at least 3% of untreated children remain carriers for as long as 1 year.[40] Another study demonstrated that 100% of 24 untreated children failed to excrete the organisms after 7 weeks.[7] More studies are needed to clarify the relationship of this organism to diarrheal disease in developing countries.

LABORATORY DIAGNOSIS

Although isolation of Campylobacter jejuni was reported in Brussels in 1973, practical techniques for demonstration or isolation of the organism were not available until several years later.[1,41–43] The lack of successful techniques for isolating the etiologic agent in Campylobacter enteritis is responsible for the small number of cases of the diarrheal disease reported as being associated with the organism in the past. The problems in culturing C. jejuni were the inability to provide appropriate microaerophilic atmosphere, an optimal temperature, and the required nutrients for growth under laboratory conditions. C. jejuni grows better at 42°C, whereas C. fetus subsp. intestinalis requires incubation at 37°C.

Microscopic Examination

Although leukocytes are found in the stools of individuals with bacterial enteritis, they are also present in a variety of other intestinal disorders.[44,45] Darkfield microscopy has been a valuable diagnostic tool in cholera for many years.[46] The characteristic darting motility exhibited by Vibrio cholerae in stool is evidence for the presence of the etiologic agent.

The use of darkfield microscopy, phase-contrast microscopy, or Gram stains has been less frequently applied in the diagnosis of Campylobacter enteritis. Presence of Campylobacter motility (CM) does have some predictive value.[44,45,47] The predictive value of any method of direct examination is greater if stools are diarrheal in consistency and contain leukocytes and erythrocytes. Although an optimal diluent for stool has not been described for demonstrating motility of campylobacters, CM has been demonstrated when stool is mixed with tryptic soy broth or Brucella broth.[47,48] Saline, however, appears to inhibit motility. A darting type of motility is also exhibited by some other organisms. Demonstration of specificity awaits development of antisera specific for C. jejuni.

Cultural Techniques

Campylobacter organisms are fastidious in their growth requirements and do not grow on basic nutrient media. The organisms will grow on Brucella agar supplemented with 5% defibrinated sheep blood, vitamin K, and hemin, or in enriched thioglycolate broth. The addition of the compounds ferrous sulfate, sodium metabisulfite, and sodium pyruvate increases the opportunity for isolation from normally sterile sites.

For isolation of campylobacters from stool specimens, it is recommended that vancomycin (10 mg), trimethoprim (5 mg), polymyxin B (2500 IU), amphotericin B (2 mg), and cephalothin (15 mg) be added to each liter of medium for inhibition of indigenous flora. Both a basic plate medium (Campy-BAP) and a thioglycolate broth (Campy-thio) are available commercially (BBL Microbiology Systems, Cockeysville, Maryland).

Either rectal swabs or 3 to 5 drops of a diarrheal stool may be used to inoculate the agar or liquid media. Solid stools can be suspended in saline and mixed prior to inoculation. An alternative method consists of inoculating media after sampling several areas of a stool specimen with a sterile swab.[13] Plates should be incubated at 42°C for 48 hours in an atmosphere of 5% oxygen and 10% carbon dioxide. An appropriate microaerophilic atmosphere can be supplied by a system known as Campy Pak II (BBL Microbiology Systems, Cockeysville, Maryland).[49] Campy-thio broths should be refrigerated overnight before plating onto Campy-BAP. The use of sterile Pasteur pipettes to withdraw subsurface growth facilitates the transfer procedure.

A control system for monitoring the microaerophilic atmosphere has been developed at the Children's Hospital of Eastern Ontario in Canada.[50] In the procedure, Pseudomonas aeruginosa, Clostridium perfringens, and C. jejuni are each streaked on a third of a blood agar plate and placed with primary plates inoculated with clinical specimens in a microaerophilic atmosphere. Growth of C. perfringens demonstrates that oxygen tension was reduced, and growth of P. aeruginosa shows that complete anaerobiosis was not obtained. Growth of a stock culture of C. jejuni indicates that optimal conditions for growth of the organism have been attained (Fig. 5–2). The use of all three organisms provides a control for appropriateness of atmospheric conditions and, in the event of a failure of the system, indicates the nature of the atmospheric aberration.

Colonies of C. jejuni are gray, flat or raised, mucoid, and nonhemolytic, measuring approximately 1.0 mm in diameter after 24 to 48 hours of incubation. Colonies of C. fetus subsp. intestinalis are often smaller, raised, opaque, and may be pale yellow.

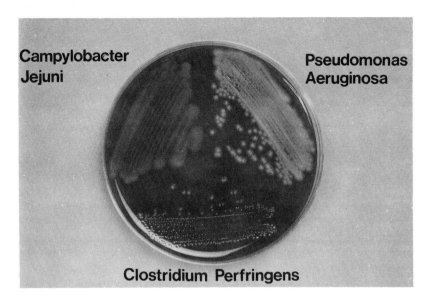

Figure 5–2. Growth of P. aeruginosa, C. perfringens, and C. jejuni on a control plate. (From Chan, F.T.H., and MacKenzie, M.R.: Enrichment medium and control system for isolation of Campylobacter fetus subsp. jejuni from stools. J. Clin. Microbiol., *15*:12, 1982.)

Table 5–1.   Biochemical characteristics of Campylobacter species.

	Campylobacter fetus		
	subsp. fetus	subsp. intestinalis	jejuni
Catalase	+	+	+
Oxidase	+	+	+
Growth			
25°C	+	+	−
35°C	+	+	+
42°C	−	±	+
Glysine 1%	−	+	+
Hippurate hydrolysis	−	−	+
Nalidixic acid (30 μg)	R	R	S
Cephalothin (30 μg)	S	R	R
Nitrate reduction	+	+	+
H$_2$S production (lead acetate)	+	+	+

Biochemical Characterization

Both C. fetus and C. jejuni are oxidase and catalase positive. For additional biochemical tests, it is recommended that an isolated colony be subcultured in Brucella broth with 0.16% agar and incubated at 37°C for 24 hours.[51] Two drops of the broth culture may be used to inoculate additional media. Typical reactions of C. fetus subsp. fetus, C. fetus subsp. intestinalis, and C. jejuni are shown in Table 5–1.

Serologic Tests

Campylobacter fetus (Vibrio fetus) was divided into three serotypes based on heat-stable antigens in 1971.[52] More recently, C. jejuni has been serotyped by a slide agglutination technique based on heat-labile antigenic factors.[37] Twenty-one serogroups were recognized, using 815 isolates from human and nonhuman sources. Serogroups 1, 2, 4, 5, 7, 9, and 11 were the most common among human isolates.

Although rough strains of C. jejuni were subcultured and treated with DNA-ase, 30 strains could not be typed because autoagglutination occurred in saline. Despite this limitation, serotyping may have diagnostic value in the epidemiology of C. jejuni. Indirect immunofluorescence may one day have practical application in serotyping, but much needs to be learned of the specificity of serologic reactions.

The heterogenicity and multiplicity of antigenic components of C. jejuni have limited the use of serodiagnosis based on antibodies in serum to those patients from whom the organism has been isolated. Agglutinating, complement-fixing, and bactericidal antibodies have been demonstrated using patients' isolates.[3,6,15,]

PROGNOSIS

In most cases of enteritis caused by Campylobacter jejuni, the illness is self-limiting. Symptoms usually disappear within 1 week. Persistent or recurrent infections have been reported and may depend on the general health of the patient.[53] A premature return to solid foods has triggered recurrences in some instances. Reactive arthritis occurring as a complication of Campylobacter enteritis lasts from 1 week to several months, but residual joint damage is minimal.[19]

Focal infections caused by C. fetus subsp. intestinalis are characterized by longer febrile periods and more frequent recurrences. The prognosis is guarded in individuals with underlying disease. Prompt institution of appropriate antibiotic therapy based on susceptibility testing is important for a favorable prognosis.

Perinatal infections in infants caused by campylobacters are usually fatal. Most often, mothers survive the illness without sequelae.

CASE REPORTS

Case 1

The patient, a 50-year-old man with end-stage chronic glomerulonephritis, was admitted to the hospital for hemodialysis in November, 1977. In March, 1978, he received a cadaver kidney transplant which was rejected after 1 month, and he was readmitted to the hospital for hemodialysis. In April, 1979, he had to be shifted to continuous ambulatory peritoneal dialysis (CAPD) for recurrent thrombosis of several arteriovenous fistulae. Since the initiation of CAPD, four episodes of peritonitis occurred, the last one, due to Streptococcus mitior, taking place 9 months before the latest admission.

On 4 October, 1981, the patient developed diarrhea with low-grade fever and abdominal discomfort. On 5 October, he was admitted to the hospital because of a cloudy peritoneal effluent. Diarrhea was still present, the temperature was 37.4°C, the heart rate was 108 beats per min, and the blood pressure was 105/85. The abdomen was diffusely tender, with generalized rebound pain, but intestinal peristaltism was present. The peritoneal fluid contained 1330 leukocytes per mm^3 and a protein level of 314 mg/dl; a Gram-stained smear of the dialysate was negative. Proper portions of stools, blood, and peritoneal effluent were obtained for culturing; SMT (80 mg of sulfamethoxazole and 16 mg of trimethoprim per liter) was added to the dialysis bags, and CAPD was carried out in the usual way. No clinical improvement followed, and the peritoneal effluent remained cloudy. On day 4, the initial peritoneal fluid culture grew C. jejuni; this bacterium was also recovered from stool cultures. SMT was replaced by gentamicin (8 mg/L) in dialysis bags, and erythromycin (3 g orally per day) was administered. Within the next 48 hours, the peritoneal fluid cleared, and gastrointestinal symptoms subsided. Three sets of blood cultures obtained upon admission remained negative. Seroconversion for C. jejuni was demonstrated 2 weeks later. A barium enema examination disclosed no abnormality.

We routinely use horse-blood agar plates and modified Lombard-Dowell broth for culturing peritoneal fluid obtained from CAPD patients. In the present case, blood plates yielded no growth, but broth cultures yielded small, gram-negative, curved rods which were further identified as C. jejuni.

For blood culture, we proceeded as follows. Ten milliliters of blood were aseptically drawn and equally distributed in 2 bottles: an anaerobic bottle (brain-heart-infusion broth containing p-aminobenzoic acid, vitamin K, hemin, and sodium polyanetholesulfonate [50 ml; GIBCO Laboratories]) and an aerobic bottle (diphasic Castaneda medium [50 ml; Pasteur Institute, Lille]). Sets of blood cultures were incubated for 10 days at 35°C. Bottles were macroscopically examined every day, and blind subcultures were systematically performed, 12 to 24 hours after the specimen was received, on chocolate agar which was incubated for 3 days in a 5% CO_2-enriched atmosphere. In the present case, a supplementary blind subculture was done on day 5 of incubation.

The antibody titer was determined by S. Lauwers (Vrij Universiteit, Brussels), who used a tube agglutination method. A formalinized antigen was prepared from strains isolated from stools and from peritoneal fluid. Similar results (titers of <1:80 upon admission and

1:2560 2 weeks later) were obtained with both antigenic preparations.*

Case 2

A 58-year-old Caucasian male was brought into the emergency room by fire rescue workers after being found on the floor of his home. He was a known alcohol abuser and appeared to have meningitis. On examination, his temperature was 103.6°F, blood pressure was 120/20, and pulse rate was 140/min and irregular. The patient was obviously septic, and because his neck was stiff in all directions, a lumbar puncture was performed after admission to the intensive care unit.

The spinal fluid obtained from the tap was purulent, with a white blood count of 7300/mm³ (92% PMNs and 8% lymphocytes). The protein was 266 mg/dl, and the glucose was 13 mg/dl. Although a resident examining the smear of CSF sediment at night saw questionable gram-negative organisms, no organisms were seen when the smear was reviewed by the microbiologist the following morning. Cultures of blood (3 sets), urine, and sputum were also obtained on admission.

Because of the possibility of gram-negative sepsis and/or meningitis, the patient was started on intravenous (IV) chloramphenicol (1 g every 4 hours), IV gentamicin (80 mg every 8 hours), and intrathecal gentamicin (5 mg). The results of the admission cultures were as follows: sputum, normal flora; urine, no growth; CSF, no growth for routine, fungus, and TB cultures; blood, initially no growth. The patient's temperature varied from 99°F to 107°F throughout his hospital stay.

Treatment with the gentamicin/chloramphenicol regimen continued. Although the CSF cleared chemically, the patient deteriorated severely. The CSF cell count dropped to 1375 WBC/mm³ and eventually came down to 3 WBC/mm³ after 4 days of antibiotic therapy. The cultures of the CSF remained negative, and the initial 3 sets of blood cultures did not reveal growth until the fourth hospital day. By the sixth hospital day, after 3 respiratory arrests, the patient lapsed into a coma and died.

The 3 sets of blood cultures were taken by inoculating approximately 5 ml of blood into each of 2 bottles of Trypticase Soy Broth with SPS and CO_2 (BBL Microbiology Systems, Cockeysville, Maryland). One bottle remained anaerobic, and the second was aerated at the time of inoculation. The bottles were subcultured at 24 and 48 hours of incubation, as well as at 7 days. The aerobic bottles were subcultured onto chocolate agar plates, and the subcultures of the

---

*From Pepersack, F., D'Haene, M., Toussaint, C., and Schoutens, E.: J. Clin. Microbiol., 16:739–741, 1982.[54]

anaerobic bottles were incubated for 48 hours in a GasPak jar (BBL Microbiology Systems) on blood agar. All 3 subcultures of the anaerobic bottles were positive after 48 hours, but the plates were not visually positive until the fourth hospital day. Smears of the colonies revealed gram-negative, pleomorphic, filamentous rods, resembling spirochetes. Smears of the bottles showed that all 6 bottles were positive.

None of the bottles subcultured aerobically and incubated in a CO_2 incubator showed growth. All 6 bottles were positive on subculture at 42°C in a reduced oxygen environment (using Marion BioBag A [Marion Scientific Corp., Kansas City, Missouri] and generator without the catalyst). The organisms grew at 37°C and 25°C, as well as at 42°C. They grew on the blood agar plates, and showed slow, slight growth on MacConkey agar as well. The biochemical characteristics were as follows: urea-negative, OF dextrose-negative, catalase-positive, oxidase-positive, resistant to nalidixic acid, NO_3 reduced to NO_2, lead acetate for H_2S-positive, and motility-positive. The organism was susceptible to chloramphenicol and gentamicin by disc diffusion. The organism was tentatively identified as Campylobacter fetus subsp. intestinalis. The identification was confirmed by the Centers for Disease Control as a "non-motile unusual" strain.

Although C. fetus subsp. jejuni is the more commonly isolated species in clinical infections with this genus, C. fetus subsp. intestinalis is also a cause of human infection. The latter has been associated with alcoholism and other underlying diseases. The source of this infection remains unknown.

The C. fetus subsp. intestinalis was clearly the cause of this patient's sepsis, and possibly the cause of his meningitis. It is interesting to wonder whether the Camplylobacter would have been recovered from the CSF if it had been cultured at 42°C in the appropriate environment. Although the organism was never recovered from the CSF, the fluid did clear after appropriate therapy. Final blood cultures taken shortly before the patient expired were negative.*

Case 3

A 28-year-old male was seen in the Long Beach Memorial Hospital clinic for the chief complaint of rectal bleeding. He stated that his illness began approximately 24 hours prior to the clinic visit and that he was experiencing crampy abdominal pain and intermittent bloody stools. Physical examination elicited no significant findings and a fecal

---

*Reprinted by permission of the publisher from Blechman, D.: Campylobacter fetus ss intestinalis sepsis and meningitis in an alcoholic. Clin. Microbiol. Newsl. *4*:94–95, 1982. Copyright 1982 by Elsevier Science Publishing Co.[25]

specimen was submitted to the laboratory for ova and parasites as well as culture.

The stool specimen received by the laboratory was characterized as watery, containing many PMNs and RBCs. Ova and parasite exams were negative. Culture of feces on the routine enterobacterial media yielded no pathogens as did culture for Neisseria gonorrhoeae. Fecal culture on Anaerobe Systems Campylobacter media at 42°C in a GasPak jar with a Campy-Pak CO_2 generator envelope (BBL) yielded growth of many colonies of an organism with microscopic morphology indicative of Campylobacter species. Subsequent testing of the organism elicited features consistent with genus Campylobacter but not consistent with any one species or group.

Based on experience with genus Campylobacter, the results indicated the organism was most likely C. fetus, despite the inconsistency of growth at 42°C and the circumstances of isolation. Because of the paucity of differential features among members of genus Campylobacter, however, the only reliable way to accurately identify this isolate was through the technique of DNA-DNA hybridization. The relevant hybridizations were performed using cold DNA from the unknown and ^{3}H-labeled DNA from C. fetus subsp. fetus (neotype strain, ATCC 27374), C. jejuni (ATCC 29428), "C. fecalis" (C-32), 'NARTC' (NCTC 11352), and C. coli (C-38). The percent relatedness figures derived from the 5 separate test hybridizations (each done in duplicate) conclusively identified the isolate as C. fetus subsp. fetus. The DNA from the unknown was 98.8% related to that from C. fetus subsp. fetus and less than 6% related to the DNA from any of the other strains.*

Case 4

This previously healthy 12-year-old white female was admitted because of oligoarthritic signs and symptoms which had become manifest 8 days after a 4-day bout of bloody diarrhea. The enteritis was characterized by abdominal colic, fever, and nausea. Past medical history and family history were noncontributory. Both knees, the left ankle and the proximal interphalangeal joint of the second left toe were red, warm, swollen, and tender. The patient was afebrile and there was no pathologic enlargement of lymph nodes, liver, or spleen. Ophthalmologic examination by a consultant was normal.

Laboratory work-up revealed hemoglobin 13.4 g/dl, white blood cell count 8600/cu mm with normal differential, platelets 571,000/cu mm, erythrocyte sedimentation rate (ESR) 82 mm/hour and C-reactive protein strongly positive. Stool culture was positive for Campylobacter species, and antibody titers against complement-fix-

---

*From Harvey, S.M., Spalsbury, M., Hardy, C., and Henke, R.: SC-ASM News *12*:4–6, 1982.[23]

ing C. jejuni antigens decreased from 1:80 at 5 weeks after onset of diarrhea to 1:40 at 12 weeks and to negative at 20 weeks. Clear, yellow synovial fluid was obtained from both knees (approximately 30 ml from each side). The WBC was 22,200/cu mm (79% polymorphonuclear cells) and Gram stain was negative for microorganisms. Bacteriologic cultures of joint fluid, including specific methods for Campylobacter, were sterile. Rheumatoid factor and antibodies against Campylobacter antigens were not detected in the aspirates from the knees. Lymphocyte typing was positive for HLA-B27. The following studies were within normal limits: examinations of bone marrow and urine; determinations of antistreptolysin O titer (75 units) and serum immunoglobulins; chest roentgenogram and electrocardiogram. Other negative results included the serum tests for rheumatoid factor, antinuclear antibodies (against DNA and RNA), circulating immune complexes and antibodies against Salmonella, Brucella, and Yersinia. Cultures for beta-hemolytic streptococci in a throat swab specimen and for Salmonella, Shigella, and Yersinia in stool were negative.

Erythromycin ethylsuccinate in a dosage of 30 mg/kg/day divided every 6 hours was given orally for 10 days. Thereafter, repeated stool cultures were negative for Campylobacter species. Salicylates given in a dosage of 70 mg/kg/day divided every 6 hours over 1.5 weeks and of 90 mg/kg/day every 6 hours over 2.5 weeks failed to relieve the arthritic symptoms. Diclofenac sodium, a new nonsteroidal antiinflammatory drug (Voltaren), was given in a dosage of 2.5 mg/kg/day divided every 12 hours and gradual improvement became manifest. This treatment together with physical therapy was continued for 4 months. Total duration of arthritic symptoms and signs was 18 weeks. At follow-up 2 weeks before and 3 months after discontinuation of antiinflammatory drug therapy, the girl was free of symptoms and all joints were completely normal with the exception of a slight enlargement of the proximal interphalangeal joint of the second left toe. Radiographs of both knees and ESR (9 mm/hour) were normal.*

SUMMARY

Campylobacter jejuni appears to be of increasing significance as a cause of enteritis. Although the enteritic infections in children are usually self-limiting, a reactive arthritis may occur several days to a few weeks following diarrhea. To adopt an appropriate therapeutic regimen, it is important to differentiate any bacterial-associated ar-

---

*From Schaad, U.B.: Pediatr. Infec. Dis. *1*:328–332. © 1982 The Williams & Wilkins Co., Baltimore.[19]

thritis from the juvenile variety of arthritis. A single case of human gastroenteritis has been reported to be caused by C. fetus.

Focal infections involving other parts of the body in compromised hosts are more often caused by C. fetus subsp. intestinalis. The severity of symptoms varies with the type of underlying disease and age of the patient. Infections in neonates are the most serious Campylobacter-associated diseases. Most neonates with campylobacteriosis do not survive.

Direct contact with infected animals, ingestion of contaminated food and water, exposure during delivery, and person-to-person transmision have been documented. Microaerophilic conditions, a temperature of 42°C, and the use of an enriched antibiotic-containing medium are critical in the isolation of C. jejuni from stool specimens. It is impossible to assess the importance of C. fetus as a cause of gastroenteritis because the routinely used temperature of 42°C and incorporation of cephalothin into commonly employed media would not permit the growth of C. fetus. Aggressive searches for the organism, using a lower temperature and no cephalothin, may reveal the incidence of C. fetus as a cause of enteric disease.

REFERENCES

1. Skirrow, M.B.: Campylobacter enteritis: A "new" disease. Br. Med. J., 2:9, 1977.
2. Sebald, M. and Véron, M.: Teneur en bases de l'ADN et classification des vibrions. Ann. Inst. Pasteur, 105:879, 1963.
3. Bokkenheuser, V.D.: Vibrio fetus infection in man: a serological test. Infect. Immun., 5:222, 1972.
4. Blaser, M.J., and Wang, W.L.: Infection of humans with Campylobacter fetus. Can. Med. Assoc. J., 119:1390, 1978.
5. Pearson, A.D., et al.: Campylobacter-associated diarrhoea in Southampton. Br. Med. J., 2:955, 1977.
6. Blaser, M.J., et al.: Campylobacter enteritis: clinical and epidemiologic features. Ann. Intern. Med., 91:179, 1979.
7. Karmali, M.A., and Fleming, P.C.: Campylobacter enteritis in children. J. Pediatr., 94:527, 1979.
8. Brown, W.J., and Sautter, R.: Campylobacter fetus septicemia with concurrent salpingitis. J. Clin. Microbiol., 6:72, 1977.
9. Dzau, V.J., Schur, P.H., and Weinstein, L.: Vibrio fetus endocarditis in a patient with systemic lupus erythematosus. Am. J. Med. Sci., 272:311, 1976.
10. Rettig, P.J.: Campylobacter infections in human beings. J. Pediatr., 94:855, 1979.
11. Lambert, M.E., et al.: Campylobacter colitis. Br. Med. J., 1:857, 1979.
12. File, T.M., Barnishan, J., and Fass, R.J.: Campylobacter fetus sepsis with mycotic aortic aneurysm. Arch. Pathol. Lab. Med., 103:143, 1979.
13. Kaplan, R.L.: Campylobacter. In Manual of Clinical Microbiology. Edited by E.H. Lennette. Washington, D.C., American Society for Microbiology, 1980.
14. Kantor, H.S.: Bacterial enteritis. In Medical Microbiology and Infectious Diseases. Edited by A.I. Braude. Philadelphia, W.B. Saunders, 1981.
15. Karmali, M.A., and Fleming, P.C.: Campylobacter enteritis. Can. Med. Assoc. J., 120:1532, 1979.
16. Gumpel, J.M., Martin, C., and Sanderson, P.J.: Reactive arthritis with Campylobacter enteritis. Ann. Rheum. Dis., 40:64, 1981.
17. Pönka, A., et al.: Carditis and arthritis associated with Campylobacter jejuni infection. Acta Med. Scand., 208:495, 1980.

18. Kosunen, T.U., et al.: Arthritis associated with Campylobacter jejuni enteritis. Scand. J. Rheumatol., *10*:77, 1981.
19. Schaad, U.B.: Reactive arthritis associated with Campylobacter enteritis. Pediatr. Infect. Dis., 1:328, 1982.
20. Olhagen, B.: Postinfective or reactive arthritis. Scand. J. Rheumatol., *9*:193, 1980.
21. Manicourt, D.H., and Orloff, S.: Immune complexes in polyarthritis after Salmonella gastroenteritis. J. Rheumatol., *8*:613, 1981.
22. Carroll, W.L., et al.: Spectrum of Salmonella-associated arthritis. Pediatrics, *61*:717, 1981.
23. Harvey, S.M., Spalsbury, M., Hardy, C., and Henke, R.: Gastroenteritis-associated Campylobacter fetus subpecies fetus. SC-ASM News, *12*:4, 1982.
24. Leuchtefeld, N.W., and Wang, W.L.L.: Campylobacter fetus subsp. jejuni in a turkey procesing plant. J. Clin. Microbiol., *13*:266, 1981.
25. Blechman, D.: Campylobacter fetus ss intestinalis sepsis and meningitis in an alcoholic. Clin. Microbiol. Newsl., *4*:94, 1982.
26. Blazevic, D.J.: Campylobacter fetus infections. Clin. Microbiol. Newsl., *1*:1, 1979.
27. Rahman, M.: Bacteremia and pericarditis from Campylobacter infection. Br. J. Clin. Pract., *33*:331, 1979.
28. Balser, M.J., et al.: Reservoirs for human campylobacteriosis. J. Infect. Dis., *141*:665, 1980.
29. Fernie, D.S., and Park, R.W.A.: The isolation and nature of campylobacters (microaerophilic vibrios) from laboratory and wild animals. J. Med. Microbiol., *10*:325, 1977.
30. Leuchtefeld, N.A., et al.: Isolation of Campylobacter fetus subsp. jejuni from migratory waterfowl. J. Clin. Microbiol., *12*:406, 1980.
31. Smith, M.V., and Muldoon, P.J.: Campylobacter fetus subspecies jejuni (Vibrio fetus) from commercially processed poultry. Appl. Microbiol. *27*:995, 1974.
32. Simmons, N.A., and Gibbs, F.J.: Campylobacter ssp. in oven-ready poultry. J. Infect. *1*:159, 1979.
33. Center for Disease Control: Campylobacter enteritis—Iowa. Morbid. Mortal. Weekly Rept. *28*:565, 1979.
34. Center for Disease Control: Waterborne Campylobacter gastroenteritis—Vermont. Morbid. Mortal. Weekly Rept., *28*:207, 1978.
35. Blaser, M.J., et al.: Outbreaks of Campylobacter enteritis in two extended families—evidence for person-to-person transmission. J. Pediatr., *98*:254, 1981.
36. Cadrenel, S., et al.: Enteritis due to "related Vibrio" in children. Am. J. Dis. Child., *126*:152, 1973.
37. Lior, H., et al.: Serotyping of Campylobacter jejuni by slide agglutination based on heat-labile antigenic factors. J. Clin. Microbiol., *15*:761, 1982.
38. Bokkenheuser, V.D., et al.: Detection of enteric campylobacteriosis in children. J. Clin. Microbiol., *9*:227, 1979.
39. Blaser, M.J., et al.: Isolation of Campylobacter fetus subsp. jejuni from Bangladeshi children. J. Clin. Microbiol., *12*:744, 1980.
40. Richardson, N.J., Loornhof, H.J., and Bokkenheuser, V.D.: Long-term infections with Campylobacter fetus subsp. jejuni. J. Clin. Microbiol., *13*:846, 1981.
41. Butzler, J.P., et al.: Related Vibrio in stools. J. Pediatr., *82*:493, 1973.
42. Karmali, M.A., and Fleming, P.C.: Campylobacter enteritis in children. J. Pediatr., *94*:527, 1979.
43. Butzler, J.P., and Skirrow, M.B.: Campylobacter enteritis. Clin. Gastroenterol., *8*:737, 1979.
44. Harris, J.C., Dupont, H.L., and Hornick, R.B.: Fecal leukocytes in diarrheal disease. Ann. Intern. Med., *76*:697, 1971.
45. Pickering, L.K., et al.: Fecal leukocytes in enteric infections. Am. J. Clin. Pathol., *68*:562, 1977.
46. Benenson, A.S., Islam, M.R., and Greenough, U.B., III.: Rapid identification of Vibrio cholerae by darkfield microscopy. Bull. WHO, *30*:827, 1964.
47. Paisley, J.W., et al.: Dark-field microscopy of human feces for presumptive diagnosis of Campylobacter fetus subsp. jejuni enteritis. J. Clin. Microbiol., *15*:61, 1982.
48. Steel, T.W., and McDermott, S.: Campylobacters isolated from hospital patients. Med. J. Aust., *2*:435, 1978.

49. Buck, G.E., et al.: Evaluation of the CampyPak II Gas Generator system for isolation of Campylobacter fetus subsp. jejuni. J. Clin. Microbiol., *15*:41, 1982.
50. Chan, F.T.H., and Mackenzie, M.R.: Enrichment medium and control system for isolation of Campylobacter fetus subsp. jejuni from stools. J. Clin. Microbiol., *15*:12, 1982.
51. Yu, K.W., and Washington, J.A., II.: Identification of aerobic and facultatively anaerobic bacteria. *In* Laboratory Procedures in Clinical Microbiology. Edited by J.A. Washington, II. New York, Springer-Verlag, 1981.
52. Berg, R.L., Jutila, J.W., and Firehammer, B.D.: A revised classification of Vibrio fetus. Am. J. Vet. Res., *32*:11, 1971.
53. Torphy, D.E., and Bond, W.W.: Campylobacter fetus infections in children. Pediatrics, *64*:898, 1979.
54. Pepersack, F., D'Haene, M., Toussaint, C., and Schoutens, E.: Campylobacter jejuni peritonitis complicating continuous ambulatory peritoneal dialysis. J. Clin. Microbiol., *16*:739, 1982.

CHAPTER 6 CRYPTOSPORIDIOSIS

Cryptosporidiosis has been recognized as a diarrheal disease in animals, especially calves, for many years.[1,2] The disease occurs in some domestic pets, such as guinea pigs, horses, rabbits, and cats, but no cases have been reported in dogs.[3–5] The infection produces gastritis in snakes and enterocolitis in calves, turkeys, and guinea pigs. More recently, cryptosporidiosis has been reported in immunologically compromised and apparently healthy human hosts.[6,7]

Human cryptosporidiosis is characterized by low-grade fever, nausea, vomiting, abdominal cramps, anorexia, 5 to 10 watery, frothy bowel movements a day, and periods of constipation. The diarrhea is self-limiting in previously healthy individuals and usually does not last more than 2 weeks.[3] The diarrhea becomes chronic in immunosuppressed individuals, and substantive weight loss may occur.[8] The seriousness of cryptosporidiosis is compounded by the lack of an effective drug for treatment of the infection.

ETIOLOGY

In studies of cryptosporidiosis in animals over the years, 11 species of the coccidian Cryptosporidium have been identified.[9] Organisms of the genus Cryptosporidium are parasitic protozoans belonging to the phylum Apicomplexa and the suborder Eimeriorina.[10] Other human pathogens classified as coccidia belong to the genera Isospora, Toxoplasma, and Sarcocystis. Although at first the species of Cryptosporidium appeared to be host-specific, recent studies have refuted the earlier observations.[11] Most evidence now supports the concept of a single species with unique adaptative abilities. Isolates of Cryptosporidium from humans and calves have produced similar infections in mice and rats.[12] The number of strains of Cryptosporidium with the potential for causing human disease is unknown.

A life cycle for the agent of human cryptosporidiosis is similar to that of other coccidia (Fig. 6–1). The one feature that distinguishes members of the genus Cryptosporidium from other coccidia is their ability to attach to the microvillar membrane of epithelial cells lining the intestine.[13] Stages of schizogony and gametogony have been observed in biopsy material and oocysts have been demonstrated in stool

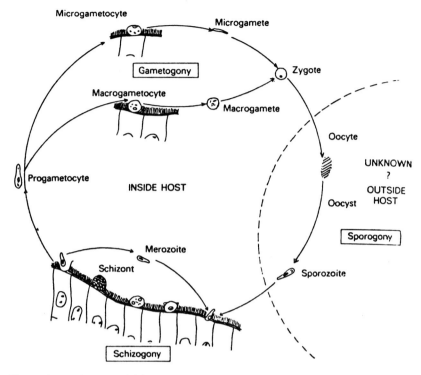

Figure 6–1. Presumed life cycle of Cryptosporidium species in human hosts. (From Bird, R.G., and Smith, M.D.: Cryptosporidiosis in man: Parasite life cycle and fine structural pathology. J. Pathol., *132*:217, 1980.)

specimens.[12] Oocysts sporulate endogenously in mice and, therefore, are infective when discharged in the feces of an infected host.[14] The typical coccidian cycle of a similar parasite, Toxoplasma gondii, occurs in domestic and wild cats.[15] Oocysts of T. gondii produce two sporocysts, which develop into sporozoites in cat feces.

Merozoites released by mature schizonts of cryptosporidial organisms develop into trophozoites. Trophozoites move between microvilli and become attached to intestinal epithelial cells. Observations made by electron microscopy indicate that penetration occurs by a process of invagination and erosion.[10] After a period of cytoplasmic proliferation, nuclear division produces schizonts. Each mature schizont contains eight merozoites, which upon their release, can attach to other epithelial cells. Other merozoites differentiate into micro- and macrogametocytes. The union of the gametocytes produces zygotes and, subsequently, the infective oocysts. Ingestion of the infective sporozoite-containing oocysts establishes the infection of a new host. The microgametocytes are distinguished from macrogametocytes by the presence of peripheral budding microgametes.

PREDISPOSING FACTORS

The single most important factor predisposing individuals to cryptosporidiosis is immunosuppression, although the disease has occurred rarely in previously healthy persons.[5,12,13] Cryptosporidial enteritis has been reported in patients with congenital hypogammaglobulinemia, individuals with IgA deficiency, and in persons undergoing chemotherapy for malignancies.[12,16] Cryptosporidiosis joins the ranks of Pneumocystis carinii pneumonia (PCP), Mycobacterium avian-intracellulare infection, human cytomegalovirus (HCV) infection, and candidiasis as a potential opportunistic infection in homosexual males with acquired immune deficiency syndrome (AIDS). Although the presence of AIDS has been reported in Haitian male immigrants without histories of homosexuality or drug abuse, only a single case of cryptosporidiosis in a Haitian victimized by AIDS occurred in the 2-year period ending in November of 1982.[6]

Because the coccidian has been identified in such a wide range of vertebrates, one might rationalize that animal handlers would be at risk of developing cryptosporidiosis, but cryptosporidiosis occurs infrequently in healthy individuals regardless of occupation. Congenital or acquired immunodeficiencies constitute more significant risk factors for cryptosporidial enteritis than does type of occupation.

The role of antecedent viral infections in providing favorable conditions for protozoal opportunists is unclear. In one case of fatal cryptosporidiosis complicated by disseminated toxoplasmosis, the patient had circulating antibodies for both HCV and Epstein-Barr virus (EBV).[8]

EPIDEMIOLOGY

The mode of transmission for the agent of human cryptosporidiosis has not been firmly established. The fecal-oral route has been suspected as the most probable mode of transmission, but the exact source of infective oocytes has not been documented.[9] In animals, contaminated food and water are believed to be the vehicles for transmission of cryptosporidiosis. It is not known whether symptom-free carriers exist. Food contaminated by mice and the possible infection of domestic pets have not been eliminated as sources of the infective agent.

The increasing number of cases of cryptosporidiosis occurring in homosexual males indicates that either an infectious agent that can promote AIDS or a Cryptosporidium species can be sexually transmitted. The occurrence of the infection in apparently healthy individuals may also mean that successful defense mechanisms are evolving in the coccidian that allow it to promote infections in human hosts. The ability of microorganisms to invade the tissue of a host is related

to both microbial and host factors. The susceptibility of other vertebrates to Cryptosporidium may help explain the emergence of the
coccidian as a human endoparasite.

LABORATORY DIAGNOSIS

In the past, diagnosis of cryptosporidiosis was made either on biopsy
or autopsy specimens of intestinal mucosa or on concentrated stool
specimens, using brightfield or electron microscopy.[11,14] Phase-contrast microscopy is particularly suitable for demonstrating the oocytes
in fecal specimens.[2,12] Electron microscopy is unparalleled in permit-
ting the observation of detailed morphology of Cryptosporidium in
tissue sections. Unfortunately, all laboratories do not have phase-contrast or electron microscopes or individuals experienced with the techniques required for their use. After an evaluation of several concentration and staining methods, a group at the University of California
at Los Angeles made recommendations for wet mounts and permanent-stained smears.[17]

Wet Mounts

Fresh stool specimens may be concentrated by flotation in Sheather's
sugar solution or by centrifugation of formalinized stool.[18] Surface
material obtained by the flotation method is transferred with a wire
loop to a glass slide. One drop of formalinized stool concentrate is
placed in 1 drop of 10% potassium hydroxide (KOH) on a glass slide.
After 1 minute (necessary for clearing), material can be examined
microscopically.

Cryptosporidium oocytes are highly refractile, measure 4.0 to 6.0
μm in diameter, and contain 1 to 6 dark granules (Fig. 6–2). Reese
and colleagues were able to document the presence of sporozoites
only after placing fecal material in 2.5% potassium dichromate
($K_2Cr_2O_7$) for 1 week at room temperature.[12]

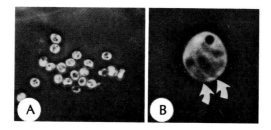

Figure 6–2. **A.** Phase-contrast micrograph of oocysts from human feces concentrated by Sheather's sugar flotation. **B.** Phase-contrast micrograph of a single
oocyst after 1 week at room temperature. (From Reese, N.C., Current, W.L.,
Ernst, J.V., and Bailey, W.S.: Cryptosporidiosis of man and calf: A case report
and results of experimental infections in mice and rats. Am. J. Trop. Hyg., 31:226,
1982.)

Permanent-Stained Smears

Permanent-stained smears are easily prepared by placing 1 drop each of a formalinized stool concentrate and 10% KOH on clean glass slides for 1 minute. After drying on a heating block maintained at 70°C, fixing in absolute methanol, and air-drying, a 1:10 dilution of Giemsa stain is recommended for staining. Best results were obtained by the California group when a 20-minute period was used for staining. Cryptosporidium oocytes stain blue, and granules appear red. Sometimes, a clear space is visible immediately inside the cell wall. Acid-fast staining of heat-fixed smears may also be used to demonstrate Cryptosporidium from stool specimens.[19,20] The organisms stain pink to deep red against a blue background. Use of both the Giemsa and acid-fast stains is recommended to detect the intestinal parasites.

Tissue Sections

Tissue specimens from human hosts, obtained by endoscopy, typically reveal the stages of schizogony of Cryptosporidium. A fibrous exudate is usually present, with evidence of inflammation. In tissue sections, the parasites stain especially well with Giemsa method, but also with toluidine blue, with hematoxylin-eosin, and with phosphotungstic acid-hematoxylin (PTAH) stains. The parasites do not stain with Gomori methenamine silver nitrate (GMSN) stain. The coccidia are attached to the border of the crypt of epithelial cells but are not found in the cytoplasm of cells (Fig. 6–3). With experience, it is possible to identify particular stages of the Cryptosporidum life cycle on electron micrographs and to observe internal morphology. Young trophozoites are enveloped by a four-unit membrane system. A nucleus, a nucleolus, and endoplasmic reticulum are often visible (Fig. 6–4).

PROGNOSIS

Human cryptosporidiosis appears to be self-limiting in previously healthy individuals, but can be rapidly fatal in immunocompromised hosts. Often the course of human cryptosporidiosis is complicated by the presence of other opportunistic infections.[5,7] In those instances, it is difficult to assess the contribution of other microorganisms in the fatal course of the disease. Until a drug proves to be effective in eliminating Cryptosporidium in the human host, the coccidian infection must be considered a serious one in immunodeficient patients.

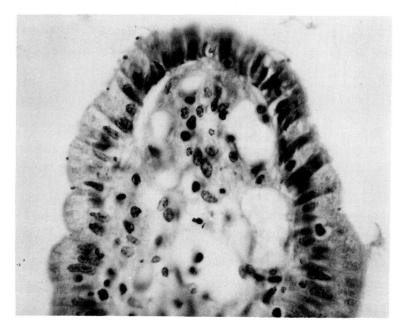

Figure 6–3. Giemsa stain of jejunal biopsy specimen, showing cryptosporidial organisms attached to the brush border of intestinal epithelial cells. (From Weisburger, W.R., et al.: Cryptosporidiosis in an immunosuppressed renal-transplant recipient with IgA deficiency. Am. J. Clin. Pathol., 72:473, 1979.)

CASE REPORTS

Case 1

A 52-year-old woman of Japanese ancestry first noticed loose bowel movements and a 20-pound weight loss 10 months prior to admission. The feces were watery in consistency without signs of steatorrhea or blood and occurred at a frequency of 1 to 4 movements a day. Prior to each bowel movement she would experience lower abdominal cramping pain, but the patient denied anorexia, dysphagia, jaundice, or fever.

As a lifelong Honolulu resident, the patient had made 1 trip to the mainland (Las Vegas, Nevada) 1 year prior to the onset of her diarrhea. She worked as a typist and had no exposure to toxins. One brother and a second cousin died of lymphosarcoma. Her only exposure to animals was to a pet dog. She had had the dog for many years and it had suffered no recent illnesses.

Other than a tonsillectomy as a child she had had no previous hospitalizations. Menopause occurred at the age of 49 years.

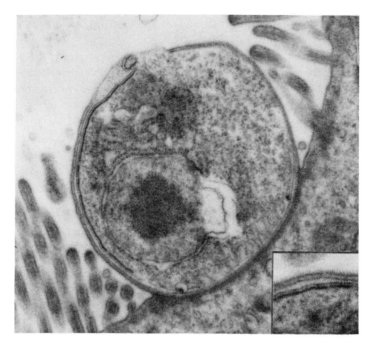

Figure 6–4. Electron micrograph of a young trophozoite of Cryptosporidium attached to an epithelial cell, showing a four-unit membrane system, a nucleus, and a prominent nucleolus. Uranyl acetate and lead citrate, × 36,000. **Inset:** A view of the membrane under higher magnification. (From Weisburger, W.R., et al.: Cryptosporidiosis in an immunosuppressed renal-transplant recipient with IgA deficiency. Am. J. Clin. Pathol., 72:473, 1979.)

The patient was admitted to the hospital on April 28, 1978. She was thin, but alert and in no acute distress. She was normotensive without orthostatic hypotension. There was no peripheral lymphadenopathy. Her abdomen was tympanitic. There was no hepatosplenomegaly.

Initial diagnostic studies indicated that she had lymphocytosis (81% of 9900/mm^3 white blood cells) and that 40% of the lymphocytes were atypical. Subsequent counts showed persistent lymphocytosis with a terminal increase in the number of white blood cells and lymphocytes.

On admission, the hematocrit value was 38% with a mean corpuscular hemoglobin concentration of 35% and a mean corpuscular volume of 107 μ. Serum glutamic oxaloacetic transaminase (SGOT) was 90 U, serum glutamic pyruvic transaminase (SGPT) was 50 U and creatine phosphokinase was normal. Alkaline phosphatase was 30 U (normal, 9 to 35 U), total bilirubin 0.6 mg/100 ml and a glutamyl transpeptidase was 20 U (normal, less than 40 U). Uric acid was 4.3 mg/100 ml, albumin 4.2 g/100 ml, and globulin 3.1 g/100 ml. Serum vitamin B_{12} was 250 pg/ml (normal, 200 to 900 pg/ml) and folate 4.1 mg/ml (normal, 4 to 20 mg/ml). Triiodothyronine resin uptake was 41.5% (normal, 35 to 45%) and thyroxine by radioimmunoassay was 8.2 µg/100 ml (normal 4.5 to 11.5 µg/100 ml). A 24-hour urine 5-hydroxyindole acetic acid determination was within normal limits. No white blood cells were seen in the stool, and an initial urinalysis did not disclose any abnormalities. Serum cholesterol was 100 mg/dl (normal, 160 to 250 mg/dl), triglyceride 59 mg/dl (normal, 10 to 160 mg/dl) and magnesium was low at 1.2 mg/dl (normal, 1.3 to 2.6 mg/dl). Serum carotene was 8 µg/dl (normal, 50 to 250 µg/dl) and prothrombin time was 60%.

Stool examinations were negative for parasites on numerous occasions, as were examinations of duodenal aspirates. A vasoactive intestinal polypeptide level was 150 pg/ml (normal, 3 to 36 pg/ml). A roentgenographic series of the small bowel showed that the proximal jejunum had an increased caliber and coarse plicae. Barium enema and protoscopy revealed no abnormalities. Computerized tomography failed to reveal enlargement of retroperitoneal lymph nodes, and a lymphangiogram was within normal limits.

A technitium sulfur colloid liver scan revealed a liver measuring 13 cm in the mid-clavicular line. Colloidal distribution was not uniform, but there were no discrete focal lesions. The spleen measured 9 cm, and the spleen to liver ratio was normal at 0.69. Hepatitis B surface antigen was not present and the liver biopsy revealed only fatty metamorphosis. A jejunal biopsy specimen showed villous atrophy. Many small parasites identified as Cryptosporidium were found on the luminal surface of the villous epithelium. These organisms were not recovered from the feces or the duodenal aspirate.

Antibodies against Toxoplasma gondii were estimated to be present at a titer of 1:512 by the indirect hemagglutination technique on May 3, 1978, and at a level of 1:256 on July 11. The antibody titers against cytomegalic virus were 1:64 on 2 occasions and against Epstein-Barr virus were 1:100 and 1:200, as estimated by the indirect fluorescent antibody technique. Evidence of an impaired immunologic status is summarized by the following abnormal findings:

Immunoglobulin G was less than 800 mg/100 ml in 4 of 5 analyses (range, 600 to 950 mg/100 ml); immunoglobulin M was more than 70 mg/100 ml in 1 of 5 analyses (range, 63 to 98 mg/100 ml); immunoglobulin A, in each of 5 analyses, was within normal limits (range 131 to 192 mg/100 ml).

The results of the lymphocyte stimulation tests are shown [in the following table]:

Results of Lymphocyte Stimulation Test*

Date	Concanavalin A	Phytohemagglutinin	Pokeweed Mitogen
April 1978	19	18	21
June 1978	19	244	14
July 1978	4	4	1
August 1978	3	4	1

*Number of mitogen events per 2.5×10^5 cells

The normal range for concanavalin A is 38 to 154 mitogen responses among 250,000 cells, for phytohemagglutinin 61 to 173, and for pokeweed mitogen 7 to 106.

The normal range for B cells is 27 to 49%. In our patient, it was 9.7 to 25%. The normal range for T cells is 36 to 60%. In our patient, the range was 36 to 60%.

In May, there was no response to Candida, dermatophytin, mumps, or purified protein derivative skin tests. In July, there was no response to mumps, varidase, and purified protein derivative skin tests. There was an erythematous reaction $(1+)$ to 2 mg DNCB sensitization; no reaction to 0.025 to 0.1 mg.

In April 1978, the third component of complement (C3c) was 63 mg/100 ml, and in May it was 65 mg/100 ml (normal range, 62 to 212 mg/100 ml). In April 1978, the fourth component of complement (C4) was 40 mg/100 ml, and in May it was 24 mg/100 ml (normal range, 20 to 50 mg/100 ml). In June 1978, total complement was 32 U/ml (CH 50; normal range, 48 to 103 U/ml). C3 activator was 5.8 mg/100 ml (normal range, 12 to 30 mg/100 ml).

The cryptosporidial infection resisted a wide variety of antibiotic agents. The antibiotic therapy may be summarized as follows: (1) Metronidazole, 250 mg, 3 times a day from April 28 to May 10. There was no response to this regimen. (2) Sulfamethoxazole, 800 mg, and trimethoprim, 160 mg, every 6 hours from May 10 to May 22. There was no clinical response although a serum sulfamethoxazole level on the third day of treatment was at normal therapeutic levels (10.2 mg/dl). (3) Pyrimethamine in an initial dose of 50 mg on May 30, followed by 25 mg daily from June 1 to June 15. A serum level on June 7 was 0.4 μg/ml—within the normal therapeutic range for this drug. (4) Sulfadiazine, 750 mg every 6 hours from May 31 to June 15. The sulfadiazine level was 8.7 mg/dl on June 7 and 9 mg/dl on June 10, again demonstrating adequate absorption and therapeutic levels. (5) Brief courses of levamisol from June 30 to July 3 and from July 13 to July 15 yielded no clinical response. (6) Amphotericin B was given intravenously from July 31 to August 23 for a total dose of 466 mg. Concomitant oral amphotericin B was given every 8 hours from August 3 to August 23 for a total dose of 549 mg. The serum amphotericin B level was measured on 2 occasions with levels of 0.32 μg/ml and 0.16 μg/ml. There was no response to this therapy.

Repeat jejunal and duodenal biopsies indicated that the cryptosporidial organisms increased in number throughout the period of antibiotic therapy. Initially, the patient was given an elemental diet, but her diarrhea did not lessen. She did not respond to the administration of cholestyramine or to a trial of an oral mixture of glucose and actively transported amino acids. Her bowel movements became so watery and explosive that eventually she could only be supported by parenteral hyperalimentation. She died in August 1978, 22 months after the onset of her loose bowel movements. Terminally, generalized lymphadenopathy, renal failure, and pulmonary insufficiency developed. She weighed 88 pounds on admission, and 1 day before her death she weighed 49 pounds. The serum creatinine level had risen from 0.7 mg/100 ml on admission to 4.4 mg/100 ml. Albumin decreased from 3.9 to 2.6, the alkaline phosphatase level had risen from 30 to 120 U, SGOT from 81 to 110 U, and the prothrombin time had decreased from 90% to 33%. The platelet count was 56,000/mm^3, but there was no laboratory evidence for disseminated intravascular coagulation. Cholesterol was stable at 119 mg/100 ml.*

Case 2

A 3½-year-old white female developed malaise and a dry cough 6 days before admission to the Vanderbilt University Hospital. Five days earlier, she was admitted to another hospital where she was vomiting everything taken by mouth and had severe watery diarrhea. Her health in the past had been excellent and development had been normal after an uneventful birth. She had received no immunizations. The patient lived in a farm house in a rural community that was supplied only with well water. The family had two cats, a dog, and nondairy cattle in a nearby field. On admission to the Vanderbilt University Hospital, her axillary temperature was 100°F and her pulse was 120. She weighed 27 pounds (several months before, she had weighed 31 pounds) and she was 40 inches tall. Physical examination showed signs of dehydration, hyperactive bowel sounds, and diffuse tenderness to deep palpation, but no distension. Her hematocrit was 43.9%. White blood count was 9600 per mm^3 with a differential of 10% juvenile, 34.5% mature polymorphonuclear leukocytes, 35.5% lymphocytes, 1.5% eosinophils, and 11.5% atypical lymphocytes. A watery stool specimen gave a positive reaction for blood (Hematest). Stool cultures and examination for ova and parasites were negative,

---

*From Stemmermann, G.N., et al.: Am. J. Med., 69:637–642, 1980.[8]

as were tuberculin and histoplasmin skin tests. The serum albumin was 4.0 g per 100 ml and the total protein was 5.9 g per 100 ml.

A chest x-ray was unremarkable. The abdominal x-ray showed large amounts of gas in the colon, and fluid levels were present in both the large and small bowel. A barium enema showed fine spiculated ulcerations, producing a markedly abnormal mucosal pattern. For 3 days after admission, she continued to be febrile, to vomit, to pass flatus and liquid stool, and to complain of crampy abdominal pain.

She was given supportive therapy that included intravenous fluids, nasogastric tube suction, and passage of a rectal tube every 3 to 4 hours. A barium enema done 4 days after admission revealed edema of the descending and sigmoid colon and rectum. This was felt to be consistent with acute colitis. Proctosigmoidoscopy performed on the fifth day showed an edematous mucosa and yellow plaques thought to be fibrinous exudate. A biopsy of the rectum was taken at this time. She subsequently continued to improve and was discharged on the ninth day of admission, afebrile and eating a full diet.

Three weeks after discharge, a follow-up sigmoidoscopy showed minimal changes that could have been caused by an enema given 40 minutes before the procedure. No biopsy was performed on this occasion. During the 18-month period since her illness, the child had an increased number of colds, and 1 year after the episode of enterocolitis she underwent a tonsillectomy. Otherwise, her health has been good and no further gastrointestinal symptoms have been present.

The diagnosis of cryptosporidiosis by light and electron microscopy was not made until long after the patient had her illness. The Cryptosporidia for the most part were attached to the crypt epithelial cells. The source of infection and mode of transmission to the child remain unidentified.*

Case 3

A 25-year-old white male contracted cryptosporidiosis approximately 3 weeks after initiating a survey of Cryptosporidium sp. in calves. Prior to the onset of clinical symptoms of cryptosporidiosis, he was in excellent health, having had no illness other than 2 mild colds during the previous 36 months. Blood samples were taken on day 8 of the illness and 3 weeks after he was fully recovered. No abnormalities were noted in the levels of serum globulins at these times, and no deficiencies in cell-mediated immune response were detected by lymphocyte blastogenesis testing. On day 1 of the illness, he experienced a low-grade fever, malaise, and nausea. During the next 4 days, he had moderate abdominal cramping, anorexia, and 5 to 10

---

*From Nime, F.A., et al.: Gastroenterol., *70*:592–598, 1976. © 1976, The Williams & Wilkins Co., Baltimore.[13]

bowel movements per day of watery, frothy feces. On days 6 to 10 of the illness, abdominal cramping was severe and he had 3 to 4 watery bowel movements per day. His appetite began to improve by day 8. He became constipated on day 11, and this condition, as well as moderate abdominal cramping, persisted for 3 days. Fourteen days after onset of the illness he was feeling well and eating a full diet.

The first fecal sample was collected approximately 56 hours after the onset of symptoms; it contained large numbers of Cryptosporidium sp. oocysts. The number of Cryptosporidium sp. oocysts in daily fecal samples remained high through day 4, decreased markedly on day 5, and remained low through day 12. No oocysts of Cryptosporidium sp. were observed in Sheather's sugar flotations of fecal samples collected on days 13 to 18.

Oocysts of the human isolate of Cryptosporidium sp. were morphologically indistinguishable from those obtained from naturally or experimentally infected calves. The appearance of Cryptosporidium sp. oocysts from calves in Giemsa-stained smears and in fecal flotations using brightfield microscopy has been described in detail. We found that phase-contrast microscopy is far superior to brightfield microscopy for detection of oocysts of Cryptosporidium sp. in fecal flotations. When observed with phase-contrast microscopy, the spherical to subspherical oocysts measured 4 to 5 μm, were highly refractile, and contained 1 to 6 prominent dark granules and numerous fine dark granules. After sporulating in 2.5% potassium dichromate for 1 week at room temperature, Cryptosporidium sp. oocysts from the human and from calves contained 4 sporozoites and a spherical residuum with 1 to 3 prominent dark granules.

All of the 1-day-old mice and rats inoculated orally with sporulated Cryptosporidium sp. oocysts of human or of calf origin were heavily infected when necropsied 6 days PI. Numerous endogenous stages of Cryptosporidium sp. were observed in the brush border of the ileum, and moderate numbers were seen in the cecum and colon of all inoculated mice and rats. Numerous oocysts of Cryptosporidium sp. were observed in Sheather's sugar flotations of intestinal homogenates of all mice and rats 6 days PI with parasites of human or of calf origin. No endogenous stages of Cryptosporidium sp. were seen in histologic sections and no oocysts were observed in intestinal homogenates of the 8 control mice and 5 control rats. Transmission electron microscopy of the ileal mucosa of 2 suckling mice 6 days PI with oocysts of human Cryptosporidium sp. revealed the presence of numerous trophozoites, schizonts, macrogametes, oocysts, and a few endogenous stages thought to be microgametocytes.

All 6 adult mice inoculated orally with sporulated oocysts of Cryptosporidium sp. of human or of calf origin became infected and passed oocysts on days 6 to 12 or 13 PI. No differences were noted in pre-patency and patency of the human and calf isolates. No oocysts of Cryptosporidium sp. were observed in daily sugar flotations of feces of 6 previously uninoculated control mice.*

SUMMARY

Human cryptosporidiosis is a recently recognized enteric disease caused by the coccidian parasite Cryptosporidium. At least 11 species have been described as causes of diarrheal enterocolitis in animals, but those organisms may represent a single species that has adapted to multiple hosts. The mode of transmission has not been definitively established. Although individuals with serious immune deficiencies are especially susceptible to the parasite, cryptosporidial enteritis can occur in previously healthy persons. Diagnosis of cryptosporidiosis is best made by finding oocysts in wet mounts or permanent-stained smears prepared from formalinized stool specimens, or by observing stages of schizogony on tissue sections prepared from biopsy or autopsy material. Abatement of human cryptosporidiosis awaits the discovery of an effective antiparasitic drug to eliminate the coccidian or to correct immune deficiencies that predispose certain individuals to the disease.

REFERENCES

1. Brownstein, D.G., et al.: Cryptosporidium in snakes with hypertrophic gastritis. Vet. Pathol., *14*:606, 1977.
2. Anderson, B.C.: Patterns of shedding of cryptosporidial oocysts in Idaho calves. J. Am. Vet. Assoc., *178*:982, 1981.
3. Vetterling, J.M., et al.: Cryptosporidium wrairi sp. n. from the guinea pig Cavia porcellus with an emendation of the genus. J. Protozool., *18*(2):243, 1971.
4. Snyder, S.P., England, J.J., and McChesney, A.: Cryptosporidiosis in immunodeficient Arabian foals. Vet. Pathol., *15*:12, 1978.
5. Inman, L.R., and Takeuchi, A.: Spontaneous cryptosporidiosis in an adult female rabbit. Vet. Pathol., *16*:89, 1979.
6. Centers for Disease Control: Cryptosporidiosis: Assessment of chemotherapy of males with acquired immune deficiency syndrome (AIDS). Morbid. Mortal. Weekly Rept., *31*:589, 1982.
7. Centers for Disease Control: Human cryptosporidiosis—Alabama. Morbid. Mortal. Weekly Rept., *31*:252, 1982.
8. Stemmermann, G.N., et al.: Cryptosporidiosis: Report of a fatal case complicated by disseminated toxoplasmosis. Am. J. Med., *69*:637, 1980.
9. Levine, N.D.: Some corrections of coccidian (Apicomplexa: Protozoa) nomenclature. J. Parasitol., *66*:830, 1980.
10. Current, W.L., et al.: Human cryptosporidiosis in immunocompetent and immunodeficient persons—Studies of an outbreak and experimental transmission. N. Engl. J. Med., *308*:1252, 1983.
11. Tzipori, S., Angus, K.W., Campbell, I., and Gray, E.W.: Cryptosporidium: Evidence for a single-species genus. Infect. Immun., *30*:884, 1980.
12. Reese, N.C., Current, W.L., Ernst, J.V., and Bailey, W.S.: Cryptosporidiosis of man

---

*From Reese, N.C., Current, W.L., Ernst, J.V., and Bailey, W.S.: Am. J. Trop. Med. Hyg., *31*:226–229, 1982. © 1982 by the American Society of Tropical Medicine and Hygiene.[12]

and calf: A case report and results of experimental infections in mice and rats. Am. J. Trop. Med. Hyg., *31*(2):226, 1982.

13. Nime, F.A., et al.: Acute enterocolitis in a human being infected with the protozoan Cryptosporidium. Gastroenterol., *70*:592, 1976.
14. Tzipori, S.: Cryptosporidiosis in animals and humans. Microbiol. Rev., *47*:84, 1983.
15. Frenkel, J.K.: Toxoplasmosis. *In* Pathology of Protozoal and Helminthic Diseases. Edited by R.A. Marcial-Rojas. Baltimore, Williams & Wilkins, 1971.
16. Lasser, K.H., Lewin, K.J., and Ryning, F.W.: Cryptosporidial enteritis in a patient with congenital hypogammaglobulinemia. Human Pathol., *10*:234, 1979.
17. Garcia, L.S., Brewer, T.C., Bruckner, D.A., and Shimizu, R.Y.: Clinical laboratory diagnosis of Cryptosporidium from human fecal specimens. Clin. Microbiol. Newsl., *4*:136, 1982.
18. Levine, N.D.: Protozoan Parasites of Domestic Animals and of Man, 2nd Ed. Minneapolis, Burgess Publ. Co., 1973.
19. Henriksen, S.A., and Pohlenz, J.: Staining of Cryptosporidia by a modified Ziehl-Neelsen technique. Acta Vet. Scand., *22*:594, 1981.
20. Garcia, L.S., Brewer, T.C., Bruckner, D.A., and Shimizu, R.Y.: Acid-fast staining of Cryptosporidium from human fecal specimens. Clin. Microbiol. Newsl., *5*:60, 1983.

CHAPTER 7 CYTOMEGALOVIRUS INFECTIONS

Although nontoxoplasmic chorioretinopathy in infants and children was described as early as 1949 in the United States, Holland, and England, it was not determined until much later that the chorioretinopathy was virus-associated.[1] In 1956 and 1957, a human cytomegalovirus (CMV) was implicated as an etiologic agent in disease of young children, including 1 case of a 3-month-old infant with jaundice, hepatosplenomegaly, cerebral calcification, and chorioretinitis.[2] The infected tissues included tissue obtained at autopsy or by biopsy of the submaxillary salivary gland, the kidney, the liver, and the adenoids. CMV has remained a significant cause of morbidity and mortality in neonates over the years. In the United States alone, it is estimated that 4000 infants every year sustain neurologic disabilities as a result of the congenital infection.[3] In England, approximately 800 cases of mental retardation annually are attributed to CMV.[1] Although statistics are not available for other countries, the virus is ubiquitous in nature and is believed to be worldwide in distribution. In recent years, the spectrum of CMV disease has been expanded to include intrapartum, postpartum, postneonatal, post-transfusion, post-transplantation, and opportunistic infections.[4-10]

NEONATAL INFECTIONS

Approximately 0.5 to 2.2% of all neonates born in the United States are infected with CMV.[11] Only about 1 in 20 infants, however, develops microcephaly, hepatosplenomegaly, cerebral calcification, or a rash.[4] It is difficult, and sometimes impossible, to distinguish CMV infections in neonates from those caused by rubella virus, herpes simplex viruses, or the protozoan of toxoplasmosis on a clinical basis. The similarity of symptoms has led to the use of the acronym TORCH for toxoplasmosis, rubella, cytomegalovirus, and herpes simplex virus in describing the infections. One characteristic that the congenital infections have in common is intrauterine growth retardation (IUGR).[12] Birth weights below the tenth percentile for gestational age have been associated with 41% of neonates with clinical CMV infection.[13] In 4 studies of unselected newborn populations, 11.4% of asymptomatic infants were below the tenth percentile for gestational age.[14-17]

POSTNEONATAL INFECTIONS

It is uncertain whether CMV infections, occurring in young children, constitute primary or reactivated infections, since, like other herpesviruses, CMV can remain in a latent state within the body for extended periods of time. The clinical manifestations of CMV infection after the neonatal period are less definitive than in the newborn. The symptoms often resemble those of infectious mononucleosis.[18] Fatigue, an elevated temperature, joint and muscle pain, general malaise, and lymphadenopathy may be present. The liver is sometimes enlarged and tender. It has been estimated that up to 10% of clinically suspected cases of infectious mononucleosis are of CMV origin. The rate of seropositivity for CMV by age 35 is about 50%.[4]

POST-TRANSFUSION INFECTIONS

The potential of blood as a vehicle for transmission of CMV has been recognized for years, but since patients are often asymptomatic, many post-transfusion CMV infections receive little attention.[19] If symptoms are present following transfusion with blood containing CMV, the symptoms are frequently indistinguishable from those of infectious mononucleosis. Fever, splenomegaly, and atypical lymphocytosis may occur 3 to 6 weeks following receipt of CMV-positive blood.[4] Post-transfusion CMV infection can be distinguished from infectious mononucleosis by the absence of heterophil antibodies.

POST-TRANSPLANTATION INFECTIONS

CMV infection following organ transplantation has received increasing attention during the last decade.[20–22] Post-transplant CMV disease is more serious than post-transfusion infection with CMV, because the required immunosuppressive therapy in transplant recipients depresses cellular immune mechanisms. In renal-transplant patients, the incidence of CMV infections is reported to be 50 to 100%.[20] Approximately one half of the cases of interstitial pneumonia known to occur in 40 to 50% of bone marrow transplant recipients are attributed to CMV.[23] CMV infections have also been reported during the first 12 weeks in heart-transplant recipients.[24]

The CMV infections in transplant recipients may constitute primary infections or be caused by reactivation of endogenous CMV. The onset of symptoms usually occurs during the first 30 to 60 days following surgery. Primary infections tend to be more serious than those associated with reactivation of latent CMV.[25,26]

Clinical features of a primary CMV infection in transplant recipients include fever, gastrointestinal bleeding, encephalitis, retinitis, leukopenia, pneumonia, hepatitis, arthralgias, and graft loss.[20,27,28] Primary CMV infection is responsible for up to 10% of the fatalities occurring in transplant recipients. Infections attributed to reactivation of latent CMV are usually asymptomatic, but preformed antibody does not prevent leukopenia.[26]

The clinical course of patients with primary CMV infection following transfusion or transplantation is often complicated by bacterial or fungal superinfections.[29] The mechanism whereby CMV potentiates superinfections remains speculative. It is also not known whether CMV infection per se has a role in allograft rejection, although recipients who are seropositive for CMV usually have fewer problems if they have received well-matched grafts.[30]

OPPORTUNISTIC CMV INFECTIONS

Cytomegalovirus (CMV) and other members of the family Herpetoviridae, which include the varicella-zoster virus (VZV), Epstein-Barr virus (EBV), and herpes simplex viruses (HSV) 1 and 2, are common causes of opportunistic infections. Patients receiving steroid or other types of immunosuppressive therapy are particularly susceptible to herpesviruses.[31]

Patients who have suffered extensive burns, or who are compromised by serious underlying disease, are prime candidates for CMV infections.[4,32,33] CMV may coexist with the protozoan Pneumocystis carinii or the yeast Candida albicans in opportunistic infections.

CMV AND OPPORTUNISTIC MALIGNANCIES

Increasingly, reports in the literature point to a role for CMV in the opportunistic malignancy known as Kaposi's sarcoma.[34-36] More than 20 cases of multicentric malignant hemangiosarcoma, characteristic of Kaposi's disease, have been reported in renal transplant recipients.[35,37] CMV appears to contribute to the immunosuppression observed in acquired immune deficiency syndrome (AIDS). In most reported cases of AIDS, elevated titers of antibodies to CMV have been demonstrated.

Another herpesvirus, the Epstein-Barr virus (EBV), is frequently found in association with Burkitt's lymphoma, a type of cancer, which is endemic in some parts of Africa. EBV is known to transform cells in vivo and in vitro, but transformation by CMV has not been observed in humans.[38] Even during CMV infections uncomplicated by immunosuppressive therapy, however, lymphocyte proliferative responses are delayed.[39]

A recent report from Tennessee of a fatal CMV infection of the skin shares some characteristics of the original description of a skin disease made by Kaposi in 1872.[40] Kaposi's sarcoma was originally considered to be a skin disease affecting the lower limbs.[41] Kaposi described skin lesions consisting of small reddish-blue macules which progressed to nodules or ulcers, some of which failed to heal. At least one type of lesion of the fatal CMV infection involving the skin was of the ulcerative variety. The patient was receiving immunosuppressive drugs for multiple myeloma. The combination of the presence of CMV infection and the receipt of immunosuppressive drugs may present the conditions required for opportunistic malignancy. The possible association of CMV and immunosuppressive drugs with Kaposi's sarcoma or similar malignancies raises some provocative questions that remain unanswered.

ETIOLOGY

Cytomegalovirus (CMV) is morphologically indistinguishable from other herpesviruses (Fig. 7–1). Herpesviruses consist of two strands of deoxyribonucleic acid (DNA) and a symmetrical protein capsid. The virion measures 180 to 200 nm. All herpesviruses possess an envelope, which is acquired upon release of the viruses from the nucleus of infected cells. Some polypeptides are associated with the DNA. Other polypeptides are contained in the envelope.[42] All strains of CMV appear to be closely related antigenically.[43]

Cells infected with CMV demonstrate 2 typical morphologic aber-

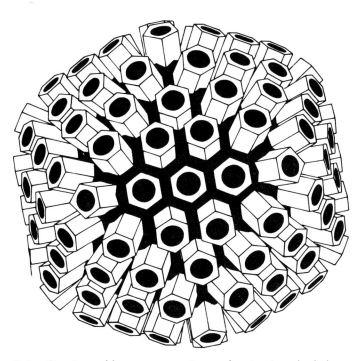

Figure 7–1. Structure of herpes group viruses showing icosahedral symmetry with five- and six-sided capsomeres. (From Horne, R.W.: Virus Structure. New York, Academic Press, 1974.)

rations. Cell rounding in early infection is followed by enlargement and development of an epithelioid appearance after 36 to 48 hours.[44] Furthermore, CMV appears to affect the molecular organization of actin but not its synthesis. Infected cells are destroyed rapidly in fulminating CMV neonatal disease. Cell death appears to be slower in postnatal infections.

CMV-infected cells can be infected with other microbial agents in vitro.[45] It appears likely that interaction between the genome of an infected cell and the virus can potentiate additional opportunism in some as yet unexplained manner. Antecedent or concurrent CMV infection in opportunistic malignancy suggests expanding roles for both virology and immunology in opportunism.

PREDISPOSING FACTORS

Since approximately 50% of all individuals either have or have had a cytomegalovirus (CMV) infection, susceptibility appears to be general; however, certain risk factors can clearly be identified with the disease for certain populations. Infection in the mother, breast feeding, and postpartum transfusion of neonates with seropositive blood constitute predisposing factors for infants. For older children and adults, the forced closeness of institutionalization, imposed by socioeconomic conditions, appears to be a risk factor. Pregnancy may predispose women to a reactivation of endogenous CMV.[46] The relationship between immune suppression in pregnancy and CMV infection is a curious one. Cellular immune responses to CMV are depressed progressively during pregnancy and return to normal gradually during the postpartum year.[47]

The receipt of renal, cardiac, or bone marrow transplants, multiple blood transfusions, or immunosuppression caused by underlying disease or drug therapy predisposes patients to CMV infection.[18] The link between multiple blood transfusions and CMV infection was publicized when the medical progress of Pope John Paul II was interrupted by such an infection after he received multiple units of blood during his hospitalization following surgery for a gunshot wound.

EPIDEMIOLOGY

Congenital CMV infections are transmitted from an infected mother across the placenta to the fetus. The infection can be acquired during birth from an infected cervix. It is estimated that approximately 20% of pregnant women in the United States harbor the virus in the cervix. The number of pregnant women infected with CMV may be higher in developing countries. In at least 1 instance, transmission of CMV from an infant with acquired infection to the mother has been documented by restriction enzyme analysis.[48] Premature twins delivered by Cesarean section from a CMV seronegative mother required multiple blood transfusions. One twin developed CMV infection at the age of 6 weeks, and the other one developed CMV infection at the age of 9 weeks. Blood was assumed to be the source of the CMV infection. CMV infection in the mother was detected 2 months after the infants were released to her care. Reactivation of CMV during a subsequent pregnancy could endanger the developing fetus. Furthermore, it is probable that CMV seronegative nursery personnel caring for CMV-infected infants are at risk of developing the disease.

CMV infection in older children and adults is transmitted by kissing, by blood transfusions, by organ transplants, and by sexual intercourse.[18] At least one study in a day-care center in the United States suggests that horizontal transmission of CMV among toddlers has occurred through shared toys.[49] Horizontal transmission of CMV in dialysis patients, unlike that of hepatitis B virus, has not been a frequent problem.[50,51]

The rate of CMV infection in young children is higher in Scandinavian countries than in the United States. This has been attributed to the greater use of day-care centers in Scandinavia.[52] The incidence of CMV infections in children in some developing countries is reported to be almost 100%. It is likely that crowded living conditions provide more opportunities for person-to-person transmission of CMV and that dietary deficiencies interfere with normal immune responses.

LABORATORY DIAGNOSIS

Because the host-cell range of CMV is wide, the virus may be present in a variety of cell types. Infections of cells are permissive lytic infections and typically produce a characteristic cytopathic effect (CPE) consisting of large cells with intranuclear or intracytoplasmic inclusions. Unlike its relative, the Epstein-Barr virus (EBV), however, it is not known whether CMV can infect lymphocytes.[38] Definitive diagnosis must be made by cultural or serologic tests.

Microscopic Examination

Biopsy material, autopsy material, throat washings, and urine are the specimens of choice for the demonstration of CMV infection. Slides made from histopathologic sections of biopsy or autopy material can be stained with hematoxylin-eosin. Throat washings can be obtained from adults by having them gargle with 10 to 20 ml of tryptose-phosphate broth and expectorate into a sterile container.[53] Swabbing the throat with 2 sterile swabs is usually more successful than gargling in young children. After the tops are broken off the swabs, the swabs can be placed in a holding medium for delivery to the laboratory. Urine not obtained by catheterization should be treated with antimicrobial agents. Final concentrations of 200 to 500 U of penicillin, 200 to 500 μg of streptomycin, and 50 to 100 U of nystatin per ml are recommended. Several specimens of fresh urine are often required, because cells may be shed only intermittently and do not remain intact for prolonged periods of time.[54] Cells may be collected on a membrane filter and stained with hematoxylin-eosin or by the Papanicolaou method. The intranuclear or intracytoplasmic inclusions in large cells are readiy observable in infected cells (Fig. 7–2). CMV can be observed by electron microscopy in the urine and oral secretions of about 30% of congenitally infected infants.[55] The virus is rarely observed in the urine of infected adults.[4]

Cultural Techniques

Cultural techniques for CMV constitute the most definitive methods for diagnosing CMV infections in infants and adults. Throat washings, multiple urine specimens, blood samples, cervical secretions, autopsy material, and tissue obtained by biopsy are most likely to yield positive results. Urine specimens should be adjusted to a pH of 7.0 with 0.1 N NaOH or 0.1 N HCl after addition of the antimicrobial agents described.

Buffy coats, obtained by sedimentation with or without dextran, from 5.0 ml of heparinized blood may be used as an inoculum after

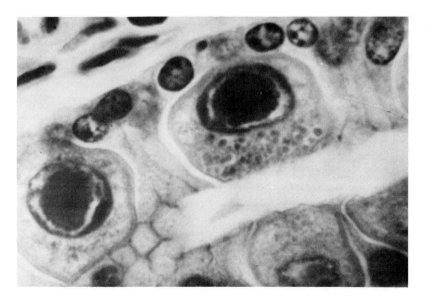

Figure 7–2. Intranuclear and intracytoplasmic inclusions in an epithelial cell infected with cytomegaloviruses. (From Bergquist, L.M.: Microbiology for the Hospital Environment. New York, Harper & Row, 1981. Courtesy, J.S. Nelson, St. Louis.)

washing twice in sterile phosphate-buffered saline (PBS) and resuspension in the same diluent. Throat or cervical secretions must be treated with the same concentrations of antimicrobial agents recommended for microscopic examination. Small pieces of autopsy or biopsy material require mincing with sterile scalpel and scissors and suspension in cell culture medium. Human fibroblast cells, such as strains of WI-38 (Microbiological Associates, Bethesda, Maryland) or Flow 2000 (Flow Laboratories, Inglewood, California) may be used to culture CMV.

Characteristic CPE can be observed frequently in less than 1 week in urine cultures from infants. Cultures should be maintained for 4 to 6 weeks, however, because only small quantities of virus may be present in some specimens. Since CMV viruria may persist for months or years after an infection, some caution should be exercised in interpretation of positive urine cultures.[4] CMV cultures may also be negative even in the presence of an infection because of intermittent shedding of CMV.[18]

Serologic Tests

Complement-fixing (CF) antibodies are readily detectable in sera of individuals infected with CMV. Most infants who acquire a congenital CMV infection have high CF antibody titers.[56] In older children and adults, the titer of CF antibodies may fluctuate, so interpretation may be difficult. Although a fourfold increase in antibody titer between acute- and convalescent-phase sera is significant in most infections, that criterion may not be reliable in CMV infections unless the first specimen is negative.[4] CMV-IgM antibodies may be present early in an active infection. Detection of CMV-IgM on fetal cord serum by radioimmunoassay made it possible to diagnose a prenatal intrauterine CMV infection.[57] An indirect fluorescent antibody (IFA) test, an anticomplement immunofluorescent-antibody (ACIF) technique, an immune adherence hemagglutination assay (IAHA), an enzyme-linked immunosorbent assay (ELISA), and a passive hemagglutination test are available, but may only be suitable for laboratories that have had considerable experience with these techniques.

PROGNOSIS

Prenatal CMV infections are associated with a wide range of disabilities and even death. Hepatomegaly, splenomegaly, jaundice, petechiae, chorioretinitis, cerebral calcification, hydrops fetalis, and mental retardation have all been reported.[1] Non-neural defects, including cardiac malformations, tetralogy of Fallot, mitral and pulmonary valve stenosis, inguinal hernias, and club feet also have been attributed to CMV infections.

Acquired or reactivated CMV infection in transplant patients or other immunocompromised individuals constitutes a serious and often life-threatening disease. Bone-marrow transplant recipients who are able to mount an antibody response to CMV or who have a high CF antibody titer to CMV have a better prognosis than either those recipients who are unable to synthesize the CMV antibodies or those with low or no CF antibodies.[58] The importance of finding seronegative CMV donors for transplant patients has been emphasized but may only partially resolve the problem since the required immunosuppressive drugs depress cellular immunity. The search for a CMV vaccine for high-risk groups is progressing, but many questions concerning its safety remain unanswered.[59]

Although the consequences of CMV infection can be serious in certain groups, most asymptomatic cases go unrecognized. Asymptomatic perinatal CMV-uria has been associated with developmental delay and hearing impairments in a limited number of individuals.[60] The greatest hazard in adults appears to be the latency of CMV, which can be reactivated when the immune mechanisms are compromised.

CASE REPORTS

Case 1

A 28-year-old rhesus-positive woman without atypical antibodies was referred at 25 weeks' gestation after ultrasonography showed a hydropic fetus. She had felt well throughout the pregnancy, denied taking any medication, and reported no relevant personal or family history. At 16 weeks' gestation, an ultrasound scan had confirmed her dates and shown no major structural abnormalities. Examination was unremarkable, with fundal height being consistent with dates. A further ultrasound scan confirmed a single fetus with gross ascites, but no other abnormalities were observed. Fetoscopy was carried out and 8 ml pure fetal blood and 260 ml ascitic fluid collected. Fetal serum showed appreciable hypoalbuminaemia of 6 g/L (normal $21 \pm$ SD 2 g/L (unpublished)). A fetal blood film showed severe erythroblastosis.

A follow-up ultrasound scan showed re-collection of the ascites. Intravascular fetal albumin infusion was planned but precluded by spontaneous premature rupture of the membranes at 27 weeks' gestation. A conservative policy was adopted but labour ensued and a 1480 g severely depressed male infant delivered. Resuscitative attempts were stopped after 20 minutes. Initial serology for cytomegalovirus on maternal sera showed an antibody titre of 32 when a complement fixation test was performed on sera collected at 21 weeks' and 25 weeks' gestation. No cytomegalovirus-specific IgM was detected in the fetal serum using indirect immunofluorescence (Electronucleonics Laboratories, Inc., Maryland, USA).

Necropsy showed non-icteric hydrops fetalis. Macroscopically, the only abnormal findings were a large liver with a finely nodular and mottled surface and massive ascites, causing gross elevation of the diaphragm with consequent pulmonary hypoplasia. Microscopy showed cytomegaly and intranuclear "owl's eye" inclusions in many organs, particularly the kidney. The appearance was typical of cytomegalic inclusion disease. The liver showed extreme active erythropoiesis. Cytomegalovirus was isolated from urine obtained at necropsy.

These findings prompted a re-examination of stored maternal and fetal cord sera. The total IgM content of the fetal serum was 0.11 g/L. This is within the normal range for a fetus of this gestation as stated by Alford, et al. Radioimmunoassay for cytomegalovirus IgM showed that the fetal serum had a titre of 4000. This is within the range seen in neonatal or cord serum from confirmed cases of symptomatic congenital cytomegalovirus. Examination of the maternal serum for cytomegalovirus-specific IgM by radioimmunoassay showed a titre of 800 in the serum taken at 21 weeks' gestation, but such IgM was absent at 25 weeks. These results were compatible with a primary infection occurring early in the pregnancy.*

Cases 2 and 3

Twins A and B were the male products of a 22-year-old gravida 2, para 3 mother and were born at 29 weeks gestation by cesarean section because of a footling breech presentation. Delivery followed spontaneous labor with rupture of the amniotic membranes occurring immediately prior to surgery. A diamniotic, monochorionic twin placenta was present at birth.

Twin A weighed 970 g at birth with Apgar scores of 1 at 1 minute and 4 at 5 minutes. He was immediately intubated and required mechanical ventilation for the initial 5 days of life. Chest roentgenograms revealed hyaline membrane disease. His hospital course was complicated by a patent ductus arteriosus, hyperbilirubinemia, apnea, and bradycardia. A perforation of his descending colon at 16 days of age required surgical repair. Management of his multiple problems necessitated blood transfusions from 21 different blood donors. After recovery, the baby was fed banked breast milk during most of his hospitalization. The infant was stabilized and grew slowly, without complications, from 6 weeks of age until the middle of the eighth week when he was noted to be extremely lethargic. An evaluation for sepsis failed to reveal any bacterial pathogens. Laboratory data included: white blood cell count 8600/mm³ with 32% polymorphonuclear leukocytes, 8% band forms, 53% lymphocytes, and 7% monocytes; hemoglobin was 11.6 g/dl; cerebrospinal fluid examination and urinalysis were unremarkable. A chest roentgenogram was unchanged

---

*From Lange, I., et al.: Br. Med. J., *284*:1673–1674, 1982. Editor S.P. Lock.[57]

from previous films. Weekly screening urine cultures revealed that the infant began excreting CMV at 9 weeks of age. All previous cultures had been CMV-negative. A CMV-CF titer at 13 weeks of age was 1:32. The infant's subsequent hospital course was unremarkable and he was discharged home at 18 weeks of age.

Twin B weighed 1020 g at birth with Apgar scores of 7 at 1 minute and 8 at 5 minutes. He was intubated shortly after delivery because of respiratory distress and apnea. Chest roentgenograms revealed severe hyaline membrane disease. The hospital course was complicated initially by hypocalcemia and then by apnea, bradycardia, and necrotizing enterocolitis. The infant required intubation until approximately 19 days of age. From 4 to 6 weeks of age, the baby was stable, and although he still required 25 to 30% oxygen, he was growing and tolerating feedings. At 6 weeks of age, the infant experienced acute respiratory failure associated with apnea, tachypnea, and cyanosis, requiring ventilatory support with an inspired oxygen of 50%. Laboratory data included a white blood cell count of 14,200/mm³ with 77% polymorphonuclear leukocytes, 5% band forms, 14% lymphocytes, 3% monocytes, and 1% metamyelocytes; hemoglobin was 11.1 g/dl. Chest roentgenogram revealed marked consolidation of both lung bases with diffusely diminished aeration. All bacterial cultures were negative for pathogens. Weekly screening urine cultures revealed that the infant began to excrete CMV during the week of his acute respiratory deterioration. All previous urine cultures had been negative for CMV. Subsequent CMV-CF titers revealed a titer rise from 1:8 to 1:64. During the infant's hospital stay he received blood transfusions from 9 different donors and was fed banked breast milk for several weeks. The infant gradually recovered and was discharged home at 13 weeks of age.

The mother of the infants was cultured for CMV at approximately 13 weeks postpartum. At that time, urine and cervical specimens were negative for CMV, and she had no detectable antibody to CMV as determined by CMV-CF, CMV-enzyme-linked immunosorbent assay and an indirect immunoperoxidase technique. Six weeks following discharge of both babies, a repeat CMV-CF titer on their mother was positive at 1:128. Although a urine culture at that time was negative for CMV, a repeat urine culture 3 weeks later grew CMV. The mother reported no clinical manifestations during this period.*

Case 4

The patient, a 29-year-old white man, presented in 1969 with asymptomatic proteinuria. Renal biopsy showed focal and segmental

---

*From Spector, S.A., and Spector, D.H.: Pediatr. Inf. Dis., *1*:405–409, 1982. © 1982 The Williams & Wilkins Co., Baltimore.[48]

sclerosis. Antihypertensive treatment was commenced in 1974. He was admitted to hospital in November, 1976, with renal failure, and renal dialysis was started. In September, 1977, a cadaver renal transplant was performed; the kidney functioned well until February, 1978, when the patient developed progressive signs of rejection despite immunosuppressive treatment with steroids, azathioprine, and at times niridazole. He developed persistent thrombocytopenia and gastro-intestinal bleeding occurred. On 25 April, the transplanted kidney was removed. It was found to be swollen and tense and showed signs of cellular rejection on histologic examination. Immunosuppressive therapy was withdrawn, apart from low-dose maintenance corticosteroids. The patient subsequently developed progressive jaundice and diffuse pulmonary infiltration with low-grade fever, while the thrombocytopenia persisted. Massive gastro-intestinal haemorrhage responded dramatically to vasopressin infusion, but he died of respiratory failure on 8 May despite intensive supportive haemodialysis and ventilation.

At autopsy, the skin was deeply jaundiced and there were numerous petechiae, ecchymoses, and a few subcutaneous nodules on the lower limbs and abdomen. There was herpes-like ulceration of the lips and mouth, and a hard submucosal nodule of tumour tissue 1 cm in diameter was found in the lower trachea. Widespread nodular masses were present throughout both lungs. The right lung had a mass of 650 g and the left lung 930 g. The mass of the heart was 310 g and there was moderate left ventricular hypertrophy. There were numerous raised nodules in the stomach, the largest 3.5 cm in diameter, each with central umbilication. These nodules extended throughout the small intestine, but were most numerous in the proximal portion, gradually diminishing in number distally, until only an occasional lesion could be seen in the large intestine. The liver (2210 g) was dark green in colour. Numerous reddish-brown specks, later shown to be tumour, could be seen in the regions of the portal tracts. The original kidneys were contracted and granular. The mass of the right kidney was 45 g and that of the left kidney 55 g. At the site of the transplanted kidney, there was a large organizing haematoma.

On histologic examination, the features of Kaposi's sarcoma were seen in the tumour masses removed from the gastro-intestinal tract, liver, lungs, trachea, and mediastinal and paratracheal lymph nodes. The liver showed numerous bile lakes, bile in the canaliculi, and acute-on-chronic cholangitis, with tumour tissue infiltrating the portal tracts. There were three parathyroid glands, which were enlarged and hyperplastic. The lungs showed cytomegalovirus infection, and metastatic calcifications were noted in the alveolar membrane. Cytomegalovirus was cultured from the kidney removed on 25 April, from a throat swab taken on 8 May, and from the lung, liver, and lymph node specimens removed at autopsy on 19 May. No cytomegalovirus was cultured from spleen and brain specimens or from blood taken post mortem. Herpesvirus hominis had previously been isolated from a throat swab taken on 3 February, 1978.*

Case 5

A 60-year-old black woman presented herself to the emergency room of Baptist Memorial Hospital on November 17, 1979, with nausea, malaise, and an eruption composed of macules and papules that had been present for several days. The eruption was believed to be drug-induced, and the patient was directed to discontinue all medications, namely, furosemide, methyldopa, hydralazine, allopurinol, and digoxin.

She returned to the hospital and was admitted on November 19 because there had been no improvement in her symptoms. Pertinent past history included the recent diagnosis 6 weeks previously of multiple myeloma, which was being treated with melphalan and prednisone. The patient's vital signs were within normal limits. Physical examination revealed, in addition to the widespread eruption, diffuse abdominal tenderness and hepatomegaly with a total span of 14 cm. Upon admission, the BUN was 121 mg/dl (normal, 10 to 20), creatinine 7.4 mg/dl (normal, 0.7 to 1.5), SGOT 112 U/L (normal, 0 to 40), LDH 426 U/L (normal, 100 to 225), SGPT 274 U/L (normal, 0 to 35), alkaline phosphatase 632 U/L (normal, 30 to 100), and total bilirubin 2.7 mg/dl (normal, 0.2 to 1.2) with direct bilirubin 2.1 mg/dl (normal, 0 to 0.4). The hematocrit was 26.9%, hemoglobin 9.3 g/dl, and white blood cell count 3000/mm³. The diagnosis at the time of admission was a toxic or viral hepatitis and a drug-induced eruption.

By November 20, the patient has developed a temperature of 101°F. Escherichia coli was cultured from her urine, and intravenous ampicillin (500 mg every 6 hours) was begun. On November 21, she developed strongly guaiac-positive profuse diarrhea for which she was given several units of packed red blood cells when a hematocrit of 22.2% was detected. By November 26, her total bilirubin had risen to 21 mg/dl with a direct component of 17.4 mg/dl, and jaundice became obvious. Purulent lesions in the perineum and on the buttocks were treated with zinc oxide applied topically. Her condition continued to deteriorate. By December 3, the total bilirubin was 45.3 mg/dl with a direct component of 34.1 mg/dl, the alkaline phosphatase was 1587 U/L, SGOT 100 U/L, and SGPT 63 U/L. Tests for hepatitis B antigen and antibody revealed a positive surface and core antibody with a negative surface antigen. By December 7, the patient was un-

*From LeRoux, F.B., Burman, N.D., and Becker, W.B.: S. Afr. Med. J., *62*:252–253, 1982.[35]

responsive, had little renal output, and at 4:25 AM she was without vital signs.

At necropsy, generalized jaundice and two distinct types of skin lesions were noted. One type of skin lesion was widespread, erythematous, and consisted of macules and papules. Histologically, this type showed vacuolar alteration at the dermal-epidermal junction with incontinence of pigment, individual necrotic keratinocytes, and a lymphohistiocytic infiltrate in the upper part of the dermis. The changes were consistent with a drug eruption. The second type of skin lesion was purulent, ulcerative, and localized to the perineum, buttocks, and upper medial portion of the thighs. The average diameter of these lesions was 0.7 cm with a depth of approximately 0.1 cm. Histologic examination of these lesions showed numerous cytomegalovirus inclusions within the nuclei of enlarged endothelial cells in blood vessels in the upper part of the dermis situated immediately beneath sites of ulceration. The inclusion bodies were typical of cytomegalovirus, being finely granular and surrounded by halos. Lymphocytes and histiocytes were present around blood vessels, but no multinucleated giant cells or nuclear or cytoplasmic inclusions in epithelial cells were seen. Cytomegalovirus inclusions were also found in mucosal cells adjacent to ulcers of the esophagus, stomach, and intestine and in hepatocytes surrounded by microabscesses. The liver was marked by extensive cholestasis, but there were no changes of viral hepatitis. Plasmacytomas were found in the 7th and 8th ribs and in the bodies of lumbar vertebrae. The cause of death was generalized infection by cytomegalovirus as a complication of multiple myeloma or its therapy.*

SUMMARY

Cytomegalovirus (CMV) infection and its potential as a life-threatening or permanently disabling disease has been recognized in infants since 1956, and has recently been associated with infections in recipients of transplants and severely compromised hosts with increasing frequency. It is estimated that CMV infection is a significant cause of morbidity in 50 to 90% of transplant recipients and may be responsible for graft failures. Post-transplant CMV infection is directly related to the use of immunosuppressive drugs. The CMV, like other herpesviruses, remains latent and the potential for reactivation awaits opportunistic circumstances in about half of the population in developed countries. Despite the serious consequences of some CMV infections, most asymptomatic infections remain undetected.

CMV diagnosis is best made by cultural or serologic methods, but some caution must be exercised in interpreting results of serologic

---

*From Walker, J.D., and Chesney, T. McC.: Am. J. Dermatopathol., *4*:263–265, 1982.[10]

tests. The presence of high titers of CMV antibodies in Americans and Europeans with Kaposi's sarcoma is particularly provocative. Although the development of vaccines holds some promise in the future for high risk groups, there remains much to be learned of the immunologic mechanisms that permit persistence of CMV in human tissue.

REFERENCES

1. Feldman, H.A.: Cytomegalovirus. *In* Obstetric and Perinatal Infections. Edited by D. Charles and M. Finland. Philadelphia, Lea & Febiger, 1973.
2. Weller, T.H.: Cytomegaloviruses: The difficult years. J. Infect. Dis., *122*:532, 1970.
3. Stagno, S., et al.: Auditory and visual defects resulting from symptomatic and subclinical congenital cytomegaloviral and toxoplasmal infections. Pediatrics, *59*:669, 1977.
4. Drew, W.L.: Cytomegalovirus. Clin. Microbiol. Newsl., *3*:105, 1981.
5. Stagno, S., Reynolds, D.W., Pass, R.F., and Alford, C.A.: Breast milk and the risk of cytomegalovirus infection. N. Engl. J. Med., *302*:1073, 1980.
6. Yeager, A.S.: Transfusion-acquired cytomegalovirus infection in newborn infants. Am. J. Dis. Child., *128*:478, 1974.
7. Spencer, E.S.: Clinical aspects of cytomegalovirus infection in kidney graft recipients. Scand. J. Infect. Dis., *6*:315, 1971.
8. Gadler, H., Tillegard, A., and Groth, C.G.: Studies of cytomegalovirus infection in renal allograft recipients. Scand. J. Infect. Dis., *14*:81, 1982.
9. Paloheimo, J.A., et al.: Subclinical cytomegalovirus infections and cytomegalovirus mononucleosis after open heart surgery. Am. J. Cardiol., *22*:624, 1968.
10. Randall, J.L., and Plotkin, S.A.: Cytomegalovirus, a model for herpesvirus opportunism. *In* Opportunistic Pathogens. Edited by J.E. Prior and H. Friedman. Baltimore, University Park Press, 1974.
11. Stagno, S., Pass, R.F., and Alford, C.A.: Perinatal infections and maldevelopment. *In* The Fetus and the Newborn. Edited by A.D. Bloom and L.S. James. New York, Alan R. Liss, 1981.
12. Primhak, R.A., and Simpson, R. McD.: Screening small for gestational age babies for congenital infection. Neonatol., *21*:417, 1982.
13. Pass, R.F., et al.: Outcome of symptomatic congenital cytomegalovirus infection: results of long-term longitudinal follow-up. Pediatrics, *66*:758, 1980.
14. Stern, H.: Isolation of cytomegalovirus and clinical manifestations of infection at different ages. Br. Med. J., *1*:665, 1969.
15. Melish, M.E., and Hanshaw, J.B.: Congenital cytomegalovirus infection. Am. J. Dis. Child., *126*:190, 1973.
16. Birnbaum, G., et al.: Cytomegalovirus infections in newborn infants. J. Pediatr., *75*:789, 1969.
17. Reynolds, D.W., et al.: Inapparent congenital cytomegalovirus infection with elevated cord IgM levels. N. Engl. J. Med., *290*:291, 1974.
18. Neumann, H.H.: The cytomegalovirus: When and how to look for it. Conn. Med., *46*:324, 1982.
19. Monif, G.R.G., Dalcoff, G.I., and Florey, L.L.: Blood as a potential vehicle for the cytomegaloviruses. Am. J. Obstet. Gynecol., *126*:445, 1976.
20. Balfour, H.H.: Cytomegalovirus: The transplant troll takes its toll. Clin. Microbiol. Newsl., *2*:1, 1980.
21. Page, Y., Seranne, C., Revillard, J.P., and Traeger, J.: Les infections à virus cytomégalique en transplantation rénale. Lyon Méd., *240*:453, 1978.
22. Ho, M.: Virus infections after transplantation in man: a brief review. Arch. Virol., *55*:1, 1977.
23. Winston, D.J., et al.: Cytomegalovirus immune plasma in bone marrow transplant recipients. Ann. Intern. Med., *97*:11, 1982.
24. Preiksaitis, J.K., Rosno, S., Rasmussen, L., and Merigan, T.C.: Cytomegalovirus

infection in heart transplant recipients: Preliminary results of a controlled trial of intravenous gamma globulin. J. Clin. Immunol., *2*(Suppl.):365, 1982.
25. Pass, R.F., et al.: Outcome of renal transplantation in patients with primary cytomegalovirus infection. Transplant Proc., 11:1288, 1979.
26. Marker, S.C., et al.: Cytomegalovirus infection: A quantitative prospective study of three hundred twenty consecutive renal transplants. Surgery, *89*:660, 1981.
27. Betts, R.F., Freeman, R.B., Douglas, R.G. Jr., and Talley, T.E.: Clinical manifestations of renal allograft derived primary cytomegalovirus infection. Am. J. Dis. Child., *131*:759, 1977.
28. Peterson, P.K., et al.: Cytomegalovirus disease in renal allograft recipients. A prospective study of the clinical features, risk factors and impact on renal transplantation. Medicine, *59*:283, 1980.
29. Rand, K.H., Pollard, R.B., and Merigan, T.C.: Increased pulmonary superinfections in cardiac-transplant patients undergoing primary cytomegalovirus infection. N. Engl. J. Med., *298*:951, 1978.
30. Diosi, P., Moldovan, E., and Rusinaru, D.: Estimation of cytomegalovirus-imposed risks on the outcome of renal transplantation. Arch. Roum. Path. Exp. Microbiol., *41*:35, 1982.
31. Cbiba, S., et al.: Active infection with cytomegalovirus and herpes-group virus in children receiving corticosteroid therapy. Tohoku. J. Exp. Med., *106*:265, 1972.
32. Nash, G.M., Asch, J., Foley, F.D., and Pruitt, B.A., Jr.: Disseminated cytomegalic inclusion disease in a burned adult. JAMA, *214*:597, 1970.
33. Foley, F.D., Greenwald, K.A., Nash, G., and Pruitt, B.A. Jr.: Herpes virus infection in burned patients. N. Engl. J. Med., *282*:652, 1970.
34. Giraldo, G., et al.: Antibody patterns to herpesvirus in Kaposi's sarcoma. II. Serological association of American Kaposi's sarcoma with cytomegalovirus. Int. J. Cancer, *22*:126, 1978.
35. LeRoux, F.D., Burman, N.D., and Becker, W.B.: Kaposi's sarcoma in a renal allograft recipient with cytomegalovirus infection. S. Afr. Med. J., *62*:252, 1982.
36. Drew, W.L., et al.: Cytomegalovirus and Kaposi's sarcoma in young homosexual men. Lancet, *2*:125, 1982.
37. Penn, I.: Kaposi's sarcoma in organ transplant recipients. Transplantation, *27*:8, 1979.
38. Ho, M.: The lymphocyte in infections with Epstein-Barr virus and cytomegalovirus. J. Infect. Dis., *143*:857, 1981.
39. Levin, M.J., et al.: Immune responses to herpesvirus antigens in adults with acute cytomegaloviral mononucleosis. J. Infect. Dis., *140*:851, 1979.
40. Walker, J.D., and Chesney, T. McC.: Cytomegalovirus infection of the skin. Am. J. Dermatopathol., *4*:263, 1982.
41. Kaposi, M.: Idiopathisches multiples Pigmensarkom der Haut. Arch. Dermatol. Syph., *4*:265, 1872.
42. Huang, E.S., Kilpatrick, H.A., Huang, Y.T., and Pagano, J.S.: Detection of human cytomegalovirus and analysis of strain variation. Yale J. Biol. Med., *49*:29, 1976.
43. Pagano, J.S., and Lemon, S.M.: The Herpesviruses. *In* Medical Microbiology and Infectious Disease. Edited by A.I. Braude, Philadelphia, W.B. Saunders, 1981.
44. Losse, D., Lauer, R., Weder, D., and Radsak, K.: Actin distribution and synthesis in human fibroblasts infected with cytomegalovirus. Arch. Virol., *71*:353, 1982.
45. Seto, D.S., and Carver, D.H.: Interaction between cytomegalovirus and Newcastle disease as mediated by intrinsic interference. J. Virol., *4*:12, 1969.
46. Huang, E.S., et al.: Molecular epidemiology of cytomegalovirus infection in women and their infants. N. Engl. J. Med., *303*:958, 1980.
47. Osborn, J.E.: Cytomegalovirus: Pathogenicity, immunology, and vaccine initiatives. J. Infect. Dis., *143*:618, 1981.
48. Spector, S.A., and Spector, D.H.: Molecular epidemiology of cytomegalovirus infections in premature twin infants and their mother. Pediatr. Infect. Dis., *1*:405, 1982.
49. Pass, R.F., August, A.M., Dworsky, M., and Reynolds, D.W.: Cytomegalovirus infection in a day-care center. N. Engl. J. Med., *307*:477, 1982.
50. Betts, R.F., Cestero, R.V.M., Freeman, R.B., and Douglas, R.G., Jr.: Epidemiology of cytomegalovirus infection in end-stage renal disease. J. Med. Virol., *4*:89, 1979.

51. Naraqi, S., Jackson, G.G., Jonasson, O., and Yamashiroya, H.M.: Prospective study of prevalence, incidence, and source of herpesvirus infections in patients with renal allografts. J. Infect. Dis., *136*:531, 1977.
52. Weller, T.H.: The cytomegaloviruses: ubiquitous agents with protean clinical manifestations (Two parts). N. Engl. J. Med., *203*:267, 1971.
53. Lennette, D.A., Melnick, J.L., and Jahrling, P.B.: Clinical virology: introduction to methods. *In* Manual of Clinical Microbiology, 3rd Ed. Edited by E.H. Lennette. Washington, D.C., American Society for Microbiology, 1980.
54. Starr, S.E. and Friedman, H.M.: Human cytomegalovirus. *In* Manual of Clinical Microbiology, 3rd Ed. Edited by E.H. Lennette. Washington, D.C., American Society for Microbiology, 1980.
55. Lee, F.K., Nahmias, A.J., and Stagno, S.: Rapid diagnosis of cytomegalovirus infection in infants by electron microscopy. N. Engl. J. Med., *229*:1266, 1978.
56. Stagno, S., et al.: Comparative serial virologic and serologic studies of symptomatic and subclinical congenitally and natally acquired cytomegalovirus infections. J. Infect. Dis., *132*:568, 1975.
57. Lange, I., et al.: Prenatal serological diagnosis of intrauterine cytomegalovirus infection. Br. Med. J., *284*:1673, 1982.
58. Winston, D.J., Gale, R.P., Meyer, D.V., and Young, L.S.: Infectious complications of human bone marrow transplantation. Medicine, *58*:1, 1979.
59. Gunby, P.: Cytomegalovirus vaccine work progressing. JAMA, *248*:1424, 1982.
60. Panjyavi, Z.F.K. and Hanshaw, J.B.: Cytomegalovirus in the perinatal period. Am. J. Dis. Child., *135*:56, 1981.

Certain biotypes of Escherichia coli were first implicated in 1923 as causing diarrhea in infants.[1] Later, specific enteropathogenic serotypes were shown to be the cause of epidemic gastroenteritis in both children and adults.[2-5] The past decade has been a period of intensive research on two enterotoxins of pathogenic strains of E. coli: a heat-labile toxin (LT) and a heat-stable toxin (ST).[6-8] More recently, a Shigella dysenteriae type 1-like cytotoxin and an LT-like toxin produced by selected strains of E. coli have been described.[9,10] Some strains of E. coli produce only one of the enterotoxins; other strains produce both LT and ST. The LT- and ST-producing E. coli have been responsible for epidemics of human diarrheal disease and for many cases of traveler's diarrhea.[11-15]

Diarrheal disease caused by LT usually has an abrupt onset of watery diarrhea, fever, chills, and cramping. It has been likened to the clinical picture of cholera, with rapid development of electrolyte imbalances.[16] Diarrheal disease associated with ST may last longer than that caused by LT, but the two entities are clinically indistinguishable. Unlike Vibrio cholerae, the colonization period of enterotoxigenic E. coli is usually not longer than 48 hours. Colonization and fluid loss may continue up to 1 week in cholera. The annoying symptoms caused by LT and ST can be relieved by fluid replacement.

ETIOLOGY

Colonization is a prerequisite for enterotoxigenic Escherichia coli (ETEC) to promote elaboration of sufficient toxin to affect mucosal cells of the intestinal epithelium. Two colonization factor antigens (CFAs), CFA/I and CFA/II, have been associated with specific serotypes of ETEC[17] (Table 8–1). Each factor consists of heat-labile hydrophobic proteins with subunits polymerized into thin peritrichous pili. The pili have an affinity for receptors on epithelial cell membranes, but the specific interaction between CFAs and receptors has not been characterized.

A single plasmid in at least one strain of ETEC encodes for LT, ST, and CFA/II.[18] The ability of the plasmid to encode for ST has been

Table 8–1.   Serotypes of CFA/I- and CFA/II-producing enterotoxigenic Escherichia coli.

Serotypes producing CFA/I	Serotypes producing CFA/II
015:H⁻	06:H⁻
015:H11	06:H16
0.25:H⁻	08:H⁻
025:H42	08:H9
049:H12	080:H9
063:H⁻	085:H7
063:H12	
078:H⁻	
078:H11	
078:H12	
0128:H⁻	
0128:H12	
0153:H12	
0148:H⁻	

From Evans, D.G., and Evans, D.J., Jr.: Colonization factor antigens of human-associated enterotoxigenic Escherichia.coli. *In* Seminars in Infectious Disease. Vol. IV: Bacterial Vaccines. Edited by J.B. Robbins, J.C. Hill, and J.C. Sadoff. New York, Thieme-Stratton, 1982.

Table 8–2.   Characteristics of heat-labile (LT) and heat-stable (ST) enterotoxins of Escherichia coli.

	LT	ST
Molecular weight	~90,000	~9,000
Immunogenicity	high	low
Action on fluid secretion	delayed	rapid
Location of genes	plasmids	plasmids

attributed to a transposon that can be integrated into a plasmid or the chromosome.

The receptor for LT on host cells has been identified as a ganglioside of intestinal mucosal cells.[19] LT stimulates the production of adenylate cyclase. The subsequent increase in intracellular levels of cyclic adenosine monophosphate (cAMP) causes alterations in the electrical potential of cell membranes. Cells lose chloride ions and fail to absorb sodium ions. ST stimulates the production of guanylate cyclase.[20] The subsequent rise in cyclic GMP stimulates secretion of chloride ions from ileal mucosal cells in a manner analogous to that initiated by increases in cyclic AMP.

No more than 20 restricted O (somatic) and H (flagellar) serotypes of E. coli have been shown to produce LT, ST, or both enterotoxins. Substantive differences exist between LT and ST[21,22] (Table 8–2). The LT-like toxin is antigenically similar to LT, but DNA of the chromosome, rather than DNA of a plasmid codes for its production.[19] In addition, there are at least two kinds of ST: STI, a methanol-soluble toxin which is detectable in the infant mouse model, and STII which is methanol-insoluble and demonstrable in ligated pig ileal loops.[23,24]

PREDISPOSING FACTORS

Although infants and young children are more susceptible to ETEC, large doses of ETEC can produce diarrhea in adults. Travel to areas of Central and South America or Southeast Asia in which bacterial diarrheal diseases are endemic is probably the most significant risk factor for adults.

EPIDEMIOLOGY

The mode of transmission for ETEC is the fecal-oral route. ETEC has been associated with the ingestion of contaminated food and water. Hands that are not washed between feedings and diaper changes are the vehicles of transmission in nurseries. Spread of the organisms by aerosols, dust, or flies remains a possibility in endemics. Healthy carriers are probably important reservoirs for ETEC. The true incidence of diarrheal disease caused by ETEC is unknown, although reports of traveler's diarrhea indicate that it is widespread.

LABORATORY DIAGNOSIS

A diagnosis of acute diarrhea requiring fluid replacement can be made clinically on the basis of history and symptoms. The self-limiting nature of the diarrheal disease makes a laboratory diagnosis of value to individual patients only in retrospect. The information obtained following outbreaks of ETEC-associated diarrhea is important in discovering common sources of the toxigenic strains of the organism. The justification for extensive laboratory investigation cannot be extended to sporadic cases of diarrhea. Some of the more technical procedures may be performed best by reference or public health laboratories with special facilities and the necessary expertise.

Microscopic Examination and Cultural Techniques

The enterotoxigenic strains of Escherichia coli are indistinguishable from strains of E. coli that comprise the normal intestinal flora on direct microscopic examination or when grown on selective media. E. coli is a gram-negative bacillus, which typically measures 0.5 by 1.0 to 3.0 μm, varying from coccoidal forms to long rods. E. coli produces colored colonies on selective media, such as eosin methylene blue (EMB) or MacConkey's (Mac) agar. The colonies are easily differentiated from the colorless colonies of Salmonella or Shigella.

Biochemical Characterization

Speciating enteric gram-negative bacilli is now practical for even small laboratories because of the commercial availability of a number of kits.[25] Identification of genus and species is possible by using a series of carbohydrates, amino acids, and other organic substrates (Table 8–3).

Serologic Tests

Identification of specific serotypes of Escherichia coli has been controversial. Serologic typing was once used extensively in E. coli-associated diarrheal disease in infants, but it appears to be of limited value in ETEC, because a given O type may or may not be toxigenic. If hemorrhagic colitis is present, serotyping can be justified. A rare serotype, 0157:H7, was associated with two outbreaks of grossly bloody diarrhea in Oregon and Michigan in 1982.[26] Epidemiologists caution that the absence of specific serotypes that are known to cause diarrhea cannot rule out other strains as the cause.

An enzyme-linked immunosorbent assay (ELISA), passive immune hemolysis, reversed passive hemagglutination, a staphylococcal coagglutination, a modified Elek test, and a latex particle agglutination test (LPAT) have been used to detect LT of E. coli.[27–32] Most of the serologic tests either have not been used extensively or are too specialized for most clinical laboratories. Most serologic techniques are not applicable for detection of ST because that toxin is not strongly immunogenic; however, a sensitive radioimmunoassay (RIA) for ST has been developed that is appealing to laboratories with the necessary equipment.[33]

Animal Test Systems

Several animal test systems exist for detecting enterotoxins produced by Escherichia coli. A rabbit intestinal loop or adaptations in other animals can be used to demonstrate LT and ST.[34,35] Differentiation of LT and ST requires additional animal testing or inoculation of cell cultures. The most widely used test for ST is the infant-mouse assay.[36,37] In the test, 3 young NMRI mice, 2 to 3 days old, are injected

Table 8–3.   Selected biochemical reactions of Escherichia coli.

Test	Typical reaction
Citrate	−
Dextrose	+
Gelatin (22°C)	−
Hydrogen sulfide	−
Indole	+
Lysine decarboxylase	−
Methyl red	+
Motility	±
O-nitrophenyl-β-D-galactosidase	+
Ornithine decarboxylase	±
Phenylalanine deaminase	−
Urease	−
Voges-Proskauer	−

intragastrically with 0.1 ml of an unconcentrated supernatant from each culture of E. coli, grown in Casamino Acids-yeast extract medium (pH 7.5), which has been incubated overnight on a shaking table (120 rpm) at 37°C and harvested by centrifugation at 4000 × G for 30 minutes.[38] One drop of 2% (wt/vol) Evans blue per milliliter of supernatant makes a convenient marker. Mice are kept for 4 hours at room temperature (20 to 22°C) and sacrificed. Intestines are removed and weighed. The ratio of intestinal weight to remaining body weight is determined. Ratios >0.090 are positive for the presence of ST. A positive infant-mouse test is accepted as definitive evidence for ST, but a negative test may not always mean that no ST has been produced by a culture of E. coli. The infant-mouse assay remains primarily an investigative tool because most laboratories do not have the time or expertise required to peform and interpret results. If an in vitro test is ever developed that can detect activation of guanylate cyclase in the presence of ST, it may be feasible for more laboratories to detect the presence of ST-producing strains of E. coli.

Cell Culture Test Systems

Several cell culture systems, including Y1 adrenal cells, Chinese hamster ovary (CHO) cells, and Vero (green monkey kidney) cells have been used to detect the presence of LT.[39–41] The LT attaches to the cells in much the same manner as it does to epithelial cells in the gastrointestinal tract and is believed to stimulate production of steroid hormones. The presence of hormones produces morphologic aberrations in cells of culture systems (Fig. 8–1).[42]

PROGNOSIS

The prognosis in enterotoxigenic Escherichia coli-associated diarrhea is excellent if lost fluid and electrolytes are restored promptly. The potential for severe dehydration and subsequent death from electrolyte imbalance is greater in young infants, but mortality rates in children with acute diarrhea have progressively declined in the United States over the past several decades.

CASE REPORTS

Case 1

On August 9, 1974, approximately 30 hours after leaving Guam, where a cholera outbreak had recently occurred, a 41-year-old male, who had been on antacid therapy for peptic ulcer experienced the onset of profuse watery diarrhea. At the time of admission to a Georgia hospital, his stool was described as clear liquid containing flecks and strings of mucus, suggesting the possibility of cholera. He was treated with intravenous fluids and made a full recovery. Rectal cul-

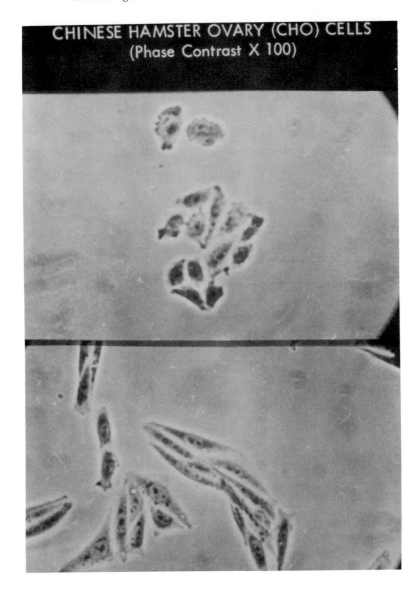

Figure 8–1. Chinese hamster ovary (CHO) cells 24 hours after exposure to the culture filtrate of nontoxigenic Escherichia coli (top) and enterotoxigenic Escherichia coli (bottom). The cells exposed to heat-labile toxin (LT) appear elongated and no longer possess knob-like projections. (Courtesy, Dr. Richard L. Guerrant, Charlottesville, Virginia.)

tures were negative for Vibrio cholerae, Vibrio parahaemolyticus, salmonella, and shigella but grew a pure culture of Escherichia coli. Ten colonies of the E. coli strain were tested for enterotoxin production in the infant-mouse assay; all 10 were positive. Filtrates of strain retested in the infant-mouse assay after boiling for 15 minutes were still positive, indicating a heat-stable enterotoxin. Tests for heat-labile toxin and mucosal invasiveness were negative.*

Case 2

The patient, a 67-year-old Indian woman living on a reserve, approximately 160 km north of Winnipeg, was in good health until September 17, 1975, when she developed voluminous yellow watery diarrhea, and was hospitalized on the same day.

Her only medication prior to this was nalidixic acid, prescribed 2 weeks previously. She had not traveled outside of Manitoba. Physical examination suggested dehydration. Her blood pressure was 105/70 mm Hg and her pulse was 120/min. The hematocrit reading was 59%, the serum potassium level was 3.9 mEq/L, and the BUN level was 13 mg/100 ml. Treatment with intravenously administered fluids and parenterally administered ampicillin and gentamicin sulfate was begun. Later the same day, she was transferred to the Health Sciences Centre (HSC), Winnipeg, where she continued to pass large amounts of watery yellow diarrhea, devoid of blood or mucus. She was afebrile and remained afebrile during her entire hospital stay. Intravenous administration of fluids was continued with bicarbonate supplementation. Antibiotics were discontinued. The initial 12-hour urine output was inadequate, and 25 gm of mannitol administered intravenously produced only slight increase in urine volume. An intravenous pyelogram showed a faint nephrogram with a normal distal urinary tract. A 24-hour creatinine clearance was (19 ml/min/sq m). On September 19, 1975 (the second hospital day), sigmoidoscopy showed normal colonic mucosa. Twenty-four-hour Levin tube and rectal tube drainage was approximately 10 liters. On the third hospital day, urine output began to increase, although diarrhea persisted for an ensuing 5 days. On the fifth hospital day, a report of an enterotoxigenic E. coli isolated from the feces, as well as the persistence of voluminous diarrhea, prompted oral therapy with trimethoprim (320 mg/day) and sulfamethoxazole (1600 mg/day). She improved thereafter, and was discharged on October 3, 1975, after 16 hospital days, in apparent good health, with renal function returning nearly to normal.

Cultures of fecal specimens were negative for Shigella, Salmonella, or Yersinia enterocolitica and electron microscopy of the initial spec-

---

*From Morbid. Mortal. Weekly Rept., 25:139, 1976.[13]

imen was negative for viral particles. From each fecal culture, up to 10 individual colonies resembling E. coli as well as 1 colonial type of all other aerobic gram-negative rods were subcultured and stored on nutrient agar. Cultures from September 17 to 24, 1975, showed a predominant growth of E. coli; while from Sept. 25 to 30, 1975, there was a paucity of Enterobacteriaceae, including E. coli. All isolates including the E. coli, Klebsiella sp., Pseudomonas aeruginosa, and Aeromonas hydrophila were tested for LT production, using the mouse adrenal-cell assay and, in some cases, for ST by the suckling-infant-mouse assay. Antibody to LT was assayed by neutralization of the morphologic change produced by LT in mouse adrenal cells as described by Sack, et al. Most E. coli isolated from the patient during her illness and up to 1 month later produced LT and ST.

The patient showed a rise in neutralizing antibody to the A. hydrophila toxin from <1:10 to 1:160.

The toxigenic strain of E. coli was 0159:H34. Both the toxigenic E. coli and A. hydrophila were resistant to ampicillin, but sensitive to the other antibiotics used, trimethoprim, sulfamethoxazole, gentamicin, and nalidixic acid.*

SUMMARY

Enterotoxigenic Escherichia coli-associated diarrhea is a mild, usually self-limiting, diarrheal disease of children and adults. The incidence is particularly high in individuals traveling in underdeveloped countries of the world. The loss of fluid and electrolytes in watery stools may require replacement therapy. A heat-labile toxin (LT) or a heat-stable toxin (ST) or both toxins are elaborated by enterotoxigenic strains of E. coli. Diagnosis can usually be made on the basis of history and clinical features. The enterotoxigenic strains of E. coli have been classically differentiated from nonpathogenic strains of E. coli by animal and cell culture test systems. Several serologic tests now available on a limited basis hold promise for rapid detection of LT. The feasibility of testing for the presence of LT and ST must be determined by individual laboratories, but testing is probably best reserved for outbreaks of diarrheal disease in which other enteric pathogens have not been identified.

---

*From Gurwith, M., et al.: Arch. Intern. Med., *137*:1461–1464, 1977. Copyright 1977, American Medical Association.[44]

REFERENCES

1. Adam, A.: Über die Biologie der Dyspepsicolia und ihre Benziehungen zur Pathogenese der Dyspepsie und Intoxikation. Jahrbuch für Kinderheilkunde *51*:295, 1923.
2. Kirby, A.C., Hall, E.G., and Coackley, W.: Neonatal diarrhoea and vomiting. Outbreak in the same maternity unit. Lancet, 2:201, 1950.
3. Ferguson, W.W., and June, R.C.: Experiments in feeding adult volunteers with Escherichia coli III, B₄, a coliform organism associated with infant diarrhea. Am. J. Hyg., 55:155, 1952.
4. Sakazaki, R., Tamura, K., and Saito, M.: Enteropathogenic Escherichia coli associated with diarrhea in children and adults. Jpn. J. Med. Sci. Biol., 20:387, 1967.
5. DuPont, H.L., et al.: Pathogenesis of Escherichia coli diarrhea. N. Engl. J. Med., 285:1, 1971.
6. Sack, R.B.: Human diarrhea disease caused by enterotoxigenic Escherichia coli. Ann. Rev. Microbiol., 29:333, 1975.
7. Sack, R.B., et al.: Enterotoxigenic Escherichia coli-associated diarrheal disease in Apache children. N. Engl. J. Med., 292:1041, 1975.
8. Clements, J.D., Yancey, R.J., and Finkelstein, R.A.: Characterization of the heat-labile enterotoxin of Escherichia. *In* Seminars in Infectious Disease. Vol. IV. Bacterial Vaccines. Edited by J.B. Robbins, J.C. Hill, and J.C. Sadoff, New York, Thieme-Stratton, 1982.
9. O'Brien, A.D., La Veck, D.G., Thompson, M.R., and Formal, S.B.: Production of Shigella dysenteriae type 1-like cytotoxin by Escherichia coli. J. Infect. Dis., *146*:763, 1982.
10. Green, B.A., Neill, R.J., Ruyechan, W.T., and Holmes, R.K.: Evidence that a new enterotoxin of Escherichia coli which activates adenylate cyclase in eucaryotic target cells is not plasma mediated. Infect. Immun., *41*:383, 1983.
11. Rosenberg, M.L., et al.: Epidemic diarrhea at Crater Lake from enterotoxigenic Escherichia coli. Ann. Intern. Med., *86*:714, 1977.
12. Rudoy, R.C., and Nelson, J.D.: Enteroinvasive and enterotoxigenic Escherichia coli occurrence in acute diarrhea of infants and children. Am. J. Dis. Child., *129*:668, 1975.
13. Merson, M.H., et al.: Traveler's diarrhea in Mexico: a prospective study of physicians and family members attending a congress. N. Engl. J. Med., *294*:1299, 1976.
14. Sack, D.A., et al.: Enterotoxigenic Escherichia coli diarrhea of travelers: a prospective study of American Peace Corps volunteers. Johns Hopkins Med. J., *141*:63, 1977.
15. Echeverria, P., Blacklow, N.R., Sanford, L.B., and Cukor, G.C.: Travelers' diarrhea among American Peace Corps volunteers in rural Thailand. J. Infect. Dis., *143*:767, 1981.
16. Carpenter, C.C.J., Jr.: Diarrheal disease caused by Escherichia coli. *In* Infectious Diseases, 3rd Ed. Edited by P.D. Hoeprich. Hagerstown, Maryland, 1983.
17. Evans, D.G., and Evans, D.J., Jr.: Colonization factor antigens of human-associated enterotoxigenic Escherichia coli. *In* Seminars in Infectious Disease. Vol. IV. Bacterial Vaccines. Edited by J.B. Robbins. J.C. Hill, and J.C. Sadoff. New York, Thieme-Stratton, 1982.
18. Penaranda, M.E., Mann, M.B., Evans, D.G., and Evans, D.J., Jr.: Transfer of a ST:LT CFA/II plasmid into Escherichia coli K-12 strain RRI by cotransformation with PSC 301 plasmid DNA.FEMS. Microbiol. Lett., 8:251, 1980.
19. Neter, I.: Enteropathogenicity: Recent developments. Klin. Wochenschr., *60*:669, 1982.
20. Field, M., Graf, L., Laird, W., and Smith, P.: Heat stable enterotoxin of Escherichia coli: in vitro effects on guanylate cyclase activity, cyclic GMP concentration, and ion transport in small intestine. Proc. Natl. Acad. Sci. U.S.A., 75:2800, 1978.
21. Hornick, R.B.: Bacterial infections of the intestine. *In* Seminars in Infectious Disease. Vol. I. Edited by L. Weinstein and B.N. Fields. New York, Stratton Intercontinental Book Corp., 1978.
22. Evans, D.G., Evans, D.J., Jr., and Pierce, N.F.: Differences in response of rabbit small intestine to heat-labile and heat-stable enterotoxins of Escherichia coli. Infect. Immun., 7:873, 1973.
23. Burgess, N.M., et al.: Biological evaluation of a methanol-soluble heat-stable Esch-

erichia coli enterotoxin in infant mice, pig, rabbits, and calves. Infect. Immun., *21*:526, 1978.

24. Hyles, C.L.: Limitations of the infant mouse test for Escherichia coli heat-stable enterotoxin. Can. J. Comp. Med., *43*:371, 1979.
25. Washington, J.A., II.:: Kits for identification of microorganisms. *In* Laboratory Medicine. Edited by G.J. Race. Hagerstown, Maryland, Harper & Row, 1979.
26. Riley, L.W., et al.: Hemorrhagic colitis associated with a rare Escherichia coli serotype. N. Engl. J. Med., *308*:681, 1983.
27. Yolken, R.H., et al.: Enzyme-linked immunosorbent assay for detection of Escherichia coli heat labile enterotoxin. J. Clin. Microbiol., *6*:439, 1977.
28. Evans, D.J., Jr., and Evans, D.G.: Direct serological assay for the heat-labile enterotoxin of Escherichia coli using passive immune hemolysis. Infect. Immun., *16*:604, 1977.
29. Kudoh, Y., et al.: Detection of heat-labile enterotoxin of Escherichia coli by reversed passive hemagglutination with specific immunoglobulin against cholera toxin. *In* Proceedings of the 14th Joint Conference of the U.S.–Japan Cooperative Medical Science Program. Edited by K. Takeya and Y. Zinnaka. Tokyo, Tokyo University, 1979.
30. Brill, B.M., Wasilauskas, B.L., and Richardson, S.H.: Adaptation of the staphylococcal coagglutination technique for detection of heat-labile enterotoxin of Escherichia coli. J. Clin. Microbiol., *9*:49, 1979.
31. Honda, T., Taga, S., Takeda, Y., and Miwatani, T.: Modified Elek test for detection of heat-labile enterotoxin of enterotoxigenic Escherichia coli. J. Clin. Microbiol., *13*:1, 1981.
32. Finkelstein, R.A., and Yang, Z.: Rapid test for identification of heat-labile enterotoxin-producing Escherichia coli colonies. J. Clin. Microbiol., *18*:23, 1983.
33. Giannella, R.A., Drake, K.W., and Luttrell, M.: Development of a radioimmunoassay for Escherichia coli heat-stable enterotoxin: comparison with the suckling mouse bioassay. Infect. Immun., *33*:186, 1981.
34. Olsson, E., and Soderlind, O.: Comparison of different assays for definition of heat-stable enterotoxigenicity of Escherichia coli porcine strains. J. Clin. Microbiol. *11*:6, 1980.
35. De, S.N. and Chatterjee, D.N.: An experimental study of the mechanism of action of Vibrio cholerae on the intestinal mucous membrane. J. Pathol. Bacteriol., *66*:559, 1953.
36. Dean, A.G., Ching, Y.C., Williams, R.G., and Harden, L.B.: Test for Escherichia coli enterotoxin using infant mice: application in a study of diarrhea in children in Honolulu. J. Infect. Dis., *125*:407, 1972.
37. Giannella, R.A.: Suckling mouse model for detection of heat-stable Escherichia coli enterotoxin. Infect. Immun., *14*:95, 1976.
38. Alderete, J.F., and Robertson, D.C.: Nutrition and enterotoxin synthesis by enterotoxigenic strains of Escherichia coli: defined medium for production of heat-stable enterotoxin. Infect. Immun., *15*:781, 1977.
39. Donta, S.T., Moon, H.W., and Whipp, S.C.: Detection of heat-labile Escherichia coli enterotoxin with the use of adrenal cells in tissue cultures. Science, *183*:334, 1974.
40. Guerrant, R.L., et al.: Cyclic adenosine monophosphate and alteration of Chinese hamster ovary cell morphology: a rapid sensitive in vitro assay for the enterotoxin of Vibrio cholerae and Escherichia coli. Infect. Immun., *10*:320, 1974.
41. Speirs, J.T., Stavric, S., and Konowalchuk, J.: Assay of Escherichia coli heat-labile enterotoxin with Vero cells. Infect. Immun., *16*:617, 1977.
42. Donta, S.T., King, M., and Sloper, K.: Induction of steroidogenesis in tissue culture by cholera enterotoxin. Nature (New Biol.), *243*:246, 1973.
43. Center for Disease Control: Cholera-like illness associated with an enterotoxigenic strain of Escherichia coli. Morbid. Mortal. Weekly Rep., *25*:139, 1976.
44. Gurwith, M., et al.: Cholera-like diarrhea in Canada—Report of a case associated with enterotoxigenic Escherichia coli and a toxin-producing Aeromonas hydrophila. Arch. Intern. Med., *137*:1461, 1977.

In 1964, the Epstein-Barr virus (EBV) was first associated with a malignant tumor known as Burkitt's lymphoma, which is endemic in some parts of Africa.[1] Four years later, EBV was demonstrated to be the cause of infectious mononucleosis.[2] Later, tumor cells in undifferentiated nasopharyngeal carcinoma were found to contain EBV.[3] The development of more sensitive diagnostic techniques has implicated EBV in an increasing number of clinical diseases.[4] Those diseases include hepatitis, encephalitis, autonomic and sensory neuropathy, Guillain-Barré syndrome, hemiplegia, myopericarditis, thrombocytopenic purpura, autoimmune hemolytic anemia, neutropenia, pancytopenia, cryoglobulinemia, vasculitis, and acute polyarthritis. In addition, polyclonal B-cell lymphoma, angioimmunoblastic lymphadenopathy, and malignant histiocytosis syndromes have been associated with EBV infections in immune deficiency states.[5,6] A definitive X-linked recessive lymphoproliferative syndrome has been described and named Duncan disease after the deaths of six boys with EBV infection in a single family.[7]

Like other herpesviruses, EBV appears to possess a potential for latency and can be associated with recrudescent disease. Decades after a primary infection, rises in EBV antibody titer and salivary shedding have been documented.[8] It is not clear whether latent infections have a role in the transmission of EBV. Primary infectious mononucleosis is a manifestation of normal immune responses to the presence of EBV in adolescents and young adults. Approximately 50% of adolescents with the infection develop overt symptoms of disease. By adulthood, about 90% of individuals have measurable antibodies to EBV.[9]

The criteria originally described for primary infectious mononucleosis pertain to most cases of the classic disease:*

---

*Adapted from Chang, R.S.: Infectious mononucleosis. Boston, G.K. Hall Medical Publisher, 1980.

Insidious onset of cervical lymphadenopathy, usually with pharyngitis.

Hematologic evidence of absolute lymphocytosis (4500/μl) with at least 52% lymphocytes, atypical lymphocytes, and persisting lymphocytosis for a duration of 2 weeks.

Serologic evidence of heterophil antibodies absorbable by beef, goat, or horse erythrocytes, but not by guinea pig kidney antigen and IgG or IgM antibody to viral capsid antigen (VCA), early antigen (EA), or EBV nuclear antigen (EBNA).

These criteria, however, exclude about 10% of the cases of primary infectious mononucleosis caused by other infectious agents. Cytomegalovirus (CMV) and the protozoan agent of toxoplasmosis have both been implicated as causes of primary infectious mononucleosis.

Factors capable of reactivating EBV are not generally well understood. EBV is usually reactivated in women during pregnancy;[10] the antibodies produced provide protection for the infant during the first 5 or 6 months of life, when a silent seroconversion occurs.

The immune deficient responses to EBV are multiple. Detailed descriptions of each clinical entity are not within the scope of this chapter. Immune deficient patients may lack the resources to mount a demonstrable EBV antibody titer, or that titer may be low. The variety of clinical and pathologic manifestations found in EBV infections is believed to be related to the status of an individual's immunocompetence.[11] A delicate balance may exist in healthy persons which allows activated EBV-containing lymphocytes to be destroyed as fast as they are generated.[12] The provocative question concerns the role of humoral and cellular immunity in controlling the expression of EBV. Whereas the B lymphocytes are the primary targets for EBV, the symptoms of primary infectious mononucleosis appear to be related to a cell-mediated immune response.[12] Furthermore, latent reservoirs of infected or transformed cells find expression only when immune responses are defective.

ETIOLOGY

Epstein-Barr virus (EBV) resembles another member of the herpesviruses, namely, the human cytomegalovirus (CMV). EBV contains double-stranded linear DNA with a molecular mass of 60 to 120 $\times$ 10^6 daltons.[13] Although EBV is primarily a pathogen of B lymphocytes, current evidence suggests that oropharyngeal epithelial cells may also support growth of the virus.[8] Once B lymphocytes are infected with EBV, the virus may produce a lytic infection, a latent infection, or a transforming infection (Fig. 9–1). Infected or transformed B lymphocytes are characterized by antigenic changes in the cell membrane. The membrane antigen is called the lymphocyte-detected membrane antigen (LYDMA) because it is recognized by T lymphocytes. The activated T lymphocytes proliferate and result in

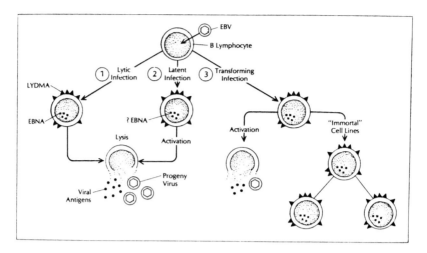

Figure 9–1. Hypothetical consequences of B-lymphocyte infection with EBV. 1. Lytic infection with subsequent lysis and release of viral antigens and progeny virus. 2. Latent infection. 3. Transforming infection with production of immortal cell lines. (From McCue, J.D.: The pathogenesis of infectious mononucleosis. Hosp. Pract. *17*:34, 1982. Artist: Nancy Lou Grahan Makris.)

the so-called atypical lymphocyte found in peripheral blood in primary infectious mononucleosis.

An Epstein-Barr nuclear antigen (EBNA) is associated with lytically infected B lymphocytes, but apparently it does not appear in latently infected cells. Once activated, latently infected B lymphocytes undergo a lytic cycle indistinguishable from that of other infected cells and release intact viruses and viral antigens. A transforming infection can be activated spontaneously in a similar manner, or part of the viral DNA can exist as circular extrachromosomal DNA in the cytoplasm of the B lymphocyte, uniquely immortalizing the cells. The transformed cells are capable of indefinite multiplication in vitro. The amount of viral DNA required for transformation of B lymphocytes has been estimated to be only one fourth of the viral genome.[14] Transformed cells contain both LYDMA and EBNA. It is currently believed that some lymphocytes are transformed in primary infectious mononucleosis and that proliferation of those lymphocytes may be prevented by control exercised by some as yet undescribed mechanisms.

The clinical course of primary infectious mononucleosis is determined by cytotoxic and suppressor activity of T lymphocytes. Depression of cell-mediated immunity and cutaneous anergy is seen early in primary infectious mononucleosis. The effect of suppressor activity may extend to inhibiting the production of antibodies against infected and transformed cells. The activity of killer T lymphocytes against B lymphocytes and the subsequent cytolysis can explain the symptoms of primary infectious mononucleosis.

PREDISPOSING FACTORS

Primary infectious mononucleosis is chiefly a disease of middle- and upper-class adolescents and young adults. Infections in children are often subclinical, but they can be associated with severe neurologic disease. EBV is reactivated during pregnancy, but rarely produces recognizable disease. Individuals with inherited or acquired immunodeficiency states are at risk of developing a wide spectrum of EBV diseases.[15–17] Immunosuppression in young recipients of transplants, accompanied by EBV infection, tends to promote polyclonal B-lymphocyte proliferation, which is often fatal.[18] Older renal-transplant patients may develop polyclonal or monoclonal malignant lymphomas.

EPIDEMIOLOGY

EBV appears to be a common virus that is worldwide in distribution.[19] Primary infectious mononucleosis is rare in densely populated developing countries with low standards of hygiene. This is in marked contrast to the incidence of primary infectious mononucleosis in countries like the United States where the case rate is estimated to be 45 per 100,000 persons annually.[20]

The salivary glands are the primary site of oropharyngeal production of EBV. Once cells of the salivary glands have been infected with EBV, an individual becomes a carrier. EBV is shed during primary infectious mononucleosis. If the latent EBV is activated later in life, protection may be afforded to the host by residual antibodies, but shedding of viruses again occurs.

It has been known for years that primary infectious mononucleosis is spread by oral contact. For that reason, the infection is commonly called the "kissing disease." The widespread incidence of the disease in adolescents and young adults is attributable both to susceptibility and to the greater degree of promiscuity in kissing habits among younger people. It is usually not possible to document transmission on a case-to-case basis. It has been reported that up to 52% of oropharyngeal excretions obtained from immunosuppressed renal-transplant patients contain EBV.[21] It is presumed that latent EBV is reactivated and causes an infectious process despite the presence of EBV antibodies.

Transfusion with fresh whole blood, packed red blood cells, plasma, and bone-marrow transplants may also constitute the means of transmission of EBV.[22–25] It is not known whether the EBV is shed from an infected individual in other body secretions or excreta to any significant extent.

LABORATORY DIAGNOSIS

For years, the finding of atypical lymphocytes on a blood smear and the demonstration of heterophil antibodies along with clinical symptoms were considered sufficient evidence for a diagnosis of primary infectious mononucleosis. Those criteria, however, would exclude about 10% of the cases because other infectious agents may be involved. Specific serologic tests have taken on increased significance in the diagnosis of EBV infections since the cytomegalovirus (CMV) and the protozoan agent of toxoplasmosis were shown to cause identical symptoms.

Microscopic Examination

The presence of atypical lymphocytes on blood smears from adolescents and young adults with fever, malaise, and lymphadenopathy, accompanied by pharyngitis, cannot be ignored. The atypical lymphocytes are often irregular in shape and may resemble monocytes.[26] The nuclei may be indented or lobated with an increased amount of chromatin (Fig. 9–2). Marked vacuolar degeneration is often present. Mononucleosis in this instance refers to an increase in lymphocytes rather than monocytes. Usually the atypical lymphocytes account for 60 to 90% of the total number of leukocytes. It is important to realize, however, that the cytologic changes described are not found exclu-

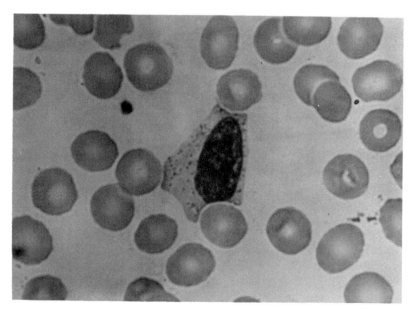

Figure 9–2. Atypical lymphocytes of peripheral blood in infectious mononucleosis. (From Radetsky, M.A.: A diagnostic approach to Epstein-Barr virus infections. Pediatr. Infect. Dis., *1*:425, 1982.)

sively in primary infectious mononucleosis. Large numbers of morphologically similar cells are found in a variety of viral infections. Unfortunately, the numbers of EBV in oropharyngeal secretions are not sufficient to detect by fluorescent antibody techniques or by electron microscopy.[27]

Cultural Techniques

No permissive cell system is known to exist for EBV, but cord-blood lymphocytes are transformed in the presence of the virus.[28,29] After sedimentation of cord-blood erythrocytes at 37°C, leukocyte-containing plasma is centrifuged at $250 \times G$ for 10 minutes. The cells are resuspended in RPMI 1640 medium, containing 20% fetal calf serum, to a final concentration of 4×10^6 to 5×10^6 cells per ml. One milliliter aliquots of the cells are placed in test tubes, capped, and incubated upright in 5% CO_2 at 37°C overnight.

Cellular or other debris is removed from throat washings or material from throat swabs by centrifugation at $1800 \times G$ for 20 minutes at 4°C. If supernatants are sufficient in quantity, they can be poured through a 0.45 μm pore-size membrane filter. In the absence of enough fluid to permit filtration, an antibiotic mixture of streptomycin (100 μg/ml) and nystatin (25 μg/ml) will inhibit growth of bacteria and fungi. After removal of the culture medium by aspiration, the cells are inoculated with 0.25 to 0.3 ml aliquots of test fluids. It is recommended that at least 4 cultures per specimen be set up and that positive and negative controls be included.

Virus adsorption is accomplished by incubating mixtures for 1½ hours at 37°C. After the addition of 0.7 ml of growth medium, cultures are maintained at the same temperature for 5 to 6 weeks. It is necessary to refeed cultures weekly. Transformation usually occurs within 35 days. The appearance of aggregates of large proliferating lymphoblastoid cells and a drop in the pH of the medium are evidence for the presence of transformed cells.

Serologic Tests

A variety of serologic techniques is available to confirm the presence of serum antibodies to EBV. Immunofluorescent antibody tests are available for (1) IgG or IgM antibody to viral capsid antigen (VCA), (2) antibody to early antigen (EA), and (3) antibody to EBV nuclear antigen (EBNA).[30] IgG antibody to VCA is present early in an infection and persists for life. IgM antibody to VCA is elevated early in primary infectious mononucleosis and in reactivated infections.[31–33] Antibody to EA is present only during the acute phase of infection. Antibody to EBNA is demonstrable within 2 to 4 weeks after onset of a primary infection and persists for life. Titers of EBNA rise when

EBV is reactivated. The availability of enzyme-labeled EBV antigens has improved the sensitivity and specificity of test procedures for the detection of EBV antibodies.[34]

In the classic fluorescent antibody tests, infected Raji cells have been used after activation of EBV with 5-bromodeoxyuridine.[35] Unfortunately, some nonspecific reactions interfere with detection of IgM antibody to EBV. The rheumatoid factor (RF) accounts for some false-positive tests for EBV-IgM.[36] It is recommended that a combination of only two simple tests be used to make a diagnosis of infection caused by EBV. A combination of the heterophil antibody test and the enzyme-labeled antigen (ELA)–IgM test for antibody to VCA appears to be reliable in detecting infection caused by EBV.

PROGNOSIS

In the absence of central nervous system (CNS) involvement, most individuals with primary infectious mononucleosis recover without consequence. In those instances of multisystem involvement, histories of patients most often reveal congenital immune deficiencies. The mortality rate in CNS involvement is estimated to be 4 to 11%.

Reactivation of EBV in acquired immune deficiencies or in the special circumstances predisposing individuals in some parts of the world to Burkitt's lymphoma or undifferentiated nasopharyngeal carcinoma, however, can produce serious sequelae. The extenuating circumstances in the induction of tumors may involve cofactors.[37] As the biology of EBV-infected cells is unraveled, the immunologic controls that keep the relationship between the host and EBV in balance may be better understood.

CASE REPORTS

Case 1

A 12-year-old boy received a maternal renal transplant for renal failure secondary to Henoch-Schönlein purpura in November, 1977. A transplant nephrectomy and splenectomy were performed 19 months later because of chronic rejection. After convalescence, the patient received total lymphoid irradiation, administered in 26 fractionated doses, for a total planned dose of 3250 rad over a 3-month period; the course was complicated by radiation sickness and mild leukopenia. A suitable cadaver for renal transplantation was not immediately available, and an additional 800 rad of total lymphoid irradiation was administered in divided doses during the next 3 months. In January, 1980, a cadaveric renal transplantation was performed, and maintenance therapy with azathioprine and prednisone was begun. One month later, an acute rejection was treated with an increase in the dose of oral prednisone. A second episode of acute rejection at 2 months was treated with prednisone and intravenous horse anti-human-lymphoblast globulin (20 mg per kilogram of body weight per day for 10 days). Ten days later, the patient was readmitted for a third episode of acute rejection and treated with intravenous methylprednisolone, an increase in the dose of oral prednisone, and a second 10-day course of anti-human-lymphoblast globulin.

Sixteen weeks after transplantation, the patient was readmitted because of a left preauricular mass and soaking night sweats. A firm, nontender left preauricular mass, 3 cm by 2 cm, and a right submandibular lymph node, 2 cm by 2 cm, were palpable. The left tonsil was grossly enlarged. All laboratory studies gave normal results, including liver-function tests and quantitation of serum immunoglobulins; heterophil antibodies were absent in the serum. No atypical lymphocytes were seen on a peripheral-blood smear. A biopsy of the left preauricular mass demonstrated a polymorphic B-cell lymphoma with surface immunoglobulin and cytoplasmic immunoglobulin of polyclonal specificity. Over 80% of the large atypical cells were positive for Epstein-Barr nuclear antigen (EBNA). Bone-marrow involvements by foci of immunoblasts were confirmed on histologic study. Azathioprine was discontinued, and the prednisone dose was reduced to maintenance levels (0.2 mg per kilogram per day), but malaise, sore throat, anorexia, and cervical lymphadenopathy progressed. Daily fever spikes to 39° or 40°C continued, and a 7-day course of intravenous acyclovir (500 mg per square meter of body-surface area every 8 hours) was begun. Within 72 hours, the patient's symptoms and fever dramatically resolved, and he resumed normal activity; the lymphadenopathy stabilized but did not resolve. A repeat trephine biopsy performed at the end of the 7-day course showed decreased involvement of the marrow with tumor cells. Within 48 hours of the cessation of acyclovir therapy, the fevers recurred, and the patient again reported malaise, generalized weakness, sore throat, and anorexia. Exacerbation of the cervical lymphadenopathy and tonsil involvement were noted. Reinstitution of acyclovir therapy led to dramatic resolution of the fever and relief of the symptoms. During the second 7-day course of acyclovir, a 50% reduction in lymphadenopathy occurred, and the tonsil lesion healed. A bone-marrow biopsy at the completion of therapy showed no evidence of marrow involvement. The patient remained afebrile and asymptomatic and was discharged 21 weeks after the transplantation. Over the next several weeks, examination revealed no further evidence of abnormal lymphoproliferation. He continued taking prednisone (0.2 mg per kilogram per day).

Twenty-seven weeks after transplantation, the patient was given azathioprine (1 mg per kilogram per day) and prednisone (2 mg per kilogram per day) for a biopsy-proved episode of acute rejection. At 31 weeks, he was readmitted with fever, sore throat, malaise, cervical lymphadenopathy, and an enlarged left tonsil. Biopsy specimens of a tonsil and a cervical lymph node were interpreted histologically as representing polymorphic B-cell lymphoma. Over 80% of the large atypical cells were EBNA-positive. Azathioprine was discontinued, and the prednisone dose was decreased to 0.3 mg per kilogram per day. A 14-day course of acyclovir was given, with some symptomatic improvement and an objective 25% reduction in lymphadenopathy, but the fever persisted. Acyclovir was continued for an additional 7 days; during this time, the symptoms and fever resolved, and the lymphadenopathy regressed. The patient was discharged 36 weeks after transplantation.

Thirty-nine weeks after transplantation, fever and sore throat were noted, and biopsies revealed a recurrence at the left base of the tongue. Four days later, a tender swelling in the left medial upper arm was noted. Acyclovir therapy was instituted, but spiking fevers continued, and the left-arm mass, from which an incisional biopsy sample was obtained, rapidly increased in size. Anemia and melena were noted. X-ray films and endoscopy of the upper gastrointestinal tract, a barium enema, and colonoscopy gave normal results. Acyclovir was discontinued. At 43 weeks after transplantation, an acute abdomen developed, and an exploratory laparotomy showed multiple tumor nodules widely scattered in the small bowel and mesenteric lymph nodes. The perforation of the ileum secondary to tumor necessitated a small-bowel resection, ileostomy, and colostomy. The patient had grand mal seizures and deteriorating neurologic function, and he died 3 weeks later. Permission for autopsy was not granted.*

Case 2

A 23-year-old white female developed the insidious onset of bifrontal headache and malaise without antecedent pharyngitis, upper respiratory infection, or lymphadenopathy. After 10 days, the headache acutely worsened, and she became disoriented and confused. On admission to the New York Hospital she was initially delirious, incoherent, agitated, and finally stuporous. The patient exhibited spontaneous conjugated roving eye movements, multifocal myoclonic jerks, and increased motor tone with paratonia more marked on the left. There was diffuse hyperreflexia with an extensor plantar response on the left. The neck was stiff. Her temperature on admission was 38.5°C. There was no pharyngitis, lymphadenopathy, or splenomegaly. The hematocrit was 38.3 and the white cell count was 6300 cells/mm³ with 36% lymphocytes and 12% atypical lymphocytes. Routine blood chemistries and liver function tests were normal. Lumbar puncture performed on admission showed an opening pressure of

---

*From Hanto, D.W., et al.: N. Engl. J. Med., *306*:913–918, 1982. Reprinted by permission of the New England Journal of Medicine.[17]

260 mm H_2O. The fluid was clear and colorless with 1 RBC/mm^3, 23 mononuclear cells/mm^3; glucose was 60 mg%, and protein was 107 mg%. The serum heterophil-antibody titer was 1:896 before and after guinea-pig-kidney absorption and negative after beef-cell absorption. The electroencephalogram was disorganized with intermittent theta and 1½ to 3 Hz delta activity seen synchronously and asynchronously from each hemisphere. Computerized tomographic brain scan prior to and after the injection of contrast medium was normal. By the third hospital day she was more responsive, able to follow commands, but was still disoriented and somewhat somnolent. There was paratonia and an extensor plantar response on the left. Repeat lumbar puncture revealed an opening pressure of 180 mm H_2O with 0 RBC/mm^3, 8 lymphocytes/mm^3; CSF glucose was 74 mg% and CSF protein was 113 mg%. Her neurologic status continued to improve and by the sixth hospital day she was alert and oriented, motor tone was normal, and she had bilateral flexor plantar responses. At this time, posterior cervical nodes were first noted to be enlarged bilaterally and the spleen tip was palpable. Lumbar puncture on the sixth hospital day (sixteenth day of illness) revealed an opening pressure 130 mm H_2O with 1 RBC/mm^3; 16 lymphocytes/mm^3; CSF glucose was 70 and CSF protein was 105 mg%. Serum heterophil titer had risen to 1:3584. Heterophil-antibody was not detectable in the CSF on either the third or sixth hospital day. The patient remained afebrile and was discharged on the fourteenth hospital day with a normal neurologic exam.

Antibody titers to the EBV-viral capsid antigen (VCA) were measured in sera and cerebrospinal fluid specimens by indirect immunofluorescence. By the sixth hospital day (sixteenth of illness), the EBV-VCA titer in serum was 1:160 and the CSF titer remained 1:10. Tests for antibodies to CMV, herpes simplex, measles, mumps, and Coxsackie B_1 to B_6 viruses were non-diagnostic in the sera and negative in the CSF.

CSF obtained on the sixteenth day of illness was tested for the presence of EBV by the leukocyte transformation assay. In order to distinguish whether virus, if present, was extracellular or cell-associated, approximately 5 ml of CSF was centrifuged to sediment the cells. Replicate cultures containing 0.4 ml of umbilical cord blood lymphocytes were inoculated with 0.1 ml of cell-free CSF or with 0.1 ml of a suspension of approximately 1.6×10^4 cells. The cultures were maintained and observed for the appearance of EBV-induced transformation for 8 weeks. Four of 4 lymphocyte cultures inoculated with CSF cells transformed while none of the 4 cultures inoculated with cell-free CSF transformed. The presence of EB viral genome in the transformed cells was confirmed by the demonstration of the EBV nuclear antigen (EBNA) in the cells.*

*From Schiff, J.A., Schaefer, J.A., and Robinson, J.E.: Yale J. Biol. Med., 55:59–63, 1982.[38]

Case 3

A 9-year-old Latin-American girl, with an unremarkable past history and current immunizations, developed a sore throat, low grade fever and maculopapular rash 1 week before admission. A throat culture obtained at that time grew normal flora and she was symptomatically treated. The fever persisted and the patient developed mild diarrhea, nausea, and vomiting 4 days prior to admission. The evening before admission she had an acute onset of left-sided weakness and a severe right parietal headache, vomiting, neck stiffness, and fever (38.8°C). Examination performed in an emergency room on the day of admission detected left-sided hemiparesis. A lumbar puncture was performed at that time and revealed clear spinal fluid which contained a "normal cell count" and a glucose of 62 mg/dl. The Gram-stained specimen of spinal fluid was negative. She was transferred to Wilford Hall USAF Medical Center where additional history revealed no recent trauma or drug ingestion other than acetaminophen. Other family members were healthy.

Physical examination revealed fever (38.6°C), lethargy, exudative tonsillopharyngitis with palatal petechiae, enlarged and tender anterior cervical nodes, and no hepatosplenomegaly. Fundoscopic examination was normal. Neurologic findings included mild left-sided hemiparesis with hyperactive deep tendon reflexes without clonus, left extensor plantar reflex, decreased sensation to pin prick on the left, and left homonymous hemianopia. There was no facial weakness.

The white blood cell count was 11,500/mm^3 with 26% lymphocytes, 8% atypical lymphocytes, 58% polymorphonuclear neutrophils, 2% band forms, and 6% monocytes. The hematocrit was 31% with a hemoglobulin of 10.4 g/dl. The peripheral smear showed microcytic and hypochromic erythrocytes (serum iron, 19 mg/dl; total iron-binding capacity, 255 mg/dl). The platelet count was 270,000/mm^3 and the erythrocyte sedimentation rate was 52 mm/hour. Serum electrolytes, aspartate aminotransferase (SGOT), blood ammonia, antinuclear antibody titer, lupus erythematosus preparation, prothrombin time, partial thromboplastin time, C3, C4, urinalysis, and chest and abdominal x-rays were normal. A Monospot test (Ortho Diagnostic Systems) using differential absorption with guinea pig kidney and beef erythrocytes was positive. Specific EBV serology documented primary infection. The cerebrospinal fluid (CSF) obtained by lumbar puncture had an opening pressure of 280 mm water and contained 63 white blood cells/mm^3 (92% mononuclear cells, 8% polymorphonuclear neutrophils); 3 red blood cells/mm^3; protein, 31 mg/dl; and glucose, 52 mg/dl, with a concurrent serum glucose of 68 mg/dl. The Gram stain of the CSF was negative. Bacterial cultures of urine, blood, and CSF were sterile. Throat culture was positive for Group A beta-hemolytic Streptococcus and the Streptozyme (Wampole Laboratories) titer was 1:800. Throat, rectal, and CSF specimens inoculated onto 5 different cell cultures (primary rhesus monkey, human embryonic kidney, rhabdomyosarcoma, VERO, and MRC-5) were negative for viruses.

An electroencephalogram showed slowing over both cerebral hemispheres with more slow wave activity over the right hemisphere. A technetium brain scan and an enhanced computer-assisted tomography scan were normal. A repeat enhanced computer-assisted tomography scan 6 days later was also normal.

The patient was treated with penicillin V and diphenylhydantoin orally. Within 12 hours there was improvement of the left-sided weakness. The patient had intermittent episodes of emesis and right-sided headache. By the fifth hospital day she appeared well, and the neurologic examination was normal. Subsequently, visual field and visual acuity examinations were normal.*

SUMMARY

The Epstein-Barr virus (EBV) has been increasingly implicated in a wide array of clinical diseases. The benign or malignant nature of the ensuing disease is related to the ability of the virus to produce a lytic infection, a latent infection, or a transforming infection of B lymphocytes. The ubiquitous EBV produces the now classic primary infectious mononucleosis in developed countries with high standards of living, but also appears to have a role in both the malignant Burkitt's lymphoma and undifferentiated nasopharyngeal carcinoma in a limited number of geographic areas. Individuals with inherited or acquired immune deficiencies are uniquely susceptible to serious, and sometimes fatal, EBV infections. The primary mode of transmission is by contact with oropharyngeal secretions. The methods of choice for diagnosis of EBV infections are serologic techniques that detect heterophil antibodies or antibodies to one or more EBV-associated antigens. The immunoregulatory mechanisms that permit a host and EBV to co-exist without clinical disease remain an enigma but may be important one day in explaining other host-virus relationships.

REFERENCES

1. Epstein, M.A., Achong, B.G., and Barr, Y.M.: Virus particles in cultured lymphoblasts from Burkitt's lymphoma. Lancet, *1*:702, 1964.
2. Henle, G., Henle, W., and Diehl, V.: Relation of Burkitt's tumor-associated herpestype virus to infectious mononucleosis. Proc. Natl. Acad. Sci. U.S.A., *59*:94, 1968.
3. Klein, G.: The relationship of the virus to nasopharyngeal carcinoma. *In* The Epstein-Barr virus. Edited by M.A. Epstein and B.G. Achong. Berlin, Springer-Verlag, 1979.

---

*From Baker, F.J., Kotchmar, G.S., Foshee, W.S., and Sumaya, C.V.: Pediatr. Infect. Dis., 2:136–138, 1983. © The Williams & Wilkins Co., Baltimore.[39]

4. Ray, C.G.: "New" syndromes due to Epstein-Barr virus infection. Infect. Dis. Newsl., *1*:4, 1981.
5. Purtilo, D.T.: Epstein-Barr virus-induced oncogenesis in immune-deficient individuals. Lancet, *1*:300, 1980.
6. Purtilo, D.T.: Immune deficiency predisposing to Epstein-Barr virus-induced lymphoproliferative diseases: The X-linked lymphoproliferative syndrome as a model. *In* Advances in Cancer Research. Edited by G. Klein and S. Weinhouse. New York, Academic Press, 1981.
7. Purtilo, D.T., et al.: X-linked recessive progressive combined variable immunodeficiency (Duncan's disease). Lancet, 1:935, 1976.
8. McCue, J.D.: The pathogenesis of infectious mononucleosis. Hosp. Pract., *17*:34, 1982.
9. Henle, W., Henle, G., and Lennette, E.H.: The Epstein-Barr virus. Sci. Am., *241*:48, 1979.
10. Sakamoto, K., et al.: Reactivation of Epstein-Barr virus in pregnant women. *In* Comparative Leukemia and Related Diseases. Edited by D. Yohn. New York, Elsevier–North-Holland, 1982.
11. Purtilo, D.T. and Sakamoto, K.: Epstein-Barr virus and human disease: Immune responses determine the clinical and pathologic expression. Hum. Pathol., *12*:677, 1981.
12. Rickinson, A.B., et al.: Long term T-cell mediated immunity to Epstein-Barr virus. Cancer Res., *41*:4216, 1981.
13. Andrewes, C.H., Periera, H.G., and Wildy, P.: Viruses of Vertebrates, 4th Ed. London, Bailliére Tindall, 1978.
14. Mark, W., and Sugden, B.: Transformation of lymphocytes by Epstein-Barr virus requires only one-fourth of the viral genome. Virology, *122*:431, 1982.
15. Purtilo, D.T.: Epstein-Barr virus-induced oncogenesis in immune-deficient individuals. Lancet, *1*:300, 1980.
16. Virelizier, J.L., Lenoir, G., and Griscelli, C.: Persistent Epstein-Barr virus infection in a child with hypergammaglobulinaemia and immunoblastic proliferation associated with a selective defect in immune interferon secretion. Lancet, *2*:231, 1978.
17. Hanto, D.W., et al.: Epstein-Barr virus-induced B-cell lymphoma after renal transplantation: Acyclovir therapy and transition from polyclonal to monoclonal B-cell proliferation. N. Engl. J. Med., *306*:913, 1982.
18. Hanto, D.W., et al.: The Epstein-Barr virus in the pathogenesis of post-transplant lymphoproliferative disorders: clinical, pathologic, and virologic correlations. Surgery, *90*:204, 1981.
19. Niederman, J.C.: Infectious mononucleosis: observations on transmission. Yale J. Biol. Med., *55*:259, 1982.
20. Stevens, D.A.: Infectious mononucleosis. *In* Medical Microbiology and Infectious Disease. Edited by A.I. Braude. Philadelphia, W.B. Saunders, 1981.
21. Strauck, B., et al.: Oropharyngeal excretion of Epstein-Barr virus by renal transplant recipients and other patients treated with immunosuppressive drugs. Lancet, *1*:234, 1974.
22. Blacklow, N.R., et al.: Mononucleosis with heterophile antibodies and EB virus infection acquired by an elderly patient in the hospital. Am. J. Med., *5*:549, 1971.
23. Turner, A.R., MacDonald, R.N., and Cooper, B.A.: Transmission of infectious mononucleosis by transfusion of pre-illness plasma. Ann. Intern. Med., *77*:751, 1972.
24. Sullivan, J.W., Wallen, W.C., and Johnson, F.L.: Epstein-Barr virus infection following bone-marrow transplantation. Int. J. Cancer, *22*(2):132, 1978.
25. Wising, P.J.: A study of infectious mononucleosis (Pfeiffer's disease) from the etiological point of view. Acta Med. Scand. (Suppl. 133), *1*:507, 1942.
26. Davidsohn, I., and Nelson, D.A.: The blood. *In* Todd-Sanford Clinical Diagnosis by Laboratory Methods. Edited by I. Davidsohn and J.B. Henry. Philadelphia, W.B. Saunders, 1969.
27. Gerber, P.: EB herpesvirus. *In* Manual of Clinical Microbiology, 3rd Ed. Edited by E.H. Lennette. Washington, D.C., American Society for Microbiology, 1980.
28. Chang, R.S., and Golden, H.D.: Transformation of human leukocytes by throat washings from infectious mononucleosis patients. Nature, *234*:359, 1971.
29. Gerber, P., Whang-Peng, J., and Monroe, J.H.: Transformation and chromosome

changes induced by Epstein-Barr virus in normal human leukocyte cultures. Proc. Natl. Acad. Sci. U.S.A., *63*:740, 1969.

30. Chernesky, M.A., Ray, C.G., and Smith, T.F.: Laboratory diagnosis of viral infections. Cumitech, *15*:1, 1982.
31. Henle, W., Henle, G., and Horwitz, C.A.: Epstein-Barr virus-diagnostic tests in infectious mononucleosis. Hum. Pathol., *5*:551, 1974.
32. Schmitz, H., and Scherer, M.: IgM antibodies to Epstein-Barr virus in infectious mononucleosis. Arch. Gesamte Virusforsch, *37*:332, 1972.
33. Nikoskelainen, J., Leikola, J., and Klemola, E.: IgM antibodies specific for Epstein-Barr virus in infectious mononucleosis without heterophil antibodies. Br. Med. J., *4*:72, 1974.
34. Schmitz, H.: Detection of immunoglobulin M antibody to Epstein-Barr virus by use of an enzyme-labeled antigen. J. Clin. Microbiol., *16*:361, 1982.
35. Gerber, P., and Lucas, S.: Epstein-Barr virus-associated antigens activated in human cells by 5-bromodeoxyuridine. Proc. Soc. Exp. Biol. Med., *141*:431, 1972.
36. Henle, G., Lennette, E.T., Alspaugh, M.A., and Henle, W.: Rheumatoid factor as a cause of positive reactions in tests for Epstein-Barr virus-specific IgM antibodies. Clin. Exp. Immunol., *36*:415, 1979.
37. Henderson, B.E., et al.: Risk factors associated with nasopharyngeal carcinoma. N. Engl. J. Med., *295*:1101, 1976.
38. Schiff, J.A., Schaefer, J.A., and Robinson, J.E.: Epstein-Barr virus in cerebrospinal fluid during infectious mononucleosis encephalitis. Yale J. Biol. Med., *55*:59, 1982.
39. Baker, F.J., Kotchmar, G.S., Foshee, W.S., and Sumaya, C.V.: Acute hemiplegia of childhood associated with Epstein-Barr virus infection. Pediatr. Infect. Dis., *2*:136, 1983.

CHAPTER 10 GASTROINTESTINAL YERSINIOSIS

Gastrointestinal yersiniosis appears to be a disease of the twentieth century, although its presence earlier may have been obscured by the inordinate attention given to isolation of the enteric pathogens that cause shigellosis or the salmonelloses. The etiologic agents are related to the organisms that cause the much feared bubonic plague, a disease that decimated entire populations in the Middle Ages.

Gastrointestinal yersiniosis was first reported in 1973 when several Japanese school children developed diarrheal disease.[1,2] The clinical manifestations of the enteritis are largely dependent on the age of the patient, numbers of organisms ingested, and the etiologic agent. By far the most common feature of the disease is an acute enteritis, which is clinically indistinguishable from diarrheal disease caused by a variety of other pathogens. Stools are typically watery and devoid of blood or mucus in small children. The enteritis is usually self-limiting, with symptoms disappearing in 5 to 10 days.

A more serious illness of shorter duration resembling staphylococcal food poisoning, with an abrupt onset of nausea, cramps, vomiting, and diarrhea, has been reported in both adults and children. In that form of the disease, mucus, blood, and leukocytes may be present in the stool. A fever is often associated with acute epidemic forms of the gastroenteritis. The illness may subside within 24 hours or may be antecedent to extraintestinal infections requiring hospitalization. Cyclic periods of acute disease and remission sometimes occur in adults.[3]

Yersiniosis in children over 5 years of age and in young adults often manifests itself as a pseudoappendicitis with lower right quadrant abdominal pain, a moderate leukocytosis, and an elevated sedimentation rate. Tenderness frequently occurs over McBurney's point, approximately 5 cm medial to the right anterior spine along the line connecting the iliac spine and the umbilicus.[4]

In numerous instances, appendectomies are performed on patients with abdominal pain only to find a mesenteric lymphadenitis or terminal ileitis.[5] The acute inflammatory process has been known to culminate in a fatal hemorrhagic necrosis of the ileocecum or entire bowel.[4]

Sequelae occurring as a result of yersiniosis in adults include septicemia, urinary tract infections, reactive arthritis, Reiter syndrome, erythema nodosum, and myocarditis.[5] Most cases of reactive arthritis have occurred in Scandinavia among men who are positive for HLA-B27.[6,7] Arthritis occurring during septicemia is believed to be an infectious process, but the reactive variety of arthritis is considered a manifestation of an allergic response.[8] Joint symptoms may be polyarticular or monoarticular, although polyarticular involvement is more common. Inflammation may persist for as long as 1 year after onset of reactive arthritis.

Neurologic complications in reactive arthritis, following a Yersinia infection, appear to be rare, but at least 3 cases have been reported.[9] In 1 case, the Miller-Fisher variant of Guillain-Barré syndrome followed a documented Yersinia infection.[10] The patient was asymptomatic in 1 year and neurologic evidence of disease has not recurred. Guillain-Barré syndrome appears to have an immunologic etiology. The peripheral neuritis experienced by patients with Guillain-Barré syndrome is believed to be related to immune complexes that destroy the myelin sheath of the axons.[11,12] It appears that Guillain-Barré syndrome can occur as a sequela following a variety of enteric infections. Often, it is impossible to document the cause of the antecedent infection.

The potential for nosocomial outbreaks of yersiniosis was demonstrated by an outbreak of the disease in hospitalized patients in Newfoundland and in Finland.[13] In a study of the outbreak of gastroenteritis in 9 patients in Newfoundland, it was determined that the index patient was asymptomatic at the time of admission, but had experienced episodes of diarrhea for the previous 6 months.[3] Unfortunately, such circumstances may be more common than are generally realized, making a thorough history with follow-up cultures important in the prevention of nosocomial outbreaks.

ETIOLOGY

The most common etiologic agent of gastrointestinal yersiniosis is the gram-negative bacillus, Yersinia enterocolitica. The organism has been recovered from a variety of domestic and wild animals. Birds, pigs, oysters, dogs, cows, sheep, horses, deer, cats, beavers, raccoons, rabbits, and chinchillas are natural reservoirs of the organism. Acute mesenteric adenitis is more frequently associated with another member of the same genus, Yersinia pseudotuberculosis.[4] Y. pseudotuberculosis was first isolated from granuloma-type lesions found in infected mammals and birds in 1883. The disease it caused was called pseudotuberculosis because the lesions resembled those of miliary tuberculosis. Despite the similarity between the two diseases, the name pseudotuberculosis for the infection caused by Y. pseudotuberculosis is probably best left to the past. Most tuberculosis today occurs as a pulmonary infection.

Recently, Y. enterocolitica has been divided on the basis of biochemical characteristics into "true" Y. enterocolitica and three additional species for whom the names, Y. kristensenii, Y. intermedia, and Y. frederiksenii have been proposed. Y. kristensenii is not a significant cause of human infection.[14] Y. frederiksenii and Y. intermedia have been isolated from skin and wound infections.[15,16]

Although strains of Y. enterocolitica and Y. pseudotuberculosis have been studied extensively, much remains to be learned about the three newly described species of Yersinia. Virulence of Y. enterocolitica has been associated with the ability of the organism to kill adult mice, invade HeLa cells, penetrate guinea pig conjunctiva, autoagglutinate when grown in tissue cultures, and produce a heat-stable enterotoxin (ST) much like that associated with some strains of Escherichia coli.[17] The presence of both a 42- and an 82-megadalton plasmid has been associated with the ability of particular strains to kill mice.[18]

PREDISPOSING FACTORS

The frequency of Yersinia enteritis in children and young adults suggests that young individuals may be more susceptible to the enteric disease than are mature healthy adults. Radiation, surgery, age, and underlying disease appeared to be predisposing factors in a nosocomial outbreak of diarrheal disease in Newfoundland.[3]

The predilection of Y. enterocolitica and Y. pseudotuberculosis for specific geographic areas has aroused the curiosity of investigators throughout the world. Reports indicate that persons living in Sweden, Finland, and Hungary may be at greater risk for developing yersiniosis than individuals living in other parts of the world.[19] In the United States, a large number of Y. enterocolitica organisms has been recovered in Wisconsin.[5] Although colder climates may enhance the virulence of the organism, it is likely that more aggressive attempts to isolate Y. enterocolitica will reveal that the incidence of enteric yersiniosis is more widespread and in more diverse geographic areas than believed.

EPIDEMIOLOGY

Gastrointestinal yersiniosis occurs as sporadic outbreaks in most countries, but in Sweden and Finland, the disease appears to be endemic.[20] In most instances, recovery of yersinias has been by laboratories aggressively seeking to isolate the organisms. Epidemiologic studies indicate that Yersinia enterocolitica is transmitted to humans by ingestion of contaminated water or food, or by contact with infected animals.[5,21–25] There is at least one published report in which Y. enterocolitica has been recovered from raw milk.[26] Y. enterocolitica is usually killed by pasteurization, but there is ample evidence that if the organisms are present in sufficient numbers, some will survive heat-processing.[27,28] The organism grows well at refrigeration temperatures, and therefore, sufficient numbers can be present in pasteurized milk to cause disease.[29]

A large interstate outbreak of enteritis caused by Y. enterocolitica occurred in the United States in 1982.[25] Persons affected in Arkansas, Tennessee, and Mississippi were found to have ingested milk pasteurized in a single Memphis plant.

The association of yersiniosis and the handling of animals is less well documented than that of illness and contaminated water or food, but European patients diagnosed as having yersiniosis frequently have had a history of either recent contact with pigs or recent ingestion of pork.[5] In 1 instance in the United States, an infection in a 4-month-old infant was associated with an infection in a dog.[30] It is not surprising that the fly has been implicated in the transmission of Yersinia enteritis since that insect has been known to be a significant vector in other enteric diseases.[31] Human-to-human transmission appears to be the primary mode of transmission in nosocomial and interfamilial outbreaks.[3,13,32]

LABORATORY DIAGNOSIS

Yersiniosis may be diagnosed in the laboratory by culturing the etiologic agent, by observing characteristic lesions in mesenteric nodes and Peyer's patches, or by demonstrating the presence of specific agglutinins. The availability of rapid identification schemes for Enterobacteriaceae and demonstration that cold enrichment may enhance recovery rates for some strains of Yersinia enterocolitica have resulted in an increased awareness of the role of yersinias in human disease. As more laboratories avail themselves of the wide array of selective media, it can be expected that recovery rates for Yersinia species will be even higher.

Microscopic Examination

The direct microscopic examination of stool is of limited value, but the presence of leukocytes may alert the laboratorian or physician that a diarrhea is of bacterial origin.[33] Erythrocytes and mucus may or may not be present. Y. enterocolitica is a gram-negative bacillus or coccobacillus that measures 1 to 2 μm in length and 0.5 to 1.0 μm in width, but it cannot be distinguished from several other morphologically similar enteric pathogens or nonpathogens. Laboratorians and physicians should work closely together in evaluating the history of the patient's illness, because it is too expensive for most laboratories to employ unlimited numbers of selective media to recover etiologic agents. A careful examination of options for collection of specimens and diagnostic procedures to follow direct microscopic examination may not only save time, but also result in more rapid isolation of enteric pathogens.

Cultural Techniques

Isolation of Yersinia species from extraintestinal sources usually presents no problems. The recovery of the organisms from stool specimens has been sometimes less that satisfactory because of the presence of large numbers of indigenous bacteria. Although a cold enrichment technique may be required for the isolation of some strains of Y. enterocolitica, the numbers of yersinias present in most cases of acute enteric disease favor recovery when MacConkey (Mac) or salmonella-shigella (SS) agar is employed directly as a plating medium. Colonies of Y. enterocolitica are light pink to peach on Mac agar and measure 1.0 to 2.0 mm in diameter. Colonies on SS agar are usually smaller and may be light pink, peach, or colorless. The use of additional selective media increases the opportunity for recovery of yersinias because some strains of Y. enterocolitica are inhibited by SS agar.[5] A medium known as CAL (cellobiose-arginine-lysine) agar, which is commercially available (Scott Laboratories, Fiskeville, Rhode Island, or Remel-Regional Media Laboratories, Inc., Lenexa, Kansas), is as sensitive as Mac agar in supporting growth of Y. enterocolitica.[34]

Colonies of Y. enterocolitica are easy to recognize on CAL agar. Because Y. enterocolitica ferments cellobiose, colonies appear red or bright burgundy on CAL agar in the presence of neutral red as a pH indicator after 36 hours of incubation at 25°C (Fig. 10–1). Colonies typically measure 0.5 to 2.5 mm in diameter. Other selective media that may prove useful in recovering Yersinia species from stool include a pectin agar, an oxalate agar, and cefsulodin-irgasan-novobiocin (CIN) agar.[35–37] Whatever plating medium is used for isolating enteric pathogens, duplicate plates should be inoculated so that one set of plates can be incubated at 37°C and the other set at 25°C, because Yersinia species grow more readily at the lower temperature.[38]

The use of cold enrichment techniques remains controversial because not all strains of Y. enterocolitica recovered in this manner have been shown to be clinically significant.[5] The technique requires that a rectal swab or one dipped in feces be placed in 5.0 ml of 0.067 M phosphate-buffered saline (pH 7.6) and be incubated at 4°C for 2 to 3 weeks before plating on selective media. The inordinate amount of time required for cold enrichment makes it of limited value. Clearly, use of selective plating media and cold enrichment needs further evaluation in diverse geographic areas before the value of the methods can be documented.

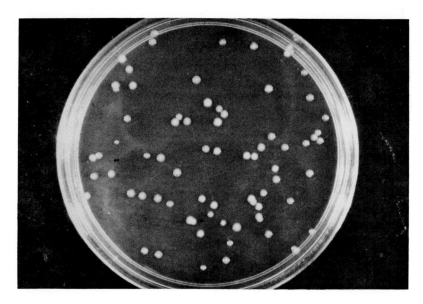

Figure 10–1. Appearance of Yersinia enterocolitica on CAL agar. (Courtesy of A.S. Weissfeld, Los Angeles.)

Table 10–1. Differentiating characteristics of selected Yersinia species.

Medium	Y. enterocolitica	Y. intermedia	Y. kristensenii	Y frederiksenii
L-rhamnose	−	+	−	+
Raffinose	−	+	−	−
Melibiose	−	+	−	−
Sucrose	+	+	−	+

Biochemical Characterization

Presumptive evidence for the presence of Yersinia species can be obtained by inoculating 4 tubes of media. Typical colonies of Yersinia can be used to inoculate 1 tube each of triple sugar iron (TSI) agar and urea agar, and 2 tubes of a motility medium. One tube of motility medium should be incubated at 25°C; the other one should be incubated at 37°C. Typically, Y. enterocolitica produces an acid butt and slant on TSI with no H_2S or gas. Y. pestis does not produce urease, but Y. enterocolitica, Y. frederiksenii, Y. kristensenii, Y. intermedia, and Y. pseudotuberculosis demonstrate urease activity. The enteric yersinias are motile at 25°C, but not at 37°C.

Y. enterocolitica can be differentiated from the three other species of enteric yersinias on the basis of L-rhamnose, raffinose, melibiose, and sucrose fermentation (Table 10–1). The API20E system may require testing with conventional media for acid production in L-rhamnose, raffinose, and melibiose since those reactions are often delayed. Sucrose-negative strains of Y. enterocolitica, Y. intermedia, and Y. frederiksenii do not appear to be enteric pathogens.[38]

Serologic Tests

Serologic diagnosis based on detection of antibodies in serum has only limited application because serum agglutinins are not universally present in individuals with gastrointestinal yersiniosis. Antigens and reference antisera are not commercially available, but the Plague Section of the Centers for Disease Control in Fort Collins, Colorado, makes a few antisera.

Serologic Typing

There are 53 somatic (O) and 19 flagellar (H) antigens associated with Y. enterocolitica.[5] Serotyping of other species of Yersinia is not yet available, and the procedure is beyond the capability of most laboratories.

Determination of serotypes has been extremely valuable in epidemiologic studies of outbreaks of diarrheal disease caused by Y. enterocolitica. Most enteric disease in Japan has been associated with serotype 0:3.[1,2] Serotypes 0:5 and 0:8 have been implicated in several outbreaks in the United States, while serotypes 0:3 and 0:9 are more common in Europe and Canada.[38]

Biotyping

Y. enterocolitica can be subdivided further into biotypes on the basis of biochemical variation of strains. Biotyping can be especially useful in the study of possible nosocomial infections caused by Y. enterocolitica. Biotype numbers are based on information obtained from a data bank containing the reactions of thousands of strains of the same organisms.

Biotypes may also be significant in assessing pathogenicity of isolates, because certain biotypes are more frequently associated with enteric disease. Assessment of pathogenicity on the basis of biotyping is complicated by an apparent geographic variation in pathogenicity of biotypes. Biotype 1 strains of Y. enterocolitica have been associated with diarrheal disease in South Africa, Canada, the United States, and Newfoundland, but rarely in Belgium.[3,39–41]

Since susceptibility of persons living in widely separated geographic areas may also differ, the presence of diarrheal disease and recovery of a biotype 1 strain of Y. enterocolitica must be considered significant. Unlike serotyping, most laboratories have the capability of determining biotypes by using conventional biochemical media or one of the commercially available systems for identification of Enterobacteri-aceae.

Phage Typing

Since most outbreaks of diarrheal disease in the United States and Europe are caused by specific serotypes of Y. enterocolitica, serotyping may have limited value in epidemiologic analyses. Phage typing has been employed in Europe in investigations of outbreaks of enteric disease caused by Y. enterocolitica;[42–45] however, the bacteriophages used do not universally lyse organisms recovered in the United States.

A new phage-typing schema was used recently in the United States to study 3 outbreaks of human and chinchilla diarrheal disease.[46] The bacteriophages used in the study were isolated from raw-sewage-treat-ment plants. A total of 24 phages, which lysed Y. enterocolitica, Y. kristensenii, Y. frederiksenii, or Y. intermedia, was recovered. Un-fortunately, only 2 phages were species specific, lysing strains of Y. kristensenii only. Despite that limitation, phage typing may be more useful in epidemiologic studies than species identification, because patterns of lysis by various bacteriophages can be determined.

Although most laboratories do not have the time, equipment, or personnel to do phage typing on Yersinia species, in the event of an outbreak of gastrointestinal yersiniosis, a reference laboratory stock-ing the bacteriophage types can be consulted. The typing phages used in the study by Baker and Farmer[46] of 3 outbreaks of Yersinia-asso-ciated diarrheal disease can be obtained from the Tennessee De-partment of Public Health, Knoxville Laboratory, Knoxville, Ten-nessee 37902.

PROGNOSIS

Gastrointestinal yersiniosis is usually self-limiting in children, but mesenteric adenitis in adults may progress to more serious disease. Young adults frequently undergo appendectomies because symptoms of acute mesenteric adenitis often mimic those of appendicitis. If sequelae to enteric infection occur, the prognosis is guarded. Yersin-iosis is a serious disease in immunocompromised hosts, and the fatality rate is high.[4] It is important to promptly initiate antimicrobial therapy, based on susceptibility testing of isolates.

CASE REPORTS

Cases 1 and 2

A 2-year-old boy from northwestern Saskatchewan developed fever, diarrhea, and vomiting. Two days later, on February 25, 1981, he was admitted to a local hospital. His temperature on admission was 40°C.

His leukocyte count was 21,400 with 76% polymorphonuclear leukocytes and 17% lymphocytes.

No localized abdominal tenderness was detected on his admission to the local hospital, and the initial diagnosis was gastroenteritis. After 3 days, an appendiceal abscess was suspected, and the boy was transferred by air ambulance to University Hospital, Saskatoon.

Two stool specimens obtained on the second and sixth days after his admission to University Hospital were negative for ova and parasites and negative for virus particles by electron microscopy. An adenovirus was isolated from both of these specimens. Cultures for Salmonella spp., Shigella spp., and Campylobacter spp. were negative. A moderate growth of Y. enterocolitica biotype 1, serotype 0:21, was obtained by direct plating on salmonella-shigella agar of stool specimens on March 6 and 9, 1981.

Fluid and electrolyte balance were maintained during the boy's stay in the hospital. He recovered without surgery and without antibiotics.

The 3-year-old sister of the boy described in case 1 was admitted to the same hospital in northern Saskatchewan on March 26, 1981. She had a high fever, decreased appetite, and abdominal tenderness. Two days after her admission to the local hospital, she developed watery brown diarrhea and vomiting. Intravenous fluids were started. Four days after her admission to the hospital, abdominal distension was evident, and a nasogastric tube was inserted. The leukocyte count ranged from 12,000 to 25,000, with a higher proportion of neutrophilic leukocytes than normal. On March 31, 1981, the child was transferred to University Hospital, Saskatoon.

An abdominal x-ray showed multiple, moderately dilated, gas-filled loops of small bowel in the mid and upper abdomen. No gas was present in the colon or rectum. Fluid appeared to be present within the peritoneal cavity.

On April 1, 1981, laparotomy was done because of the suspected peritonitis. At surgery, the presence of acute ileitis with peritonitis was confirmed. The appendix had a slight degree of inflammation and was removed. The terminal ileum was very inflamed and edematous. Treatment was started with gentamicin and clindamycin.

Microscopic examination of the appendix showed mucosal ulceration and purulent exudate in the lumen. Fibrinous exudate was present on the surface. The deeper layers of the appendix were edematous, congested, and infiltrated by polymorphonuclear neutrophils and polymorphonuclear eosinophils.

Aerobic and anaerobic cultures of the peritoneal fluid showed no growth. Culture of a biopsy of a lymph node of the small bowel near the terminal ileum grew Escherichia coli. The strain was resistant to ampicillin but sensitive to gentamicin. Cold enrichment of the lymph node tissue for 3 weeks failed to yield Y. enterocolitica. Blood and spinal fluid cultures were negative for Y. enterocolitica.

Two days after surgery, rectal washings were obtained for culture, since the child was no longer passing stool. After cold enrichment for 18 days in selenite F medium, Y. enterocolitica biotype 1, serotype 0:21, was isolated from this specimen. A serum sample obtained on April 3, 1981, gave an agglutination titer of 1/100 with the homologous strain of Y. enterocolitica serotype 0:21.

Between April 2, 1981, and her death on May 13, 1981, the child developed progressive multisystem failure, including hepatic and renal failure, metabolic encephalopathy, thrombocytopenia, and severe gastrointestinal hemorrhaging.

An autopsy revealed a retroperitoneal hematoma, with intraperitoneal hemorrhage and cutaneous ecchymoses, indicating a degree of disseminated intravascular coagulation.*

Case 3

A 7-year-old female was seen at the emergency department with a 3-day history of general malaise, headache, intermittent fever, and increasing periumbilical and lower abdominal pain. She had not had a bowel movement for 2 days.

On examination, the child looked flushed, but was not in acute distress. The temperature was 39.2°C, and the heart rate was 100 beats/min. Examination of the abdomen showed tenderness on deep palpation in the right lower quadrant. There was no guarding or rebound tenderness. Normal bowel sounds were heard. No other abnormalities were noted on examination. The leukocyte count was slightly elevated at 13.7×10^9 cells/L.

The patient was admitted for observation with a diagnosis of possible appendicitis. Subsequently, when her signs and symptoms worsened, she was operated on through a McBurney incision for acute appendicitis. A small quantity of clear peritoneal fluid was present. The appendix looked grossly normal, but the terminal ileum was red and inflamed with some nearby enlarged lymph nodes. An appendectomy was performed. The child had an uneventful postoperative course and was discharged well 7 days later. Bacteriologic culture of the appendix stump yielded a heavy growth of Y. enterocolitica. Histology of sections of the appendix showed "a focus of neutrophil infiltrate in the lamina propria which extends through the epithelium and is associated with exudate of neutrophils in the lumen. The appearance is that of mild early appendicitis."

Five days after discharge from the hospital, the patient was read-

---

*From Martin, T., Kasian, G.F., and Stead, S.: J. Clin. Microbiol., *16*:622–626, 1982.[47]

mitted with a complaint of soreness and swelling around the abdominal incision site, and fever with a temperature of 38.1°C. Examination showed redness around the incision site and a fluctuant swelling beneath the skin. The wound was reopened, and a collection of pus was noted. This was drained and examined bacteriologically. Culture of the pus gave a heavy pure growth of Y. enterocolitica. The wound was managed by drainage and local irrigation with a sodium hypochlorite solution (Hygeol). Antibiotic therapy was withheld. The wound infection resolved satisfactorily, and the patient was discharged 4 days later.

A stool sample was obtained during the second admission. Culture yielded a heavy growth of Y. enterocolitica. The patient lived in a small rural community about 150 miles north of Toronto. She had arrived in Toronto 2 days before the onset of her symptoms. An 8-year-old cousin and a 10-year-old brother had also developed abdominal pain and fever at around the same time as our patient. However, it was not possible to perform early bacteriologic studies on these patients.

The 2 isolates of Y. enterocolitica from the appendix stump and wound were obtained in pure culture on blood agar and bile salts medium. The isolate from the stool was found to be the predominant colony type among mixed aerobic fecal flora on blood agar, Mac-Conkey medium, and salmonella-shigella agar. All 3 isolates had features typical of Y. enterocolitica biotype 3 (G. Wauters, Ph.D. thesis, Vander, Louvain, Belgium, 1970) and were negative for salicin and esculin. They were found to be serotype 0:21. A serum sample obtained from the patient about 3 weeks after the onset of symptoms had an agglutinating titer of 800 against the strain of Y. enterocolitica isolated from the appendix.

The strains were examined by one of us (D.A.S.) in various laboratory in vivo and in vitro systems used for evaluating pathogenicity. Representative colonies from 2 strains were autoagglutinable by the method of Laird and Cavanaugh. Further tests of pathogenicity were performed only on the stool isolate of Y. enterocolitica. Representative colonies showed a high index of infectivity in a HeLa cell culture system, produced heat-stable enterotoxin in the infant mouse assay system, produced conjunctivitis in guinea pigs, and were unable to grow on magnesium oxalate agar at 35°C. When tested in the mouse diarrhea model, the stool isolate produced diarrhea and subsequently death.*

———————————
*From Karmali, M.A., Toma, S., Schiemann, D.A., and Ein, S.H.: J. Clin. Microbiol., *15*:596–598, 1982.[48]

Case 4

A 4-month-old girl had swelling of the right labium. She was examined by a local physician and treated first with intramuscular penicillin and later with oral ampicillin. The swelling was unresponsive, and the child was referred for hospitalization.

Throughout her illness, the child had had no history of fever, irritability, vomiting, anorexia, diarrhea, or vaginal discharge. The mother's pregnancy had been uncomplicated. There was a history of a brief mild diaper rash during the first 2 weeks of life. There was no history of trauma to the perineal area.

On admission, she had a rectal temperature of 40°C. The physical examination was normal except for the genitals; the right labium was erythematous and tender, had a slightly milky discharge from an externally draining sinus, and was markedly swollen. Inguinal nodes of both sides were large, firm, and tender, with ecchymosis of the skin above the nodes. The white blood cell count was 18,800 with 39% lymphocytes, 52% polymorphonuclear leukocytes, and 9% mononuclear cells. An aspirate of the right inguinal node grew an organism identified as Y. enterocolitica. Initial treatment was intravenous ampicillin and gentamicin, which was changed to gentamicin intramuscularly. The infant responded within 5 to 6 days. A stool specimen obtained during hospitalization failed to grow Y. enterocolitica on blood agar. She was discharged on the sixth hospital day and has continued to do well.

The day before the onset of the patient's symptoms, the family moved from the house they had occupied for 6 months. According to the history, the infant had been fed only commercially prepared and preserved foods; she was bathed in her own bathing tub and did not share washcloths or towels, and only disposable paper diapers were reportedly used. (It was noted on a visit to the house during the investigation, however, that she was wearing a makeshift diaper from an old dishtowel.)

None of 15 immediate and extended family members gave any history of diarrheal disease, abdominal pain, arthritis, or fever within the preceding 4 months.

The month before the child's illness, the family's pet dog whelped 11 puppies. Eight of these puppies died with what was described as "wasting away." The puppies that died had no evidence of diarrhea. There were no farm animals or other pets in the immediate vicinity of the child's home.*

---

*From Wilson, H.D., McCormick, J.B., and Feeley, J.C.: J. Pediatr., *89*:767–769, 1976.[30]

SUMMARY

Gastrointestinal yersiniosis is usually a self-limiting disease that occurs most frequently in children and young adults. The illness typically manifests itself as a gastroenteritis or acute mesenteric lymphadenitis. Extraintestinal yersiniosis is believed to be rare, but, when present, constitutes a life-threatening or disabling internal disease. The enteric form of the disease has occurred in nosocomial outbreaks in immunocompromised hosts. Although Yersinia gastroenteritis was first reported in Japan, the etiologic agent appears to have a greater predilection for cold climates of the northern European countries. The organism is transmitted by contaminated water or food or by contact with infected animals. The availability of selective media for Yersinia species has made it feasible for most laboratories to recover the organism directly from stool specimens.

REFERENCES

1. Asakawa, Y., et al.: Two community outbreaks of human infection with Yersinia enterocolitica. J. Hyg. (Lond.), *71*:715, 1973.
2. Zen-Yoji, H., et al.: An outbreak of enteritis due to Yersinia enterocolitica occurring at a junior high school. Jpn. J. Microbiol., *17*:220, 1973.
3. Ratnam, S., et al.: A nosocomial outbreak of diarrheal disease due to Yersinia enterocolitica serotype 0:5, biotype 1. J. Infect. Dis., *145*:242, 1982.
4. Keusch, G.T.: Yersinia enteritis. *In* Medical Microbiology and Infectious Diseases. Edited by A.I. Braude. Philadelphia, W.B. Saunders, 1981.
5. Weissfeld, A.S.: Yersinia enterocolitica. Clin. Microbiol. Newsl., *3*:91, 1981.
6. Ahvonen, P., Sievers, K., and Aho, K.: Arthritis associated with Yersinia enterocolitica infection. Acta Rheumatol. Scand., *15*:232, 1969.
7. Aho, K., Ahvonen, P., and Lassus, A.: HL-A antigen 27 and reactive arthritis. Lancet, *2*:157, 1973.
8. Spira, T.J., and Kabins, S.A.: Yersinia enterocolitica associated with septic arthritis. Arch. Intern. Med., *136*:1305, 1976.
9. Farag, S.S., and Gelles, D.B.: Yersinia arthritis and Guillain-Barré syndrome. N. Engl. J. Med., *307*:755, 1982.
10. Asbury, A.K.: Diagnostic considerations in Guillain-Barré syndrome. Ann. Neurol., *9*(Suppl):1, 1981.
11. Prineas, J.W.: Pathology of the Guillain-Barré syndrome. Ann. Neurol., *9*(Suppl):6, 1981.
12. Cook, S.D., and Dowlins, P.C.: The role of autoantibody and immune complexes in the pathogenesis of Guillain-Barré syndrome. Ann. Neurol., *9*(Suppl):70, 1981.
13. Toivanen, P., et al.: Hospital outbreak of Yersinia enterocolitica infection. Lancet, *1*:801, 1973.
14. Bercovier, H., et al.: Yersinia kristensenii: a new species of Enterobacteriaceae composed of sucrose-negative strains (formerly called Yersinia enterocolitica or Yersinia enterocolitica-like). Curr. Microbiol., *4*:219, 1980.
15. Bottone, E.J.: Yersinia enterocolitica: a panoramic view of a charismatic microorganism. Crit. Rev. Microbiol., *5*:211, 1977.
16. Brenner, D.J.: Speciation in Yersinia. Contrib. Microbiol. Immunol., *5*:33, 1974.
17. Nunes, M.P., and Ricciardi, I.D.: Detection of Yersinia enterocolitica heat-stable enterotoxin by suckling mouse bioassay. J. Clin. Microbiol., *13*:783, 1981.
18. Kay, B.A., Wachsmuth, K., and Gemski, P.: New virulence-associated plasmid in Yersinia enterocolitica. J. Clin. Microbiol., *15*:1161, 1982.
19. Fallon, R.J.: Yersinia enterocolitica epidemiology and antibiotic susceptibility. J. Antimicrob. Chemother., *5*:241, 1979.
20. Winblad, S.: Yersiniosis enterocolitica. Läkkartignengen, *70*:270, 1973.

21. Lassen, J.: Yersinia enterocolitica in drinking water. Scand. J. Infect. Dis., *4*:125, 1972.
22. Keet, E.E.: Yersinia enterocolitica septicemia. Source of infection and incubation period identified. N.Y. State J. Med., *74*:2226, 1974.
23. Black, R.E., et al.: Epidemic Yersinia enterocolitica infection due to contaminated chocolate milk. N. Engl. J. Med., *298*:76, 1978.
24. Lee, W.H.: An assessment of Yersinia enterocolitica and its presence in foods. J. Food Protect., *40*:486, 1977.
25. Centers for Disease Control: Multi-state outbreak of yersiniosis. Morbid. Mortal. Weekly Rept., *31*:505, 1982.
26. Vidon, D.J., and Delmas, C.L.: Incidence of Yersinia enterocolitica in raw milk in eastern France. Appl. Environ. Microbiol., *41*:355, 1981.
27. Francis, D.W., Spaulding, P.L., and Lovett, J.: Enterotoxin production and thermal resistance of Yersinia enterocolitica in milk. Appl. Environ. Microbiol., *40*:174, 1980.
28. Hughes, D.: Isolation of Yersinia enterocolitica from milk and a dairy farm in Australia. J. Appl. Bacteriol., *46*:125, 1979.
29. Morris, G.K., et al.: Isolation and identification of Yersinia enterocolitica. Public Health Laboratory, *35*:217, 1977.
30. Wilson, H.D., McCormick, J.B., and Feeley, J.C.: Yersinia enterocolitica infection in a 4-month-old infant associated with infection in household dogs. J. Pediatr., *89*:767, 1976.
31. Fukushima, H.: Role of the fly in the transport of Yersinia enterocolitica. Appl. Environ. Microbiol., *38*:1009, 1979.
32. Gutman, L.T., et al.: An interfamilial outbreak of Yersinia enterocolitica enteritis. N. Engl. J. Med., *288*:1372, 1973.
33. Harris, J.C., DuPont, H.L., and Hornick, R.B.: Fecal leukocytes in diarrheal disease. Ann. Intern. Med., *76*:697, 1972.
34. Michael, M.V., and Shotts, E.M., Jr.: Medium for isolation of Yersinia enterocolitica. J. Clin. Microbiol., *10*:180, 1979.
35. Bowen, J.H., and Kominos, S.D.: Evaluation of a pectin agar for isolation of Yersinia enterocolitica within 48 hours. Ann. J. Clin. Pathol., *72*:586, 1979.
36. Soltesz, L.V., Schalen, C., and Mardh, P.: An effective selective medium for Yersinia enterocolitica containing sodium oxalate. Acta Pathol. Microbiol. Scand., *B 88*:11, 1980.
37. Schiemann, D.A.: Synthesis of a selective agar medium for Yersinia enterocolitica. Can. J. Microbiol., *25*:1298, 1979.
38. Sack, R.B., Tilton, R.C., and Weissfeld, A.S.: Laboratory diagnosis of bacterial diarrhea. Cumitech, *12*:1, 1980.
39. Robins-Browne, R.M., et al.: Yersinia enterocolitica biotype 1 in South Africa. S. Afr. Med. J., *55*:1057, 1979.
40. Marks, M.I., et al.: Yersinia enterocolitica gastroenteritis: a prospective study of clinical, bacteriologic, and epidemiologic features. J. Pediatr., *96*:26, 1980.
41. Weissfeld, A.S., and Sonnenwirth, A.C.: Yersinia enterocolitica in adults with gastrointestinal disturbances: need for cold enrichment. J. Clin. Microbiol., *11*:196, 1980.
42. Van Noyen, R., Vandepitte, J., and Wauters, G.: Nonvalue of cold enrichment of stools for isolation of Yersinia enterocolitica serotypes 3 and 9 from patients. J. Clin. Microbiol., *11*:127, 1980.
43. Mollaret, H.H., and Nicolle, P.: Sur la fréquence de la lysogénie dans l'espèce nouvelle Yersinia enterocolitica. C.R. Acad. Sci., *260*:1027, 1965.
44. Nicolle, P.: Lysotypie und ander spezielle epidemiologische Laboratoriums—methoden. Edited by H. Rische. Jena, East Germany, VEB Gustav Fisher Verlag, 1973.
45. Nicolle, P., Mollaret, H.H., and Brault, J.: Sur une parenté lysotypique entre des souches humaines de des souches porcines de Yersinia enterocolitica. Symp. Ser. Immunobiol. Stand., *9*:357, 1968.
46. Baker, P.M., and Farmer, J.J.: New bacteriophage typing system for Yersinia enterocolitica, Yersinia kristensenii, Yersinia frederiksenii, and Yersinia intermedia; Correlation with serotyping, biotyping, and antibiotic susceptibility. J. Clin. Microbiol., *15*:491, 1982.

47. Martin, T., Kasian, G.F., and Stead, S.: Family outbreak of yersiniosis. J. Clin. Microbiol., *16*:622, 1982.
48. Karmali, M.A., Toma, S., Schiemann, D.A., and Ein, S.H.: Infection caused by Yersinia enterocolitica serotype 0:21. J. Clin. Microbiol., *15*:596, 1982.

CHAPTER 11 HEPATITIS B

It has long been recognized that so-called viral hepatitis consists of at least two clinically distinct human diseases, formerly designated as "infectious hepatitis" and "serum hepatitis." MacCallum proposed in 1947 that the names hepatitis A and hepatitis B be used to designate the viral-associated liver diseases.[1] Since that time, a third type of viral hepatitis, known as non-A, non-B hepatitis, has emerged as a significant cause of human disease.[2-4] The number of reported cases of hepatitis B and non-A, non-B hepatitis is increasing, whereas the number of reported cases of hepatitis A is decreasing in the United States (Fig. 11–1).

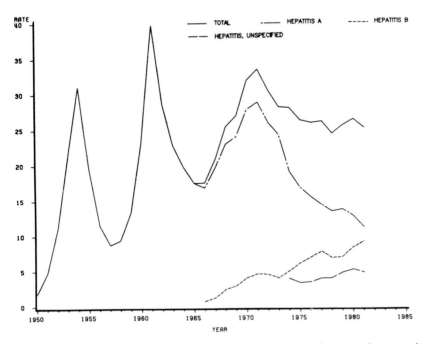

Figure 11–1. Reported cases of hepatitis per 100,000 population in the United States, 1950 to 1981. (From Centers for Disease Control: Morbid. Mortal. Weekly Rept., Annual Summary 1981, 30:43, 1982.)

Although a huge worldwide reservoir of hepatitis B virus (HBV) exists, hepatitis B is usually a relatively mild disease.[5] Most individuals do not require hospitalization. In those individuals in whom complications occur, however, the consequences can be serious. Potential complications include arthritis, acute polyneuritis, and vasculitis.[6-8] The mortality rate approximates 1%; however, 6 to 10% of young adults having an HBV infection become carriers. Approximately one fourth of the carriers can be expected to develop chronic active hepatitis, which may progress to cirrhosis or HBV-related cancer of the liver.

Hepatitis A and hepatitis B are clearly distinct from one another, but do have some characteristics in common (Table 11–1). As information on non-A, non-B hepatitis emerges, it appears that it may also be endemic and responsible for both acute and chronic disease.

The onset of initial acute hepatitis B is usually insidious and occurs 60 to 160 days after exposure to hepatitis B virus (HBV). Although the hallmark of hepatitis is often jaundice, most initial infections caused by HBV produce nonicteric disease. The time of incubation is related to the dosage of viruses. Higher doses are associated with shorter incubation times. During the icteric phase of the disease, patients frequently complain of extreme fatigue. Approximately 10 to 20% of individuals with icteric hepatitis have a skin rash, urticaria, arthralgias, and even arthritis before onset of liver disease.[9]

Immune complexes are believed to have a primary role in producing extrahepatic manifestations of hepatitis B. The symptoms most often disappear without residual damage within 1 week. Rare outbreaks have been reported in which a fulminating hepatitis B has been responsible for death.[5] In at least 1 outbreak of fulminating hepatitis B, patients were taking multiple drugs.[10]

Chronic infections of HBV are usually asymptomatic, but both hepatomegaly and splenomegaly can occur. Transient elevations in

Table 11–1. Characteristics of hepatitis A and hepatitis B.

Characteristic	Hepatitis A	Hepatitis B
Incubation period	15 to 40 days	60 to 160 days
Onset	abrupt	insidious
Target organ	liver	liver
Clinical hallmark	jaundice	jaundice
Fever	present	absent
Malaise	present	present
Gastrointestinal symptoms	present	absent
Severity	mild to moderately severe	moderate to severe
Serum transaminases	elevated	elevated
Type of infection	acute	acute to chronic
Carrier state	absent	present
Immunologic sequelae	absent	present

serum glutamic-oxaloacetic transaminase (SGOT) and serum glutamic-pyruvic transaminase (SGPT) can persist for years. Chronic infections are frequent in infants and the elderly. Progression to more serious diseases rarely occurs, but if it does, the entity is called active chronic hepatitis.

In active chronic hepatitis, jaundice may or may not be present. Elevations in SGOT and SGPT accompany the necrosis that follows an inflammatory response. Each year, about 4000 Americans succumb from HBV-associated cirrhosis.[11] In addition, at least another 800 die from HBV-related cancer.

In children, the onset of hepatitis is abrupt, and abdominal pain and vomiting, accompanied by fever, are often present. The duration of jaundice and fever tends to be briefer in children than in adults. Immune complex disease is manifested more often as dermatitis or glomerulonephritis in children than as the arthritic complications seen in adults.

Although there is no recognized treatment for HBV infections, the recent availability of an inactivated HBV vaccine for individuals at risk of contracting the virus is expected to substantially reduce the reservoir of carriers of HBV and, therefore, the number of HBV infections.

ETIOLOGY

The discovery by Blumberg and his colleagues of Australia (Au) antigen, at first thought to occur only in Australian aborigines, turned out to be an important step in understanding the etiology of hepatitis B.[12] When the Au antigen was also discovered in the sera of 20% of individuals with hepatitis, it became known as the hepatitis-associated antigen (HAA). The antigen was also found to occur in 10 to 14% of patients with leukemia and in some apparently healthy people of South East Asia.[13]

In 1968, HAA was detected in the blood of a patient during the incubation period of post-transfusion hepatitis.[14] It was apparent in subsequent studies that the antigen can persist in the blood of persons who have had hepatitis B for 1 to 20 years.[15]

Three virus-like particles have been identified in the blood of individuals who have or have had hepatitis B: (1) spherical particles that are 20 nm in diameter; (2) filamentous particles that measure up to 10 nm or longer and 20 nm in diameter; and (3) spherical Dane particles that measure 45 nm in diameter (Fig. 11–2).[16–18] The core component of the Dane particle contains the antigens HBcAg and HBeAg, DNA polymerase, and double-stranded DNA.

Surface antigen HBsAg is the antigen once called HAA. The HBsAgs of all three particles are identical. Purified preparations of HBsAg contain 4 polypeptides and 4 glycoproteins, with molecular

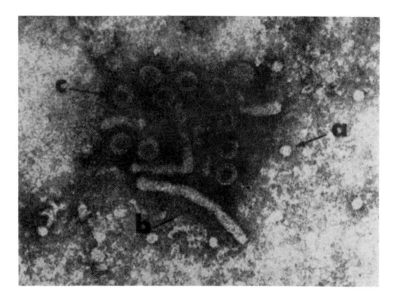

Figure 11–2. Electron micrograph of serum, showing three viruslike particles: (a) small spherical particles; (b) filamentous particles; and (c) large spherical particles (Dane particles). (From Hollinger, F.B., and Dienstag, J.L.: Hepatitis viruses. *In* Manual of Clinical Microbiology, 3rd Ed. Edited by E.H. Lennette. Washington, D.C., American Society for Microbiology, 1980.)

Table 11–2. Major and minor subtypes of HBsAg.

Major	Minor
ayw1	q
ayw2	x
ayw3	f
ayr	t
adw2	j
adw4	n
adr	g
adwy	
adyr	

From Hirschman, S.Z.: Hepatitis viruses. *In* Medical Microbiology and Infectious Diseases. Edited by A.I. Braude. Philadelphia, W.B. Saunders, 1980.

masses ranging from 22,000 to 68,000 daltons. The Dane particle, now considered to be the HBV, can be differentiated from the smaller spherical forms or core particles by additional chemical and physical characteristics.

At least eight antigenically distinct major subtypes and seven minor subtypes of HBsAg have been recognized (Table 11–2). The antigenic type adw2 is found more frequently in the United States, whereas antigenic types ayw2 and ayw3 are more common in Africa and the

Middle East. Determination of subtypes may be useful in epidemiologic studies and can explain partial identity in immunodiffusion tests.

HBcAg appears in the blood approximately 4 weeks after exposure to HBV. In another week, HBeAg and DNA polymerase activity are the most important markers for viral replication. In a limited study of 20 carriers of HBV in Japan, viral replication was related in part to hepatic cell necrosis but did not seem to be responsible for progression to liver cirrhosis.[19] Understanding remission or progression of HBV-associated disease awaits the clarification of the long-term host-parasite relationship.

PREDISPOSING FACTORS

The Immunization Practices Advisory Committee of the Centers for Disease Control has placed individuals at risk of developing hepatitis B into three groups based on prevalence of serologic markers (Table 11–3). Immigrants or refugees from areas to which hepatitis B is endemic constitute the group at highest risk for developing HBV infection. Also included in the high-risk group are institutionalized mentally retarded individuals, homosexually active males, users of illicit parenteral drugs, and patients undergoing frequent hemodialysis. Household contacts of HBV carriers and health care personnel who routinely handle blood specimens are also at risk. The now rou-

Table 11–3. Expected hepatitis B virus prevalence in various population groups.

	Prevalence of serologic markers of HBV infection	
	HBsAG (%)	All markers (%)
High risk		
Immigrants/refugees from areas of high HBV endemicity	13	70–85
Clients in institutions for the mentally retarded	10–20	35–80
Users of illicit parenteral drugs	7	60–80
Homosexually active males	6	35–80
Household contacts of HBV carriers	3–6	30–60
Patients of hemodialysis units	3–10	20–80
Intermediate risk		
Prisoners (male)	1–8	10–80
Staff of institutions for the mentally retarded	1	10–25
Health-care workers		
Frequent blood contact	1–2	15–30
Low risk		
Health-care workers		
No or infrequent blood contact	0.3	3–10
Healthy adults (first-time volunteer blood donors)	0.3	3–5

From Centers for Disease Control: Inactivated hepatitis B virus vaccine. Morbid. Mortal. Weekly Rept., *31*:318, 1982.

tine screening of blood that is to be used for transfusion for HBsAg no longer appears to make individuals receiving multiple transfusions at risk for the development of hepatitis B.

EPIDEMIOLOGY

Although hepatitis A and hepatitis B became separately reportable diseases in the United States in 1966, the difficulty in differential diagnosis of the clinical entities, until the availability of HBsAg testing, probably renders the accumulated statistics of limited value. Certain trends, however, can be seen. The incidence of viral hepatitis is increasing in metropolitan areas, occurring more frequently in males than in females, and no longer associated with a seasonal variation.[9] Although hepatitis B is known to be endemic throughout the world, statistics of its true incidence are not available.[20]

HBV was once thought to be transmitted only by the parenteral route, but percutaneous, perinatal, and sexual transmission have been demonstrated in recent years.[21-24] Infections in neonates born to HBsAG-positive mothers can be modified by the administration of hepatitis B immune globulin (HBIG).[25] HBsAg can be detected in urine, saliva, tears, semen, and impetiginized skin lesions of infected persons.

LABORATORY DIAGNOSIS

Specimens suspected of containing HBV should be handled with extreme care. Disposable gowns and gloves should always be worn when working with possible infectious products or specimens. Rigid attention should be given to hand washing. Eating, drinking, smoking, and mouth pipetting should be avoided. Samples should be kept at 4°C until the tests can be performed.

Microscopic Examination

Direct examination, using electron microscopy, immunofluorescence, and immunoperoxidase staining, has been used successfully to detect the three particles associated with HBV infections, but the techniques are primarily investigative tools.[26,27] HBcAg-containing particles are usually found within the nuclei of liver cells, whereas HBsAg-containing particles are seen exclusively in the cytoplasm of hepatocytes.[28] Direct examination is not a method of choice for rapid diagnosis of hepatitis B.

Cultural Techniques

No cell system has been found to support growth of the HBV for any substantive period of time. Chimpanzees are susceptible to induced HBV infection, but the limited availability of the primates has precluded their use except in investigative studies.[29]

Serologic Tests

A large number of serologic techniques is available for detection of HBV antigens and antibodies (Table 11–4). Laboratory workers should become familiar with the limitations and idiosyncrasies of particular procedures. The choice of tests depends on the expertise of laboratory personnel and available facilities. Interpretation of serologic markers requires familiarity with the time of appearance of specific antigens and antibodies (Table 11–5). The presence of HBsAg or HBcAg in serum indicates a current active acute or chronic infection. HBcAg is often associated with more serious liver dysfunction, a high rate of infectivity, and a poorer prognosis. Anti-HBc is the first antibody to appear and may be detectable for several years. It is of no value, however, if HBsAg is present in detectable amounts. Anti-HBe appears 10 or more days after anti-HBc, but does not reach the levels of anti-HBc. Anti-HBs is the last antibody to appear and is associated with immunity to HBV infections. Paired sera for detection

Table 11–4. Serologic techniques used to detect hepatitis B antigens and antibodies.

Technique	Relative sensitivity
Agarose gel diffusion	Low
Counterimmunoelectrophoresis	Intermediate
Complement fixation	
Reverse passive latex agglutination	
Hemagglutination	
Enzyme-linked immunosorbent assay (ELISA)	High
Radioimmunoassay (RIA)	

Table 11–5. Time of appearance and interpretation of HBV serologic markers in hepatitis B.

Marker	Time of appearance	Interpretation
HBsAg	~ 40 to 60 days after exposure	Active hepatitis B infection acute or chronic
HBeAg	~ 50 to 60 days after exposure	Active hepatitis B infection acute or chronic Possibly enhanced infectivity
Anti-HBc	~ 60 to 90 days after exposure	Active hepatitis B infection acute or chronic* or carrier state
Anti-HBe	~ 100 to 120 days after exposure	Active hepatitis B infection acute or chronic** or carrier state
Anti-HBs	~ 30 to 60 days after disappearance of HBsAg	Immunity to HBV infection

*A test for anti-HBc is of value only if HBsAg levels are not present in detectable levels.
**A fourfold or greater rise in titer between acute and convalescent sera occurs in active HBV infections.

of anti-HBc or anti-HBe titers are required to distinguish between active acute or chronic hepatitis B infections and the carrier states.

Detection of Antigens

Agarose gel diffusion is the least sensitive method for detecting HBsAg, but it is useful in obtaining patterns of identity, partial identity, or nonidentity. The 2-dimensional micro-Ouchterlony immunodiffusion tests require a 24- to 72-hour incubation period at 37°C for the development of precipitin lines.

Discontinuous counterimmunoelectrophoresis or counterelectrophoresis has been used extensively in subtyping HBsAg and in evaluation of antigens associated with non-A, non-B hepatitis. HBsAg migrates toward the anode in an electric field under alkaline conditions. The accuracy of the test is dependent on a balance between antigen and antibody. False negative results may be obtained, if either antigen or antibody is present in excess.[30]

Reverse passive latex and erythrocyte agglutination are both simple and rapid techniques for detecting the presence of HBsAg.[31,32] The passive latex agglutination requires rotation of guinea pig anti-HBsAg with serum samples in a humidified chamber for 30 minutes. Observations for agglutination must be made within 5 minutes. The erythrocyte agglutination test requires a 3-hour incubation period at room temperature. Like many other agglutination tests, the presence of rheumatoid factor, lipemia, autoimmune or heterophil antibodies, and albumin-globulin imbalances may cause false positive reactions.[28]

The enzyme-linked immunosorbent assay (ELISA) employs disks coated with horse serum anti-HBsAg and alkaline phosphatase or horseradish peroxidase.[33,34] An incubation period of $2\frac{1}{2}$ to 4 hours is required after adding diluted serum samples. The temperature of incubation depends on the test procedure employed. The ELISA tests are sensitive and reliable, with a minimum of false positive reactions.

The radioimmunoassay (RIA) continues to be the most sensitive and specific method for testing of all HBV markers.[35] Both the double-antibody RIA procedure and the solid-phase "sandwich" RIA technique are commonly employed to detect HBsAg. The methods employ ^{125}I-labeled purified HBsAg. Unlabeled antigen competes against labeled antigen for binding sites on a fixed amount of antibody. The antigen-antibody complexes are precipitated in the presence of anti-IgG in the double-antibody RIA procedure. In the solid-phase "sandwich" RIA technique, free antigen is separated from bound antigen by the addition of an adsorbent. The amount of antigen present in a sample is determined by comparing the bound radioactivity with the radioactivity bound in solutions containing known amounts of antigen on a gamma counter. The RIA tests do require expensive equipment and both safe handling and disposal of hazardous materials.[36]

Detection of Antibodies

Antibodies to the various HBV antigens can be detected by agarose gel diffusion, counterelectrophoresis, reverse passive latex or erythrocyte agglutination, complement-fixation, enzyme-linked immunosorbent assays (ELISA), and radioimmunoassay (RIA). The late appearance of antibodies in hepatitis B may make the tests of value only in retrospect. A fourfold or greater rise in anti-HBe titer in acute and convalescent sera can be used to differentiate between acute disease and either the asymptomatic carrier state or passive chronic state. In a few instances, when levels of HBsAg are undetectable, anti-HBcAg may be found in measurable amounts.[27] Anti-HBcAg is present in all HBsAg carriers. Therefore, it is of value in testing donor blood in which HBsAg levels may not be detectable.

PROGNOSIS

Acute hepatitis B is usually a benign self-limiting infection. In those individuals with fulminating disease resulting in rapid death, it is assumed that an immune deficiency may contribute to the progression of the disease. It is estimated that 10% of individuals with acute hepatitis B may become carriers. It has been suggested that the carrier state and chronic hepatitis B may represent 2 stages of chronic infection.[37] It is estimated that from 10 to 20% of patients with chronic hepatitis B infections enter a state of remission each year. In the asymptomatic carrier states, direct markers of HBV disappear and anti-HBe appears in the blood. Long-term HBsAg carriers are at risk of developing primary hepatocellular carcinoma.[38] Although HBV-DNA can be found in both tumorous and nontumorous liver cells, the significance of its presence is not clear.[38-41] Carriers are susceptible to other forms of liver disease. Acute infections caused by the virus of hepatitis A have been reported in carriers of HBeAg.[42-44] Reactivation from the carrier to the chronic stage has been associated with chemotherapy or immunosuppressive agents.[45]

A unique relationship between an RNA virus called delta and HBsAg can promote acute or chronic hepatitis.[46] The virus requires HBsAg for replication and becomes encapsidated by HBsAg. The interaction of the replicative cycle of HBV and the host's immunologic responses to viral products appear to affect the prognosis following an acute infection of hepatitis B.

It is the hope of public health officials that use of an inactivated hepatitis B virus vaccine made from HBsAg for high-risk groups will reduce the incidence of hepatitis B within the next several years. The primary adult vaccination consists of 3 intramuscular doses of 1.0 ml of vaccine (20 μg/1.0 ml) each. For children under 10 years of age, 3 doses of 0.5 ml (10 μg/0.5 ml) are recommended. Three 2.0 ml doses (40 μg/2.0 ml) are recommended for immunosuppressed patients or individuals on hemodialysis.[47] The cost of the vaccine for widespread use is currently a limiting factor.

CASE REPORTS

Case 1

This female infant was the product of a term pregnancy complicated by a "flu-like" illness during the eighth month of gestation. Delivery and neonatal course were unremarkable; the child was breast fed. Growth and development were normal. Three days prior to admission at the age of 8 months, she developed the sudden onset of vomiting and diarrhea and was admitted to the Children's Hospital and Health Center for intravenous hydration and observation. The remainder of her medical history was noncontributory.

On physical examination, the child was alert, afebrile, and moderately dehydrated. Blood pressure was 160 mm Hg by palpation. The liver span was 10 cm and the spleen tip was palpable. Admission laboratory values included: WBC: 27,800/mm³, 43% poly, 13% band, 37% lymphocytes, 7% monocytes; Westergren sedimentation rate 40 mm/hour. Urinalysis showed specific gravity 1.023, pH 6, 3+ blood, 1+ protein, no cells. Serum electrolyte values were normal; blood urea nitrogen 54 mg/dl, creatinine 1.6 mg/dl, SGOT 4740 IU/L (normal, 5 to 27), SGPT 1681 IU/L (normal, 1 to 29). LDH 10 400 IU/L (normal, 100 to 190), CPK 1 660 IU/L (normal, 150 to 160), total bilirubin 1.1 mg/dl, direct bilirubin 0.7 mg/dl, alkaline phosphatase 295 IU/L, amylase 274 IU/L (normal, 5 to 81), and lipase 48 mg/dl (normal, 4 to 24). Serologic studies gave the following results: C_3 74 mg/dl (normal, 90 to 239), C_4 6 mg/dl (normal, 13 to 35), CH 10 U/ml (normal, 40 to 60), hepatitis B surface antigen positive. Maternal serum was also positive for hepatitis B surface antigen. Intravenous pyelogram and renal scan showed 2 small functioning kidneys.

The child was thought to have hepatitis B infection with associated vasculitis. She was treated with antihypertensive medications and her blood pressure became normal. Further diagnostic work-up was refused and she was discharged on treatment with hydralazine, propranolol, and furosemide, with improved renal and liver function.

She was readmitted 2 months later following a seizure. Her blood pressure was 180/110 mm Hg. A renal arteriogram showed necrotizing arteritis and microinfarcts. Renal vein renin values were markedly elevated: vena cava 26 ng/ml/hour; right renal vein 36 ng/ml/hour; left renal vein 36 ng/ml/hour (normal supine, 0.2 to 1; normal upright, 0.9 to 4.5). An open liver biopsy showed chronic aggressive hepatitis with mild periportal fibrosis. There were many sclerotic glomeruli in the kidney biopsy and abnormalities of most blood vessels, with endothelial proliferation and scattered areas of inflammatory infiltrate. Immunofluorescence of the kidney tissue was negative. Prednisone therapy, 2 mg/kg, was begun. Because her blood pressure was poorly controlled, guanethedine was added to her antihypertensive medications. Nevertheless, over the next 4 months, she had 3 admissions for malignant hypertension with blood pressure as high as 200/100 mm Hg. Left ventricular hypertrophy developed on electrocardiogram and chest film. She was begun on minoxidil therapy, and had marked improvement of blood pressure. She has been maintained for 20 months on treatment with minoxidil, propranolol, furosemide, and prednisone 5 mg/day. Her serum chemistry values are stable: SGOT 50 to 60 IU/L, SGPT 50 to 60 IU/L, BUN 10 mg/dl, and creatinine 0.5 mg/dl. Her serum complement values are normal. She continues to be hepatitis B surface antigen positive, as does her mother, who now also has chronic aggressive hepatitis on liver biopsy. To date, the child has had some growth and developmental delay but there have been no exacerbations of liver or kidney disease.*

Case 2

A 61-year-old man had a 3-week history of weakness in his legs. Numbness in the distal portion of his lower extremities began 2 days prior to admission. He denied pain in his back or limbs, paresthesias, and diplopia. Malaise had developed 1 month before the weakness. He had no fever, icterus, nausea, or abdominal pain. Examination revealed a well-developed, well-nourished man with normal vital signs. There was no scleral icterus, hepatic tenderness, hepatomegaly, or splenomegaly. Cranial nerve function was normal, but there was symmetric weakness of the lower extremities, greatest distally with areflexia. He had a broad-based, steppage gait. Neither fasciculations nor atrophy was present. Sensory examination revealed minimally decreased pinprick, temperature, and light touch sense, and moderately decreased vibration and position sense in the distal portion of the lower extremities.

On admission, the patient's hemoglobin value was 16 g/dl and the WBC count was 8200/cu mm, with a normal differential cell count. Serum electrolyte, calcium, phophorus, BUN, glucose, creatinine, uric acid, and urinalysis values were all normal. A VDRL test was negative. Pertinent laboratory values were as follows: SGOT, 279 units/ml (normal, 3 to 20 units/ml); SGPT, 800 units/ml (normal, 3 to 15 units/ml); alkaline phosphatase, 92 IU/ml (normal, 20 to 90 IU/ml); direct bilirubin, 0.3 mg/dl; total bilirubin, 0.7 mg/dl; albumin, 4.4 g/dl; and total protein, 9.0 g/dl. Prothrombin time was normal. A differential

*From Reznik, V.M., Mendoza, S.A., Self, T.W., and Griswold, W.R.: J. Pediatr., *98*:252–254, 1981.[48]

absorption test (Monospot) was negative, as were screening tests for heavy metals. The CSF was clear and colorless, with an opening pressure of 110 mm H_2O. It was acellular with a glucose value of 87 mg/dl and a protein value of 93 mg/dl. The CSF γ-globulin level was increased at 17.6%.

On admission, hepatitis-associated antigen and antibody were positive and negative, respectively. Liver biopsy revealed hepatocellular disarray, necrosis of liver cells, and periportal inflammatory infiltrate compatible with the diagnosis of acute viral hepatitis. Two weeks after hospitalization, hepatitis-associated antibody was detected.

During the month of hospitalization, results of liver function studies returned to normal, although hepatitis-associated antigen remained positive. Motor and sensory functions improved and 4 months after hospital discharge were normal. He remained areflexic.*

Case 3

A 28-year-old laboratory technician had been in excellent health until November, 1981, when she complained of nausea, anorexia, and malaise. Investigation showed raised serum alanine aminotransferase activity (serum ALT; SGPT). There was no history of hepatitis, drug abuse, transfusion, or shellfish ingestion. None of her family had had hepatitis. Her husband, a doctor in a haemodialysis unit, proved negative for markers of hepatitis B virus but positive for anti-hepatitis A virus IgG. Results of radioimmunoassay of the patient's serum were positive for hepatitis B surface-antigen, hepatitis Be antigen (HBeAg), and anti-hepatitis B core IgM (anti-HBc IgM) and negative for anti-hepatitis Be antigen, anti-hepatitis B surface antigen, and anti-hepatitis A virus for both IgG and IgM classes. The clinical and laboratory features supported the diagnosis of acute B viral hepatitis. She refused admission to hospital.

At the end of December, because of an increase in serum ALT and aspartate transamine (serum AST; SGOT) activity and the onset of jaundice, she was admitted to hospital. The liver was tender and slightly enlarged. Serum ALT activity was 1260 IU/L at 37°C (normal value up to 42 IU), serum bilirubin concentration 154 μmol/L (9 mg/100 ml), and prothrombin time 80% normal. Packed cell volume, white cell count, differential cell count, and peripheral blood smear were normal. Serum protein concentration was 57.5 g/L (albumin, 32 g/L), and ammonia, glucose, and nitrogen values were normal.

Radioimmunoassay for markers of hepatitis B virus and hepatitis A virus showed the following results: hepatitis B surface antigen positive, hepatitis Be antigen positive, anti-hepatitis Be negative, anti-

---

*From Berger, J.R., Ayyar, D.R., and Sheremata, W.A.: Arch. Neurol., *38*:366–367, 1981. Copyright 1981, American Medical Association.[7]

hepatitis B core IgM positive, anti-hepatitis B surface negative, anti-hepatitis A virus IgM positive, anti-hepatitis A virus IgG positive. Tests repeated after 12 days yielded the same results. Double infection with hepatitis B virus and hepatitis A virus was evident.

Antibody titers against cytomegalovirus and herpes 1 and 2 were 1/32, 1/16, and 1/8, respectively, on paired serum samples taken at an interval of 15 days; antibody against Epstein-Barr virus was undetectable by indirect fluorescent antibody tests.

Hyperammonaemia appeared on the twenty-sixth hospital day and the liver was greatly reduced in size. Despite supportive treatment, she gradually entered coma, and 2 days later she died from massive intestinal bleeding.*

SUMMARY

Hepatitis B has been a major public health problem throughout the world. Its true dimension can only be estimated since many of the cases are not reported. Once thought to be transmitted only parenterally, it is now recognized that hepatitis B can be transmitted in a variety of ways. Diagnosis of hepatitis B has been facilitated by the availability of antisera to specific HBV markers. Although acute hepatitis B is a mild, usually benign disease, chronic hepatitis and its sequelae, including cirrhosis and hepatocellular carcinoma, occur in some carriers. It will take many years to assess the true efficacy of the recently available inactivated HBV vaccine. The duration of protection and possible need for boosters remain to be determined.

REFERENCES

1. Krugman, S.: Viral hepatitis. *In* Human Diseases Caused by Viruses. Edited by H. Rothschild, F. Allison, and C. Howe. New York, Oxford University Press, 1978.
2. Seeff, L.B., Wright, E.D., McCollum, R.W.: The VA Hepatitis Studies Group. VA cooperative study of post-transfusion hepatitis, 1969–1974: incidence and characteristics of hepatitis and responsible risk factors. Am. J. Med. Sci., *270*:355, 1975.
3. Goldfield, M., et al.: The consequences of administering blood pretested for HBsAg by third generation techniques: a progress report. Am. J. Med. Sci., *270*:335, 1975.
4. Berman, M.: The chronic sequelae of non-A, non-B hepatitis. Ann. Intern. Med., *91*:1, 1979.
5. Center for Disease Control: Hepatitis B—New Bern, North Carolina. Morbid. Mortal. Weekly Rept., *28*:373, 1979.
6. Wands, J.R., et al.: The pathogenesis of arthritis associated with acute hepatitis B surface antigen positive hepatitis. J. Clin. Invest., *55*:930, 1976.
7. Berger, J.R., Ayyar, D.R., and Sheremata, W.A.: Guillain-Barré syndrome complicating acute hepatitis B. A case with detailed electrophysiological and immunological studies. Arch. Neurol., *38*:366, 1981.
8. Sargent, J.S., Lockshin, M.D., Christian, C.L., and Gocke, D.J.: Vasculitis with hepatitis B antigenemia. Medicine, *55*:1, 1976.
9. Robinson, W.S., and Greenberg, H.: Hepatitis B. *In* Infectious Diseases, 3rd Ed. Edited by P.D. Hoeprich. Hagerstown, Maryland, Harper & Row, 1983.

---

*From Piazza, M., Guadagnino, V., Orlando, R., and Picciotto, L.: Br. Med. J., *284*:1913–1914, 1982. Editor, S.P. Lock.[44]

10. Dougherty, W.J., and Altman, R.: Viral hepatitis in New Jersey, 1960–1961. Am. J. Med., *32*:704, 1962.
11. Quinn, J.P.: Inactivated hepatitis B vaccine. Clin. Microbiol. Newsl., *5*:33, 1983.
12. Blumberg, B.S., Sutnick, A.I., London, W.T., and Millman, I.: The discovery of the Australia antigen and its relation to viral hepatitis. Perspect. Virol., *7*:223, 1971.
13. Blumberg, B.S., Alter, H.J., and Visnich, S.A.: A 'new' antigen in leukemia sera. JAMA, *191*:541, 1965.
14. Prince, A.M.: An antigen detected in blood during incubation period of serum hepatitis. Proc. Natl. Acad. Sci. U.S.A., *60*:814, 1968.
15. Giles, J.P., McCollum, R.W., Berndtson, L.W., Jr., and Krugman, S.: Viral hepatitis—Relation to Australia-SH antigen to the Willowbrook MS-2 strain. N. Engl. J. Med., *281*:119, 1969.
16. Bayer, M.E., Blumberg, B.S., and Werner, B.: Particles associated with Australia antigen in the sera of patients with leukemia, Down's syndrome and hepatitis. Nature, *218*:1057, 1968.
17. Hirschman, R.J., et al.: Virus-like particles in sera of patients with infectious and serum hepatitis. JAMA, *208*:1667, 1969.
18. Dane, D.S., Cameron, C.H., and Briggs, M.: Virus-like particles in serum of patients with Australia-antigen-associated hepatitis. Lancet, *1*:695, 1970.
19. Kinoshita, R., et al.: Chronic hepatitis B: Correlation between viral replication and clinical course. J. Infect. Dis., *144*:303, 1981.
20. Mosely, J.W.: Hepatitis types B and non-B. Epidemiologic background. JAMA, *233*:697, 1975.
21. Pattison, C.P., et al.: Epidemic hepatitis in a clinical laboratory: possible association with computer card handling. JAMA, *230*:854, 1974.
22. Pattison, C.P., Maynard, J.E., Berquist, K.R., and Webster, H.M.: Epidemiology of hepatitis B in hospital personnel. Am. J. Epidemiol., *101*:59, 1975.
23. Hersh, T., Melnick, J.L., Goyal, R.K., and Hollinger, F.B.: Nonparenteral transmission of viral hepatitis type B (Australia antigen associated serum hepatitis). N. Engl. J. Med., *285*:1363, 1971.
24. Szmuness, W.I., et al.: On the role of sexual behavior in the spread of hepatitis B infection. Ann. Intern. Med., *83*:489, 1975.
25. Chin, J.: Prevention of chronic hepatitis B virus infection from mothers to infants in the United States—13 States. Pediatrics, *71*:289, 1983.
26. Huang, S., Minassian, H., and More, J.D.: Application of immunofluorescent staining on paraffin sections improved by trypsin digestion. Lab. Invest., *35*:383, 1976.
27. Ray, M.B.: Hepatitis B Virus Antigens in Tissue. Baltimore, University Park Press, 1979.
28. Hollinger, F.B., and Dienstag, J.L.: Hepatitis viruses. *In* Manual of Clinical Microbiology, 3rd Ed. Edited by E.H. Lennette. Washington, D.C., American Society for Microbiology, 1980.
29. Barker, L.F., et al.: Viral hepatitis, type B, in experimental animals. Am. J. Med. Sci., *270*:189, 1975.
30. Dreesman, G.R., Hollinger, F.B., and Melnick, J.L.: Detection of hepatitis B antigen by counter-immunoelectrophoresis: enhancing role of homologous serum diluents. Appl. Microbiol., *24*:1001, 1972.
31. Kachani, Z.F., and Gocke, D.J.: An agglutination-flocculation test for rapid detection of hepatitis B antigen. J. Immunol., *111*:1564, 1973.
32. Hollinger, F.B., Wasi, C., Dreesman, G.R., and Melnick, J. L.: Subtyping hepatitis B antigen using monospecific antibody-coated cells. J. Infect. Dis., *128*:753, 1973.
33. Halbert, S.P., and Anken, M.: Detection of hepatitis B surface antigen (HBsAg) with use of alkaline phosphatase-labeled antibody to HBsAg. J. Infect. Dis., *136* (Suppl.):318, 1977.
34. Wolters, G.L., Kuijpers, P.C., Kacaki, J., and Scheuirs, A.H.W.M.: Enzyme-linked immunosorbent assay for hepatitis B surface antigen. J. Infect. Dis., *136* (Suppl.):311, 1977.
35. Hollinger, F.B., Vordam, V., and Dreesman, G.R.: Assay of Australia antigen and antibody employing double-antibody and solid-phase radioimmunoassay tech-

niques and comparison with passive hemagglutination methods. J. Immunol., *107*:1099, 1971.

36. Chernesky, M.A., Ray, C.G., and Smith, T.F.: Laboratory diagnosis of viral infections. Cumitech, *15*:1, 1982.
37. Hoofnagle, J.H.: Chronic type B hepatitis. Gastroenterology, *84*:422, 1983.
38. Beasley, R.P., Hwang, L.W., Lin, C.C., and Chien, C.S.: Hepatocellular carcinoma and hepatitis B virus. A prospective study of 22,707 men in Taiwan. Lancet, *2*:1129, 1981.
39. Chen, D.S., et al.: Detection and properties of hepatitis B viral DNA in liver tissues from patients with hepatocellular carcinomas. Hepatology, *2*:42S, 1982.
40. Shafritz, D.A., and Kew, M.C.: Identification of integrated hepatitis B virus DNA sequences in human hepatocellular carcinomas. Hepatology, *1*:1, 1981.
41. Brechot, C., et al.: Detection of hepatitis B virus DNA in liver and serum. A direct appraisal of the chronic carrier state. Lancet, *2*:765, 1981.
42. Hindman, S.H., et al.: Simultaneous infection with type A and B hepatitis viruses. Am. J. Epidemiol., *105*:135, 1977.
43. Goldstein, J.: Concurrent acute infection with hepatitis A and B. JAMA, *249*:727, 1983.
44. Piazza, M., Guadagnino, V., Orlando, R., and Picciotto, L.: Acute B viral hepatitis becomes fulminant after infection with hepatitis A virus. Br. Med. J., *284*:1913, 1982.
45. Hoofnagle, J.H., et al.: Reactivation of chronic hepatitis B virus infection by cancer chemotherapy. Ann. Intern. Med., *96*:447, 1982.
46. Rizzetto, M.: Biology and characterization of the delta agent. *In* Viral Hepatitis, 1981 International Symposium. Edited by W. Szmuness, H.J. Alter, and J.E. Maynard. Philadelphia, Franklin Institute Press, 1982.
47. Centers for Disease Control. Inactivated hepatitis B virus vaccine. Morbid. Mortal. Weekly Rept., *31*:317, 1982.
48. Reznik, V.M., Mendoza, S.A., Self, T.W., and Griswold, W.R.: Hepatitis B-associated vasculitis in an infant. J. Pediatr., *98*:252, 1981.

CHAPTER 12 HERPES GENITALIS

Genital herpes infection has been recognized as a venereal disease since 1883 when it was described in prostitutes of Hamburg.[1] It is now one of the major sexually transmitted infections in the world and, probably, the most important venereal disease. The disease can occur as a primary exogenous infection or as a recurrent endogenous infection resulting from activation of a latent herpesvirus in the sacral sensory ganglia. External lesions appear in a majority of patients with primary or recurrent herpes genitalis (Fig. 12–1). In females, vesicles and ulcers appear primarily in the cervix, vulva, and vagina. The surrounding skin of the perineum, buttocks, and thighs may also be affected. In males, lesions tend to occur on the glans penis, and less frequently, on the scrotum or perineum. The lesions in both sexes are painful and accompanied most often by fever, dysuria, and bilateral inguinal lymphadenopathy. A few patients remain asymptomatic.

The number of consultations with private physicians for genital herpes infection increased from 29,560 in 1966 to 260,890 in 1979 (Fig. 12–2). Neonatal and nosocomial infections have also been reported. Transplacental infections are rare, but can be acquired in the event of herpes simplex viremia in the mother.[2] Herpes genitalis is common in pregnant women. If lesions are present at birth during vaginal delivery, a significant chance exists that the infant will contract the disease. No doubt, the greater sexual freedom of the last decade has placed an increasing proportion of the population at risk. The trend can be expected to continue into the next decade or longer. The rise in numbers of cases of herpes genitalis has brought about a resurgence of interest in the epidemiology and clinical course of the disease.

ETIOLOGY

The primary etiologic agent of herpes genitalis is herpes simplex virus 2 (HSV-2), although in an increasing number of instances, herpes simplex 1 (HSV-1) is implicated. A 1979 study of genital herpes in coeds in the United States reported that as many as 35% of the infections were caused by HSV-1.[3] Epidemiologists are speculating that HSV-1 and HSV-2 may one day be isolated with about the same

152

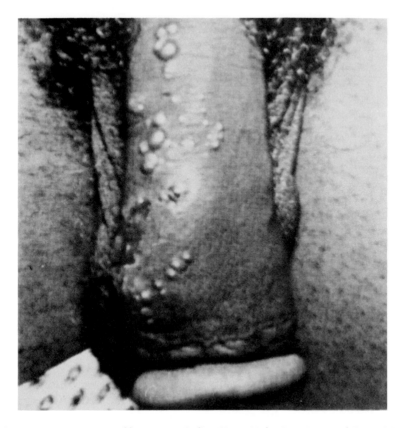

Figure 12–1. Lesions of herpes genitalis. (From Nahmias, A.J., and Starr, S.E.: Infections caused by herpes simplex viruses. *In* Infectious Diseases, 3rd Ed. Edited by P.D. Hoeprich. New York, Harper & Row, 1983.)

frequency from genital lesions. The increase in oral-genital sex is presumed responsible for the changing etiology. As might be expected for the same reason, HSV-2 has been isolated in some cases of herpetic gingiostomatitis and pharyngotonsillitis. The viruses are 2 of the 5 types of herpesviruses affecting humans. All of the herpesviruses, including HSV-1 and HSV-2, are characterized by their ability to remain latent in a host for indefinite periods and to be activated when homeostatic mechanisms are compromised. HSV-1 is most usually associated with a latent infection of the trigeminal ganglion, whereas HSV-2 remains dormant in the sacral ganglia.

The herpesviruses cannot be distinguished from one another by electron microscopy. All of the herpesviruses contain double-stranded DNA and are approximately 180 to 200 nm in diameter. The virion is pleomorphic, and the nucleocapsid demonstrates icosahedral symmetry (see Fig. 7–1). The herpesviruses are unique among the DNA

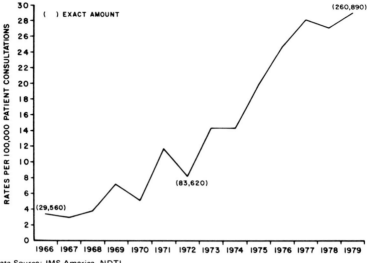

*Data Source: IMS America, NDTI.

Figure 12–2. Estimated rate of patient consultations* with private physician for genital herpes infections in the United States, 1966 to 1979. (From Genital herpes infection—United States, 1966–1979. Morbid. Mortal. Weekly Rept., *31*:137, 1982.)

viruses in that they possess an envelope acquired by budding from the nucleus or cytoplasm of host cells during maturation. Loss of the envelope results in diminished infectivity. At least 33 surface polypeptides of the virion or envelope have been identified. Additional polypeptides, which may control the expression of viral genes, are found in the core of the virion. None of these polypeptides is an enzyme, per se, but they do code for several virus-specific enzymes.[4]

PREDISPOSING FACTORS

Exposure to HSV-1 occurs during birth or very early in life. Antibody to HSV-2 can seldom be demonstrated before the age of 15. That observation supports the long-held view that HSV-2 is transmitted sexually. Although most primary infections are asymptomatic, neonates are more susceptible to symptomatic infections. Primary genital herpes infection is more common in adolescents and young adults of lower socioeconomic groups. Genital herpes infections are common during pregnancy. The high incidence of the disease in pregnancy is ascribed to impaired mechanisms of cell-mediated immunity.[5] Recurrent herpes genital infection can occur at any age.[6] Ultraviolet light, x-ray, heat, cold, hormonal imbalance, immunosuppressed state, or emotional disturbances may induce viral multiplication and recurrent disease. Hormonal changes preceding menses may trigger recurrent infections in some women.[7] Herpetic paronychia constitutes an occupational hazard for persons caring for patients with HSV-1 or HSV-2.[8] The infections can be painful and can be complicated by systemic symptoms, including acute membranous pharyngitis.

EPIDEMIOLOGY

Humans are the only major reservoirs of HSV-1 and HSV-2. The herpesviruses have often been called the "viruses of love" since both kissing and intercourse have been implicated in their transmission. The viruses can survive at room temperature on toilet seats, towels, rubber gloves, and surgical instruments for 4 to 72 hours.

No vectors for herpesviruses have ever been demonstrated. Long recognized as endemic in nature, genital herpes infection has existed in epidemic proportions since 1966 in the United States according to statistics collected by the National Disease and Therapeutic Index (NDTI) in a stratified, random sample (Fig. 12–2). The number of cases of genital herpes infections in the United States is not known, but the disease is occurring with greater frequency than ever before. It is estimated that 15 to 20 million individuals in the United States have had genital herpes infections and that the disease will occur with increasing frequency unless an effective treatment or vaccine becomes available.

The role of herpesviruses as opportunistic pathogens in nosocomial infections is well recognized. Most hospitals make serious attempts to protect immunocompromised patients from exposure to any potentially infectious agent. The now popular, and sometimes necessary, practice of personnel rotation and liberal visitation privileges in hospitals would appear to be ongoing risk factors.[9] The incubation period of primary HSV-1 or HSV-2 infection varies from 2 to 12 days. Infections caused by HSV-1 and HSV-2 stimulate cellular and humoral immune responses. The magnitude of the responses, however, is not sufficient to prevent recurrent disease in the presence of activating factors.

For many years, attempts have been made to link HSV-2 infections with cancer of the cervix. Approximately 80% of women in the United States with cancer of the cervix have antibodies against the genital virus. The incidence of cervical cancer is high among women who have had sexual experiences early in life and who have had multiple sex partners. The relationship between cervical cancer and HSV-2 remains obscure, however.

LABORATORY DIAGNOSIS

Although a presumptive diagnosis of genital herpes infection can be made without the aid of the laboratory, HSV infection can sometimes be confused with other infections. An increasing number of laboratory tests is available for detecting the presence of HSV infection. The availability of what are hoped to be specific antiviral chemotherapeutic agents makes it important to confirm a diagnosis in the laboratory.

Microscopic Examination

Scrapings, obtained from the base of fresh lesions, can be submitted for cytologic studies. If Tzanck smears are air-dried and stained with Giemsa or Wright stains, multinuclear giant cells, but no intranuclear inclusions, may be observable. Papanicolaou smears require immediate fixing in 95% alcohol before staining and may reveal intranuclear inclusions and multinucleated giant cells if HSV infection is present. It is not possible to differentiate between HSV-1 and HSV-2 infections by microscopic examination of scrapings from lesions. Unfortunately, the cytologic changes are similar for measles and the varicella-zoster viruses; however, the lesions associated with measles are not typically vesicular.

Punch biopsies may be valuable in demonstrating cytologic alterations induced by HSV. It is recommended that Bouin's solution, instead of formalin, be used as a fixative to demonstrate Cowdry Type A intranuclear inclusions stained with hematoxylin-eosin; however, intranuclear inclusions are not consistently present in either HSV or varicella-zoster infections.

A direct immunofluorescent technique can be used for the identification of HSV antigens in clinical specimens. Some experience is required in the interpretation of observations made on clinical specimens because nonspecific fluorescence occurs with frequency. In laboratories having electron microscopes, HSV can be detected in vesicular fluid.[10] HSV can be differentiated from other herpesviruses by applying immune electron microscopy to vesicular fluid or ferritin peroxidase techniques to tissue sections.

Cultural Techniques

A variety of animals and tissues can be used to grow HSV-1 or HSV-2. At one time, rabbit corneas, suckling mice, and chorioallantoic membranes of embryonated chicken eggs were used to culture the viruses from clinical material. The commercial availability of cell cultures that support growth of herpesviruses has limited the usefulness of animal inoculations. HSV will grow in human embryonic fibroblasts and primary or secondary rabbit kidney cells. Leibovitz-Emory transplant medium (LEM) is recommended as a transport medium for storing or shipping.[11] HSV will survive chilling, but not freezing; however, virus titers do decrease with time.

Typical cytopathic effect (CPE) in tissue cultures is often observable within 24 hours after inoculation and incubation at 37°C (Fig. 12–3).

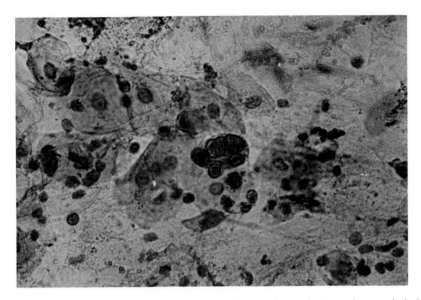

Figure 12–3. Multinucleation and intranuclear inclusion bodies of an epithelial cell infected with HSV. (From Shah, S.M., Schaefer, R.F., and Araoz, E.: Cytologic diagnosis of herpetic esophagitis. Acta Cytologica, *21*:109, 1977. © 1977 by International Academy of Cytology.)

Cytoplasmic granulation and ballooning of cells are usually followed by production of rounded forms with a refractile quality. Multinucleated cells may not appear in monolayer tissue cultures.

Typing of Isolates

HSV isolates can be typed by the following immunologic techniques:*

1. Complement fixation
2. Countercurrent immunoelectrophoresis
3. Cross immunoelectrophoresis
4. Immunofluorescence
5. Immunoperoxidase
6. Inhibition passive hemagglutination
7. Neutralization
8. Radioimmunoassay
9. Staph protein A assay

Indirect immunofluorescence has been widely applied to distinguish between HSV-1 and HSV-2 after separating infected cells from cul-

---

*Adapted from Nahmias, A.J.: The laboratory diagnosis of herpes simplex infection— Prospects and problems. Diagnostic Horizons, *1*:1, 1977.

ture medium by centrifuging at 200 × G for 10 minutes and resuspending cells in phosphate-buffered saline containing 2% fetal bovine serum to a density of 10^6 cells per ml.[12] Aliquots containing approximately 0.05 ml of resuspended cells are transferred to clean microscope slides, air-dried, and fixed in cold acetone for 10 minutes. After rinsing smears in phosphate-buffered saline, HSV-1 antiserum and HSV-2 antiserum are applied to separate smears. The antisera are allowed to react during a 30-minute incubation time at 37°C, and washed 3 times in phosphate-buffered saline. After cover-slipping, slides are examined under a fluorescence microscope.

Serologic Tests

Total humoral antibodies to HSV-1 and HSV-2 can be detected by a variety of serologic techniques, including complement-fixation, indirect immunofluorescence, neutralization, inhibition of passive hemagglutination, indirect hemagglutination, radioimmunoassay, enzyme immunoassay, and indirect immunoperoxidase staining.[13–20] The detection of type-specific antibodies requires sera adsorbed with heterologous antibodies.[21] The sensitivity of some tests is dependent on whether the infection is primary or recurrent and on the stage of the lesions.[22] In primary infections, a zero to fourfold increase in complement-fixing and neutralizing antibody can be demonstrated. No further increases are likely to be detected in recurrent infections.

PROGNOSIS

Herpes genitalis in otherwise healthy individuals, despite its severity, is usually self-limiting. In some instances, however, the dissemination of lesions and intense pain may require hospitalization. Complete healing usually occurs in 3 to 5 weeks, but females may shed the etiologic agent for weeks after symptoms have disappeared.[23] Superinfections are rare. Primary infections are more severe in neonates and compromised hosts. The mortality in neonates approximates 50%, and surviving infants may have serious sequelae, including neurologic, ocular, or other organ-system disease. Once acquired, HSV-1 or HSV-2 remains within the host in a latent state. One recent estimate places the recurrence rate at 55%.[24] Recurrent genital herpes infection is often of shorter duration, but can be extremely painful and emotionally debilitating. The lesions heal in approximately 10 days. No specific treatment can prevent recurrences of genital herpes infection, although acyclovir may help to abate a primary infection. Acyclovir is a cyclic nucleoside analog, which has an affinity for herpes-infected cells.[25] The drug is phosphorylated by a thymidine kinase and inhibits the action of viral DNA polymerase.

CASE REPORTS

Case 1

B. H. was a 29-year-old married white woman who was hospitalized because of a progressively severe headache and stiff neck for 3 days. About 10 days before admission, a number of painful lesions developed on her vulva. The lesions quickly ulcerated and were associated with a large amount of somewhat foul-smelling vaginal discharge. She did not seek medical care for these problems until nearly a week later when she decided they were not responding to self-medication. She saw her gynecologist who diagnosed genital herpes and prescribed symptomatic treatment. Shortly after this, about 3 days before admission, a generalized headache developed, progressed in severity, and became associated with increasing neck pain and stiffness, causing her to return to her gynecologist who admitted her to the hospital.

On admission, she was a well-developed and nourished young woman who appeared acutely ill and in moderate distress from headache. Temperature was 38°C by mouth but other vital signs were normal. The neck was quite stiff. There were 1 to 1.5 cm tender lymph nodes in both inguinal areas. There were multiple punched-out, superficial ulcerations, particularly numerous over the posterior fourchette, labia minora, and the anterior vaginal wall. Peripheral blood white cell count was 9100 with a normal differential. Cerebrospinal fluid was clear but contained 825 white cells, 80% of which were mononuclear. The spinal fluid protein was 145 mg per 100 ml and the glucose was 44 mg per 100 ml. Virus culture of the genital lesions grew HSV type 2, but similar culture of the spinal fluid was negative. A genital Pap smear did not show herpes-type changes. In a serum sample obtained on day 10 of illness, herpes simplex virus complement-fixing antibody could not be detected, but 1 month later, the herpes simplex virus antibody titer was greater than 512.*

Case 2

S.G. was a 26-year-old, single white man, who first developed genital herpes about 1 year prior to our first contact. During that year, he had a recurrence every 2 to 3 weeks. The young woman with whom he was living had been found to have genital herpes. This young man was in an allied medical profession and had read a great deal about herpes simplex virus infection. He had tried a number of local therapies to no avail, and, 6 months before he was seen, he had removed some material from a penile lesion and had used it to inoculate the skin over his left shoulder in an effort to enhance his immunity and prevent recurrence. Following this "vaccination," he experienced re-

---

*From Rosenthal, M.S.: Primary Care, 6:517–528, 1979.[26]

current lesions on his left shoulder along with the genital recurrences. At the time he was first seen, he had been given 8 or 9 smallpox vaccinations on an every other week schedule with no benefit.

At his initial visit, all the lesions he had were nearly healed and consisted of a half-dozen, 1 to 2 mm erythematous papules on the middle of the penile shaft from which herpes simplex virus could not be recovered. In discussing things that might be triggering his recurrences, it was noted that he wore tight-fitting jockey shorts, and it was suggested that he try wearing loose-fitting underwear. He called back 7 weeks later to say that he had not had a recurrence since be began to wear boxer shorts right after his initial visit. He was convinced he had not experienced so long a recurrence-free interval since his trouble started. He was disappointed that a virus was not recovered and said that if he remained recurrence-free for another month, he would start wearing jockey shorts in an effort to trigger a recurrence from which virus might be recovered. About 6 weeks later, he called again to say that he had started wearing his jockey shorts about a week previously because there had been no recurrence since his previous call. After 5 days in jockey shorts, recurrent lesions had developed on his penis and shoulder, and he wanted to come in for cultures. A day later, both penile and shoulder lesions were cultured and yielded herpes simplex virus type 2. He then went back to wearing boxer shorts and has not been heard from since.*

Case 3

A 23-year-old black woman, gravida 4, para 1, aborta 2, was admitted at 36 weeks gestation because of premature rupture of membranes 3 days earlier. Her prenatal course had been essentially unremarkable until the membranes ruptured, after which she experienced occasional sharp pain in her vagina.

The obstetrical history included a normal delivery of a 7 lb female infant in 1972 and 2 voluntary abortions at gestational ages of 6 and 8 weeks. The patient denied any history suggestive of herpes progenitalis nor did she complain of a painful vaginal or vulvar lesion at any time. Her past medical and surgical history were negative.

On admission, she was alert and her vital signs were normal except for a temperature of 38.6°C, a pulse rate of 140, and a respiratory rate of 22. Head, neck, eyes, nose, throat, and chest including the chest wall, breasts, heart, and lungs were negative on physical examination.

The abdomen was enlarged, compatible with a 32 to 33 weeks' gestation and the uterus was not tender. The fetal heart rate was

---

*From Rosenthal, M.S.: Primary Care, 6:517–528, 1979.[26]

slightly tachycardic with 160 beats per minute, but regular. On pelvic examination, the periurethral tissues and the anterior portion of the vulva were intensely congested and tender to the touch. The patient was complaining of piercing pain in the same areas. The cervix was 20% effaced, 2 cm dilated, and on speculum examination, clear amniotic fluid oozed from the cervical os. At this time, endocervical, cervical, vaginal, urine, and blood specimens were obtained for culture.

A Gram stain of the amniotic fluid showed mixed bacteria consisting of predominantly gram-positive cocci, and few polymorphonuclear leukocytes were seen. A complete blood count revealed a hematocrit of 32%, WBC of 12,000 with 86% polymorphonuclear leukocytes. Internal monitoring and pitocin induction were started immediately.

After 4 hours of pitocin stimulation, severe variable decelerations were noted. Because of this, prolonged rupture of the membrane, and apparent deterioration of the clinical condition of the mother, in terms of looking toxic with rising temperature, a low transverse cesarean section was performed under general anesthesia. Amniotic fluid and uterine content revealed no gross evidence of intrauterine infection. Aerobic and anaerobic cultures were obtained from the uterine cavity, and a piece of the membranes as well as the surgeon's gloves were part of a study protocol.

On careful questioning, the patient revealed that 2 weeks prior to her admission, her husband had observed multiple vesiculo-ulcerative lesions of the penis. He did not seek any medical advice and the lesions disappeared spontaneously after 2 weeks. A Pap smear of the mother taken 2 months prior to her admission did not show any evidence of Herpes simplex changes. At this time, vaginal and cervical swabs were negative for Herpes virus hominis. The herpes antibody titer at 10 weeks of pregnancy was 1:16 and was 1:64 3 weeks after the delivery.

The newborn weighed 4 lb, 4 oz, and his Apgar scores were 10 at 1 and 10 at 5 minutes. He was active, alert, and in no distress. The physical examination was negative. He continued to do well and was started on oral feedings. On day 6, he became lethargic, refused feedings, and was transferred to the intensive care nursery; he was mildly icteric and in mild respiratory distress. The liver was palpable 2 cm below the right costal margin, while the spleen was not enlarged on clinical examination.

On day 7, he began to bleed and hematomas developed around puncture sites. In spite of blood exchange and platelet transfusions, he continued to bleed from skin sites, the gastrointestinal tract, and the endotracheal tube. He developed seizures and died at the age of 8 days.

The autopsy revealed a generalized hemorrhagic diathesis with multiple focal hemorrhages in the myocardium, lungs, brain, renal pelvices, and the pancreas. The liver was slightly enlarged and markedly congested. There were numerous miliary yellowish-white foci representing coagulation necrosis of hepatocytes without any significant inflammatory reaction. Hepatocytes at the periphery of these necrotic foci were frequently multinucleated, and the individual nuclei were enlarged and occupied by acidophilic homogeneous material surrounded by marginated chromatin. The adrenal glands showed extensive focal necrosis and nuclear changes similar to those seen in the liver. The spleen was the site of occasional foci of necrosis. Herpes simplex virus was cultured from liver, adrenal, lung, and brain tissues. The latter two organs, however, did not show morphologic evidence of Herpes simplex infection.*

SUMMARY

Genital herpes infection has been occurring in epidemic proportions in the United States for almost 20 years. Both HSV-1 and HSV-2 have been implicated as etiologic agents. Primary genital herpes infection can be fatal in neonates or immunocompromised hosts. Recurrent infection may be of exogenous or endogenous origin. It is difficult, if not impossible, to prevent recurrent infection because of the latency potential of both HSV-1 and HSV-2. Prevention of herpes genitalis awaits development of appropriate therapy or immunization.

REFERENCES

1. Hutfield, D.C.: History of herpes genitalis. Br. J. Vener. Dis., *42*:263, 1966.
2. Hanshaw, J.B.: Herpesvirus hominis infections in the fetus and the newborn. Am. J. Dis. Child., *126*:546, 1973.
3. Kalinyak, J.E., Fleagle, G., and Docherry, J.J.: Incidence and distribution of herpes simplex virus-1 and -2 from genital lesions in college women. J. Med. Virol., *1*:175, 1979.
4. Pagano, J.S., and Lemon, S.M.: The herpesviruses. *In* Medical Microbiology and Infectious Disease. Edited by A.I. Braude. Philadelphia, W.B. Saunders, 1981.
5. Dini, D., Alrenga, D.P., and Freese, U.: Perinatal herpes virus infection: Report of a case indicating the paternal role. J. Natl. Med. Assoc., *72*:1193, 1980.
6. Rawls, W.E., and Campione-Piccardo, J.: Epidemiology of herpes simplex virus type 1 and type 2 infections. *In* The Human Herpesviruses. Edited by A.J. Nahmias, W.R. Dowdle, and R.E. Schinazi. New York, Elsevier, 1981.
7. Guinan, M.E., et al.: The course of untreated recurrent genital herpes simplex in 27 women. N. Engl. J. Med., *304*:759, 1981.
8. Rosaro, R.E., Rosato, E.F., and Plotkin, G.A.: Herpetic paronychia—an occupational hazard of medical personnel. N. Engl. J. Med., *283*:804, 1970.
9. Nahmias, A.J., and Starr, G.E.: Infections caused by Herpes simplex viruses. *In* Infectious Diseases, 3rd Ed. Edited by P.D. Hoeprich. New York, Harper & Row, 1983.
10. Nahmias, A.J.: The laboratory diagnosis of herpes simplex virus infection—Prospects and problems. Diagnostic Horizons, *1*:1, 1977.
11. Nahmias, A.J., et al.: Transport media for herpes simplex virus types 1 and 2. Appl. Microbiol., *22*:451, 1971.

---

*From Dini, M., Alrenga, D.P., and Freese, U.: J. Natl. Med. Assoc., *72*:1193–1195, 1980.[5]

12. Rawls, W.E.: Herpes simplex viruses. *In* Manual of Clinical Microbiology, 3rd Ed. Edited by E.H. Lennette. Washington, D.C., American Society for icrobiology, 1980.
13. Skinner, G.R.B., Hartley, C., and Whitney, J.E.: Detection of type-specific antibody to herpes simplex virus type 1 and 2 in human sera by complement-fixation tests. Arch. Virol., *50*:323, 1976.
14. Hanna, L., Keshishyan, H., Jawetz, F., and Coleman, V.R.: Diagnois of Herpesvirus hominis infections in a general hospital laboratory. J. Clin. Microbiol., *1*:318, 1975.
15. Back, A.F., and Schmidt, N.J.: Typing Herpesvirus hominis antibodies and isolates by inhibition of the indirect hemagglutination reaction. Appl. Microbiol., *28*:400, 1974.
16. Stewart, J.A. and Herrmann, K.L.: Herpes simplex virus. *In* Manual of Clinical Immunology. Edited by N.R. Rose and H. Friedman. Washington, D.C., American Society for Microbiology, 1980.
17. Forghani, B., Schmidt, N.J., and Lennette, E.H.: Solid-phase radioimmunoassay for identification of Herpesvirus hominis types 1 and 2 from clinical materials. Appl. Microbiol., *28*:661, 1974.
18. Gilman, S.C., and Docherty, J.J.: Detection of antibodies specific for herpes simplex virus in human serum by the enzyme-linked immunosorbent assay. J. Infect. Dis. (Suppl.), *136*:286, 1977.
19. Vestergaard, B.F., Grauballe, P.C., and Spangaard, H.: Titration of herpes simplex virus antibodies in human sera by the enzyme-linked immunosorbent assay (ELISA). Acta Pathol. Microbiol. Scand., Sect. B., *85*:466, 1977.
20. Benjamin, D.R.: Rapid typing of herpes simplex virus strain using the indirect immunoperoxidase method. Appl. Microbiol., *28*:568, 1974.
21. Plummer, G., et al.: Herpes simplex viruses: discrimination of types and correlation between different characteristics. Virology, *60*:206, 1974.
22. Moseley, R.C., et al.: Comparison of viral isolation, direct immunofluorescence, and indirect immunoperoxidase techniques for detection of genital herpes simplex virus infection. J. Clin. Microbiol., *13*:913, 1981.
23. Adams, H.G., et al.: Genital herpetic infection in men and women: Clinical course and effect of topical application of adenine arabinoside. J. Infect. Dis., *133*:A151, 1976.
24. Strassburg, M.A.: Recurrent genital herpes: Reinfection or reactivation? N. Engl. J. Med., *305*:1586, 1981.
25. Serota, F.T., et al.: Acyclovir treatment of herpes zoster infections. JAMA, *247*:2132, 1982.
26. Rosenthal, M.S.: Genital herpes simplex virus infections. Primary Care, *6*:517, 1979.

13 INFANT BOTULISM

Botulism is a life-threatening neuroparalytic disease that has classically been associated with the ingestion of preformed toxin contained in improperly preserved food. In vivo production of botulinum toxin has been reported in the clinical entities "wound botulism" and "infant botulism."[1,2] Wound botulism is rare, but infant botulism appears to be increasing (Fig. 13–1).[3] Only 27 cases of wound botulism have been reported in the United States since 1943.[4] Constipation is often the first symptom exhibited in infant botulism. In addition, babies dem-

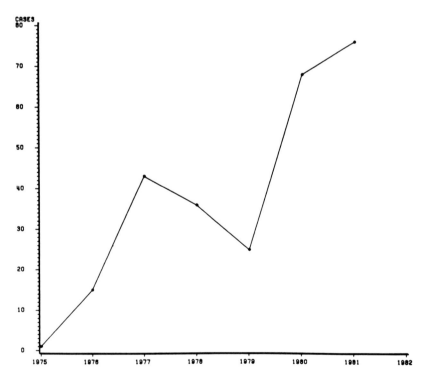

Figure 13–1. Reported cases of infant botulism in the United States, 1975 to 1981. (From Centers for Disease Control: Morbid. Mortal. Weekly Rept., Annual Summary 1981, Atlanta, 1982.)

onstrate listlessness, hypotonia, difficulty in swallowing, pooled oral secretions, pupils that respond poorly to light, poor anal sphincter tone, and absence of the gag reflex.[5-7] Infant botulism ranges from a mild toxinogenic disease to a rapidly fulminating or even fatal illness and may be one cause of the enigmatic sudden death syndrome.

ETIOLOGY

Infant botulism is caused by a toxin of the gram-positive spore-forming anaerobic bacillus, Clostridium botulinum. The spores of C. botulinum are abundant in soil. Ingested spores subsequently germinate and the vegetative forms multiply and elaborate toxin in the intestines of the infant. Seven types of botulinum toxin (A through G) have been identified.[8] Most cases of infant botulism have involved type A or type B toxin. At least one case has been attributed to type F toxin.[9] The impairment in neuromuscular transmission in those three forms of botulism is related to the irreversible "binding" of toxin to efferent nerve endings. The bound toxin blocks the release of acetylcholine.

PREDISPOSING FACTORS

The term "infant botulism" is descriptive because one of the most obvious characteristics of the disease is the limited range of susceptibility. Ninety-five percent of the cases have occurred during the first 6 months of life. A prerequisite for infant botulism is the ingestion of spores during the first weeks or months of life.[5] A cross section of racial and ethnic groups has been affected. The syndrome has occurred in both sexes and in both bottle- and breast-fed babies.

EPIDEMIOLOGY

Clostridium botulinum is ubiquitous in soil, but in certain soils, particular toxigenic types may predominate. For example, most organisms found west of the Mississippi River produce type A toxin. In soils east of the Mississippi, there is a preponderance of organisms that produce type B toxin. Infant botulism has been recognized in Canada, England, Australia, and in 22 states of the United States.[5] To date, the greatest number of cases has been reported from California. Most hospitalized cases of infant botulism in that state have occurred in infants 6 months of age or less and have not been limited to any one racial or ethnic group. The actual incidence of infant botulism is unknown because the disease may easily be confused with myasthenia gravis, poliomyelitis, encephalitis, meningitis, or Guillain-Barré syndrome. No preformed toxin has been identified in food ingested by infants. Raw honey, vacuum cleaner dust, and soil have been implicated as sources of the spores of C. botulinum.

LABORATORY DIAGNOSIS

Classic botulism is usually diagnosed clinically on the basis of symptoms and recent history of consuming suspected food. A diagnosis of infant botulism is supported by electromyography. Typical patterns consist of brief, abundant unit-action potentials of small amplitude (Fig. 13–2).[10] Confirmation of a diagnosis of infant botulism is made by demonstrating the presence of botulinal toxin in sera or stool samples or the presence of C. botulinum in stool samples. Most hospital laboratories are not equipped to handle specimens from patients suspected of having botulism. If questions arise, local or state public health laboratories can be of service. The Centers for Disease Control in Atlanta, Georgia, also maintain a 24-hour telephone service to provide epidemiologic aid and laboratory services in emergencies.

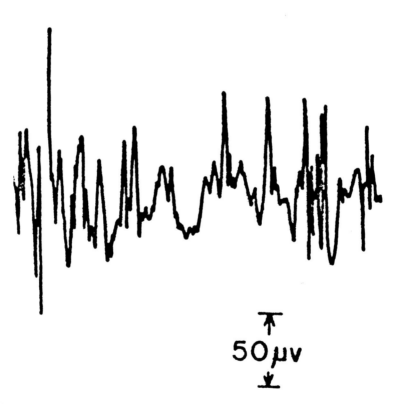

$$\bar{\top}$$
50 μv
$$\underline{\bot}$$

Figure 13–2. Small amplitude and brief polyphasic motor unit potentials from voluntary contraction of the deltoid characteristic of infant botulism. (From McKee, K.T., Kilroy, A.W., Harrison, W.W., and Schaffner, W.: Botulism in infancy. Am. J. Dis. Child., *131*:857, 1977. Copyright 1977 American Medical Association.)

Cultural Techniques

If infant botulism is suspected, as much passed stool as possible should be sent to the laboratory. Suspensions can be made by mixing approximately equal volumes of stool and physiologic saline (0.85%).

It is customary to inoculate 2 tubes of an enriched broth, such as peptone-yeast-glucose (PYG)-starch broth, with 2 drops each of the fecal suspension.[11] One tube of inoculated broth is heated in an 80°C water bath for 10 minutes to kill vegetative cells. Both inoculated tubes of PYG-starch broth are incubated anaerobically at 37°C for 24 hours.

Egg yolk agar (EYA) is the medium of choice for subculturing from heated and unheated tubes of PYG-starch broth containing growth of Clostridium botulinum. An anaerobic incubation period of 48 hours is usually sufficient to produce colonies, but prolonged incubation at 37°C up to 7 days may be required for detection of lipase activity. C. botulinum and C. sporogenes produce lipase, causing the appearance of an oily, irridescent film or sheen on EYA on the surface of the colonies or in the medium below colonies.[12] The only test that will distinguish C. botulinum from C. sporogenes is a toxin assay, because the 2 organisms are biochemically identical.

Microscopic Examination

Smears and Gram strains may be made from colonies demonstrating lipase activity or from boiled PYG-starch broth cultures. C. botulinum is a large gram-positive bacillus, measuring 1.0 to 1.5 μm by 4.0 to 8.0 μm, which produces oval subterminal spores. Gram stains, made from any suspected food, are of limited value. Supernatants of broth, serum, or stool must be proved toxinogenic to laboratory mice to support a diagnosis of infant botulism.

Toxin Assay

Homogenized food samples, serum, gastric contents, or toxin-containing broth may be used to inject white mice intraperitoneally. The mice usually exhibit neurologic symptoms and die within several hours. Sometimes trypsin is used to pretreat suspected toxin-containing material to enhance toxin activity. The type of botulinal toxin can be ascertained by neutralization experiments in mice. Since food extracts and biologic specimens may contain lethal factors not related to botulism, care must be taken in interpreting results of animal inoculations. Mouse neutralization tests are performed by some state public health laboratories and by the Centers for Disease Control in Atlanta, Georgia. All specimens should be sent to the laboratory in insulated containers maintained at -4°C.

PROGNOSIS

If babies with infant botulism are hospitalized on onset of symptoms and supportive care in the form of gavage feeding and mechanical ventilation is instituted promptly, the prognosis is excellent.[5] Deaths are rare, and most infants recover without neurologic sequelae. In some cases, antibiotics have been employed, but their efficacy is not certain. Since the only available antitoxin is equine in origin and is associated with side effects, including sensitization to horse serum, its use cannot be recommended.[13]

CASE REPORTS

Case 1

A 2-month-old boy had diffuse weakness of short duration. He was the product of an unremarkable gestation, labor, and delivery. At birth, examination was normal; he had a vigorous suck. He was breast-fed and received only vitamin preparations. Growth and development were normal until he was 6 weeks old, when over a period of 2 days he was unable to suck or swallow, and became weak. A chest radiograph demonstrated "an infiltrate," and he received ampicillin (170 mg/kg/day) and gentamicin (7 mg/kg/day) for 4 days. The weakness became more severe, and the infant was referred to University of California, San Francisco, 2 weeks later. He had received no other medication, and there was no snake bite. He had no stool for 1 week.

The infant was profoundly weak. He had mild bilateral ptosis, and the pupils were dilated and reacted sluggishly to light. The extraocular movements were full, but there was a paucity of facial movement. The gag reflex was diminished. He lay without movement. There was a severe decrease in tone and no head control. Muscle bulk was normal, stretch reflexes decreased, and plantar responses were extensor. The infant appeared to perceive touch and painful stimuli. The general examination was normal.

Routine blood and urine studies, creatine phosphokinase, cerebrospinal fluid, serum calcium, magnesium, and manganese were normal. Urine toxicology screen was negative for heavy metals. In a search for botulinal toxin, blood and stool specimens were sent for assay. Type A botulinal toxin and C. botulinum organisms were identified in the stool; no toxin was found in the serum.

Seven days after admission, his cranial-nerve function and general strength had improved; he was discharged 3½ weeks after admission in a mildly weak state. The physical examination and chest radiograph 2 weeks later were normal. Type A botulinal toxin and organisms were recovered from the stool as late as 6 weeks following diagnosis. No antitoxin was given. The toxin source remains unknown.*

Case 2

A 3-month-old boy was admitted for evaluation of weakness of 7 days' duration. He was the product of an unremarkable gestation, labor, and delivery, and the newborn examination was normal. He was an active newborn and sucked vigorously. The infant received breast milk, bananas, orange "pop," and apple juice.

Over 1 day, the infant became limp and weak. He had difficulty in supporting his head and was unable to suck well. He was thought to have a "strep throat" and was given penicillin. Swallowing was so reduced that a nasogastric feeding tube was placed. Because of increasing weakness, the infant was referred to University of California, San Francisco, for evaluation. He had no stool for 1 week. The infant received no other known medication, except for a negative Tensilon (edrophonium chloride) test, and he had not been bitten by a snake.

The infant lay without movement and was severely hypotonic, without head control. There was bilateral ptosis, the pupils were widely dilated and reacted sluggishly to light. The extraocular movements were full. There was a paucity of facial movements, and the gag reflex was depressed. Stretch reflexes were reduced or absent; plantar responses were extensor. The infant responded to touch and noxious stimuli. The general examination was normal.

Routine blood and urine studies, routine chest radiograph, creatine phosphokinase, serum calcium, magnesium, and manganese were normal. Urine toxicology screen for heavy metals was negative. Serum and stool specimens were submitted for identification of botulinal toxin; Type B toxin was identified in the stool but not the serum.

Ten days after admission the ptosis disappeared, the suck and swallow improved so that the nasogastric tube was removed, and he could support his head. The tone and muscle power returned to normal over a 3-week period. The toxin source is unknown. He received no antitoxin treatment.*

Case 3

The patient was a male term product of a 19-year-old gravida 1 woman whose pregnancy and breech delivery were uncomplicated. The child was vigorous from birth. He was well until the twenty-second day of life when he became irritable and was treated with a penicillin preparation for "sore throat and ears." Symptoms persisted,

*From Pickett, J., Berg, B., Chaplin, E., and Brunstetter-Shafer, M.: N. Engl. J. Med., *295*:770–771, 1976. Reprinted by permission of the New England Journal of Medicine.[2]

with constipation and mild weakness noted the following day. The next morning, weakness had increased in severity, and swallowing became difficult. The infant was taken to a clinic, where he experienced a cyanotic episode in the waiting room. He was resuscitated by vigorous stimulation and promptly admitted to a hospital. No other family members were ill, and there was no history of traumatic wound, snakebite, or household poison exposure. Physical examination at that time revealed an afebrile infant with profound weakness and hypotonia. Areflexia, ptosis, sluggish pupillary responses to light, and limitation of extraocular movements to 15° lateral gaze were noted. Scattered rhonchi were present on auscultation of the chest. The WBC count was 13,900/cu mm, with the differential cell count, hemoglobin level, serum electrolyte levels, calcium level, and results of urinalysis all within normal limits. Lumbar puncture was traumatic, with 2340 RBCs and no WBCs per cu mm of CSF. The CSF protein level was 140 mg/100 ml and the glucose level, 33 mg/100 ml. Gram's stain, India ink examination, and culture of CSF were negative. Skull and chest roentgenograms were normal. Serum amino acid pattern was unremarkable, and tests for drugs in the urine using both gas and thin-layer chromatography were negative. Bacteria did not grow from blood cultures obtained at admission. Electromyography (EMG) was performed and demonstrated occasional low-amplitude complexes that did not appear unusually brief in duration; however, well-formed motor complexes were never recorded. An equivocal result was obtained on edrophonium chloride challenge, but repeat examination with physostigmine was negative. After 5 days without improvement, the child was transferred to Vanderbilt Children's Hospital.

Physical examination on arrival at Vanderbilt revealed an afebrile infant with watery diarrhea who was hypotonic, but not obtunded. The pupils were equal, large, and reacted only slowly to light. No voluntary extraocular movements were noted, although oculocephalic reflexes (doll's eyes) were demonstrable bilaterally. There was bilateral facial weakness and ptosis, absent gag reflex, and a weak cry. Generalized weakness and areflexia were present, but sensation appeared intact. Muscle mass was normal. There was no wound and the umbilical stump was well-healed. The remainder of the findings from the physical examination were normal.

Laboratory values were essentially unchanged from those obtained previously. Lumbar puncture yielded clear CSF with 1 mononuclear cell and no RBCs per cu mm. Protein level was 90 mg/100 ml, and glucose level 38 mg/100 ml (simultaneous serum glucose level was 76 mg/100 ml). Gram's stain, countercurrent immunoelectrophoresis (against pneumococcal, meningococcal, and Haemophilus influenzae antisera), and cultures were negative. Blood and urine cultures were negative, and no Salmonella or Shigella grew from stool cultures. Electroencephalography was normal.

The infant was treated for 3 days with ampicillin sodium, 200 mg/kg/day and gentamicin sulfate, 5 mg/kg/day until cultures were returned as negative. Diarrhea subsided the day after admission.

Two days later, stool samples were collected by means of a tap water enema, and sent with serum specimens to the laboratories of the Tennessee Department of Public Health and the Enteric Diseases Division, Bureau of Epidemiology, Center for Disease Control, Atlanta, for anaerobic culture and analysis for botulinus toxin. Mouse neutralization assay in both laboratories confirmed the presence of Type B botulinus toxin in fecal specimens, while serum specimens were negative. Stool cultures revealed the presence of Clostridium botulinum type B.

Electromyography was performed on admission to Vanderbilt Children's Hospital. The right median nerve showed normal motor conduction velocity and distal motor latency with, however, an abnormally small compound muscle action potential of 1 μV. There was no significant decrementing response on 2 per second stimulation. A more complete study 6 days later showed, after 10 seconds of tetanic stimulation to the right median nerve, a posttetanic facilitation to 152%, assuming pretetanic amplitude as 100%. Needle examination of the right deltoid and right quadriceps muscles in both studies showed occasional fibrillations at rest. On voluntary contraction, the motor unit potentials were of decreased amplitude, up to 175 μV, and many were of brief duration and polyphasic form. These findings were consistent with those of botulism.

By the fifth day of illness, the child had begun to improve clinically, with slow but steady progress thereafter. By 2 weeks' time, hypotonia and weakness (including impaired extraocular function) had virtually resolved, and there were no apparent focal neurologic residua.

Details of the feeding history in this infant disclosed that he had been fed only canned formula of a single standard, commercial type from birth, with the exception of 2 packets of dry formula mix 2 weeks prior to the onset of symptoms. Additionally, the infant had received occasional doses of milk of magnesia, acetaminophen drops, and water with corn syrup. Culture and toxin analysis of all products done in the laboratories of the Food and Drug Administration were unrevealing.*

---

*From McKee, K.T., Kilroy, A.W., Harrison, W.W., and Schaffner, W.: Am. J. Dis. Child., *131*:857–859, 1977. Copyright 1977, American Medical Association.[6]

SUMMARY

Infant botulism is now recognized as a form of botulism and is associated primarily with toxin serotypes A and B of Clostridium botulinum. The disease occurs only in infants who are presumed to have ingested spores of the organism in the first few weeks or months of life. Infant botulism is deserving of consideration in the differential diagnosis of causes for constipation, hypotonia, and listlessness in children under 1 year of age. The specific conditions that permit colonization of C. botulinum in the intestinal tract of infants remain to be elucidated. Observations in animal models suggest that infants may not have acquired competing intestinal microorganisms indigenous to adults. If lack of certain indigenous microorganisms or their products proves to be a contributory factor in infant botulism, it is likely that a counterpart of the disease could occur in adults as a consequence of antimicrobial therapy.

REFERENCES

1. Center for Disease Control: Botulism in the United States, 1899–1977. Handbook for epidemiologists, clinicians, and laboratory workers. Atlanta, Georgia, 1979.
2. Pickett, J., Berg, B., Chaplin, E., and Brunstetter-Shafer, M.: Syndrome of botulism in infancy: Clinical and electrophysiologic study. N. Engl. J. Med., 295:770, 1976.
3. Centers for Disease Control: Botulism—United States, 1979–1980. Morbid. Mortal. Weekly Rept., 30:121, 1981.
4. Centers for Disease Control: Wound botulism associated with parenteral cocaine abuse—New York City. Morbid. Mortal. Weekly Rept., 31:87, 1982.
5. Midura, T.F.: Infant botulism. Clin. Microbiol. Newsl., 2:1, 1980.
6. McKee, K.T., Kilroy, A.W., Harrison, W.W., and Schaffner, W.: Botulism in infancy. Am. J. Dis. Child., 131:857, 1977.
7. Arnon, S.S., and Chin, J.: The clinical spectrum of infant botulism. Rev. Infect. Dis., 1:614, 1979.
8. Peterson, D.R., Eklund, M.W., and Chinn, N.M.: The sudden infant death syndrome and infant botulism. Rev. Infect. Dis., 1:630, 1979.
9. Centers for Disease Control. Type F infant botulism—New Mexico. Morbid. Mortal. Weekly Rept., 29:85, 1980.
10. Arnon, S.S., et al.: Infant botulism; Epidemiological, clinical and laboratory aspects. JAMA, 237:1946, 1977.
11. Rosenblatt, J.E.: Anaerobic bacteria. In Laboratory Procedures in Clinical Microbiology. Edited by J.A. Washington. New York, Springer-Verlag, 1981.
12. Allen, S.D., and Siders, J.A.: Procedures for isolation and characterization of anaerobic bacteria. In Manual of Clinical Microbiology, 3rd Ed. Edited by E.H. Lennette. Washington, D.C., American Society for Microbiology, 1980.
13. Merson, M.H., et al.: Current trends in botulism in the United States. JAMA, 229:1305, 1974.

CHAPTER 14 KAWASAKI SYNDROME

Kawasaki syndrome was first recognized as a clinical entity in 50 Japanese children by Dr. Tomisaku Kawasaki in 1967.[1] The syndrome, which is still sometimes called mucocutaneous lymph node syndrome, was thought to be relatively rare, benign, and self-limiting. Since that time, however, the syndrome has been reported with increasing frequency in Japan and other countries.[2-6] Kawasaki syndrome was first recognized in the United States in Hawaii in 1971.[7] Since that time, more than 25,000 cases of the enigmatic syndrome have been recorded in 6 nationwide surveys. In one instance, the disease appeared to occur 3 times in the same patient.[8] The fatality rate, which approximates 2%, is associated with sudden death or coronary artery aneurysms.[9]

Kawasaki syndrome is a multisystem disorder, and diagnosis depends not only on satisfying 5 of 6 criteria, but also on ruling out other multisystem disorders. The diagnostic criteria for Kawasaki disease are as follows:*

A. Fever of 5 or more days
B. Presence of 4 of the following 5 conditions
    1. Bilateral conjunctival injection
    2. One or more changes in the mucous membranes of the upper respiratory tract, such as:
       injected pharynx
       injected lips
       dry, fissured lips
       "strawberry" tongue
    3. One or more changes in the peripheral extremities, such as:
       peripheral edema
       peripheral erythema
       desquamation
       periungual desquamation
    4. Rash, primarily truncal; polymorphous but nonvesicular
    5. Cervical lymphadenopathy
C. Illness cannot be explained by other known disease process

---

*From Centers for Disease Control: Kawasaki disease—New York. Morbid. Mortal. Weekly Rept., 29:61, 1980.

The most prominent features of Kawasaki disease are arteritis of medium-sized arteries and palmar and solar erythema of a deep purple-red. Fever, however, is the first sign of illness. Temperatures ranging from 101°F to 104°F have been reported in the acute febrile phase, which may last from 6 to 25 days. Conjunctival alterations usually consist of easily recognized vascular injection of bulbar and palpebral conjunctivae. Less frequently, follicular palpebral conjunctivitis is present. Strawberry tongue and oropharyngeal erythema are similar to those associated with streptococcal disease. Dryness of the lips often reults in cracks, fissures, crusting, or even bleeding.

Another characteristic associated with Kawasaki syndrome is that the skin appears to be tightly stretched over the hands and feet in a manner resembling the induration of acute scleroderma. A concomitant fusiform swelling of the fingers and toes is painful and often interferes with a child's ability to grasp objects or to stand in an erect position. An erythematous rash is usually diffuse, but is frequently observed on the extremities and on the trunk. The lesions are morbilliform, urticarial, polymorphous, or scarlatine in form. No vesicular, bullous, or petechial lesions are seen.

At least 90% of patients with Kawasaki syndrome exhibit fever, conjunctival injection, erythema of the mouth, palms, and soles, and an erythematous rash during the first week of illnes. Lymphadenopathy has been reported in 75% of Japanese patients and in at least 50% of the patients in the United States. Cervical lymph nodes are most frequently enlarged. The lymph node involvement is usually unilateral. Lymph node masses must measure more than 1.5 cm in diameter to meet the diagnostic criterion. Lethargy, irritability, emotional instability, and anorexia are additional features associated with the acute febrile phase of Kawasaki syndrome.

In the subacute phase of Kawasaki syndrome, the fever begins to subside and lymph nodes return to normal. The desquamation of palms and soles that occurs is not unlike that observed in patients with toxic shock syndrome. Arthritis, arthralgias, and cardiac disease are complications of the subacute phase of the syndrome. Cardiac complications occur in approximately 20% of patients with Kawasaki syndrome.[10,11]

Other complications that can occur during the acute febrile or subacute phases demonstrate features of multisystem disease. The associated features of Kawasaki syndrome in their order of frequency are as follows:*

---

*From Melish, M.E.: Kawasaki syndrome (The mucocutaneous lymph node syndrome). *In* Medical Microbiology and Infectious Diseases. Edited by A.I. Braude. Philadelphia, W.B. Saunders, 1981.

Pyuria and urethritis
Arthralgia and arthritis
Aseptic meningitis
Diarrhea
Abdominal pain
Obstructive jaundice
Hydrops of gallbladder
Myocardiopathy
Pericardial effusion
Acute mitral insufficiency
Myocardial infarction

A self-limiting liver dysfunction occurs in about 10% of patients. Gallbladder distention, verifiable by ultrasound, is observed in approximately 3% of the patients.[12]

The duration of the subacute phase of Kawasaki syndrome varies, but usually lasts at least 2 weeks in the absence of complications. The convalescent phase begins when no signs of illness are detectable and lasts until the sedimentation rate has returned to normal. The convalescent phase may last for 6 to 8 weeks.[13]

ETIOLOGY

Although Kawasaki syndrome resembles an infectious disease, it has not been associated with a particular microorganism. Initially, a group A β-hemolytic Streptococcus was suspected as the probable cause, but the streptococci have been ruled out as the etiologic agent of Kawasaki syndrome by extensive cultural and serologic studies. More recently, similarities between toxic shock syndrome (TSS) and Kawasaki syndrome have led to a consideration of an exotoxin-producing Staphylococcus aureus as the etiologic agent of Kawasaki syndrome. Although S. aureus has been isolated in at least 20% of cases of the syndrome, the rate of colonization is not higher than in some healthy groups of individuals.[2] Attempts to isolate viruses, rickettsiae, and leptospires from patients with Kawasaki syndrome have yielded inconsistent results.

PREDISPOSING FACTORS

In one study, children who developed Kawasaki syndrome were reported to have had previous episodes of pharyngitis, eczema, urticaria, or allergic rhinitis.[3] In a limited number of cases, antecedent infections with parainfluenza viruses have occurred.[14,15] In all studies made to date, boys have appeared to be more susceptible than girls to Kawasaki syndrome. Some caution must be exercised in interpreting data, however, because of the limited number of cases.

EPIDEMIOLOGY

Data obtained since 1974 indicate that Kawasaki syndrome is worldwide in distribution, occurring in both developed and developing countries. The multisystem entity has been recognized most frequently in Japan and Hawaii. Surveillance studies in Japan have documented a steady increase in numbers of cases of the syndrome reported since 1971. More than 25,000 cases have occurred in that country, primarily in endemic form. No striking geographic or seasonal differences in incidence have been evident, but cases of the disease in boys have outnumbered those in girls by a ratio of 1.5 to 1. No common-source outbreaks have surfaced, and person-to-person transmission appears to be rare.[3]

Data from the Centers for Disease Control show an over-representation of children of Oriental ancestry among reported cases when compared with Caucasian children.[9] The reason is not clear. A genetic predisposition to Kawasaki syndrome has been suspected, but no one HLA antigen has been common to all cases.

LABORATORY DIAGNOSIS

The diagnosis of Kawasaki syndrome is based on the clinical criteria described earlier in the chapter. The laboratory abnormalities are nonspecific.[9] The white blood cell count is elevated, with a preponderance of polymorphonuclear cells, during the first week of illness. C-reactive protein and sedimentation rate are elevated for 6 to 10 weeks. An increase in circulating platelets is universal after 10 days and averages 800,000/mm[3]. Although elevation of serum glutamic-oxaloacetic transaminase (SGOT), serum glutamic-pyruvic transaminase (SGPT), and alkaline phosphatase can occur, they are by no means universal findings. The continuing search for a microbial-associated etiology may one day reveal the value of additional laboratory tests in Kawasaki syndrome.

PROGNOSIS

Kawasaki syndrome is self-limiting in most patients. A 2% mortality rate has been reported for the syndrome in Japan. Deaths in Japanese children have occurred during the third or fourth weeks following onset, when recovery was expected.[8] In most instances, death was caused by myocardial infarction associated with coronary thrombosis. A total of approximately 20% of patients with Kawasaki syndrome in Japan develop cardiac disease.[7]

Manifestations other than myocardial infarction include myocarditis, mitral insufficiency, aneurysms, and arrhythmias. Risk factors for aneurysms include a history of cardiogenic shock on onset of the disease, mitral insufficiency, cardiomegaly, or myocardial infarction.[10,11] Other risk factors of less significance for predicting cardiac complications are age of less than 1 year, male sex, recrudescent fever, or initial fever for more than 14 days, history of arrhythmias, or other ECG abnormalities. Long-term follow-up studies will be required to determine the incidence of premature arteriosclerosis or morbidity associated with coronary artery disease.

CASE REPORTS

Case 1

A 3-year-old black boy spent several hours in close contact with his first cousin during his cousin's first day of fever. The boys had not played together during the preceding 10 days, nor were they together during the subsequent month. Fourteen days after playing with his ill cousin, the patient became febrile (temperature, 39°C) and was hospitalized with an almost confluent macular rash over the upper trunk and arms, a flushed face with very red, dry lips, bilateral conjunctival injection, and 3 enlarged cervical nodes, the largest measuring 2 cm. By the fourth day of illness, a supraclavicular node, swollen fissured lips, and erythema of palms and soles were noted. The total duration of fever was 8 days. The boy's rash had faded, and peeling of his fingers and palms began on day 11 of the illness. The ESR was 122 mm/hr; WBC count, 17,500/cu mm; platelet count, 655,000/cu mm; and IgE level, 34 units/ml. There was pyuria; an ASO titer was normal and a slide test for infectious mononucleosis heterophil antibody was negative. Multiple cultures of blood and urine were negative; a throat culture yielded normal bacterial flora; and no viruses were isolated from throat or stool. A chest roentgenogram showed mild cardiac enlargement; the ECG and echocardiogram were normal. Immune-adherence hemagglutination titers to parainfluenza type 3 rose from below 1:8 on the third day of illness to 1:32 on the 28th day. Parainfluenza type 1 titers in these specimens were both below 1:8.

Seroconversion could not be demonstrated against the following agents: leptospirae (12 antigens), Epstein-Barr virus, Legionella pneumophila, influenza A or B, measles, herpes simplex, adenovirus, varicella-zoster, Mycoplasma pneumoniae, Chlamydia, cytomegalovirus, or respiratory syncytial virus. Tissue culture media used were sensitive for parainfluenza and other respiratory viruses. The child recovered uneventfully.

The patient had not had any illnesses, immunizations, or medications within 1 month before onset of KS. Other than the sibling of the cousin, no playmates or household contacts of either patient became ill within 2 to 3 weeks before or after the onset of KS. The patient's and cousin's mothers are biologic sisters. There is no known

family history of illness resembling KS, early cardiac death, or autoimmune or collagen vascular disease. Parental permission could not
be obtained for an evaluation of family genetic relationships.*

Case 2

The patient is a 26-year-old female pathologist. On the day of onset
she awoke with malaise, nausea, vomiting, and diffuse headache. She
had fever and chills with temperature reaching 39.6°C. Aspirin produced defervescence and diaphoresis. She felt better over the next 2
days, even though she was fatigued and experienced occasional periods of tachycardia. Three days after onset the patient awoke with
generalized arthralgia, profound asthenia, severe muscle pain, and
headache. She had abdominal pain, and nausea and vomiting, but no
diarrhea. She had fever, chills, and diaphoresis. Her urine output was
diminished. A nonpruritic erythematous indurative rash developed
over her palms and soles. She took 2 or 3 doses of erythromycin, 250
mg. Four days after onset she was seen by one of us (John H. Vaughan,
M.D.) and was admitted to the Green Hospital of Scripps Clinic. New
symptoms at this time included a mild cough, palpitations, tachycardia, and dysuria. She appeared pale and acutely ill. The temperature
was 39.4°C, the pulse 100, and the respirations 20. The blood pressure
was 70/40 mm Hg. Posterior cervical and axillary nodes were small
but tender. The conjunctivae were injected. The tonsils and posterior
pharynx were erythematous. The neck was supple. The chest was
clear. The heart was not enlarged; a grade I/VI early systolic ejection
murmur was heard at the apex; a faint 2-component rub was heard
along the left sternal border; an S sound was present. The abdomen
was flat and diffusely tender, and there was no enlargement of the
liver or spleen. There was diffuse muscle pain. Marked erythema was
present over the palms and soles. The neurologic examination was
normal.

The urine had a specific gravity of 1.024. There was 2+ protein,
and the sediment contained 3 to 5 erythrocytes, 25 to 30 leukocytes,
and some granular casts per high-power field. The hematocrit was
39%; the leukocyte count was 19,800/mm³ with 57 segmented neutrophils, 35 band forms, 3 lymphocytes, 3 monocytes, and 2-meta-
myelocytes. The electrolytes, the platelets, and the prothrombin time
were normal. The glutamic oxaloacetic transaminase level was greater
than 300 mU/ml (normal, 7 to 40 mU/ml) and total bilirubin was 2
mg/dl. Two days later the bilirubin was normal and the serum glutamic
oxaloacetic transaminase was 78 IU/L (normal, 8 to 30 IU/L), the
alkaline phosphatase was 12.7 IU/dl (normal, 4.5 to 11.0 IU/dl), and

---

*From Schnaar, D.A., and Bell, D.M.: Am. J. Dis. Child, *136*:554–555, 1982. Copyright
1982, American Medical Association.[15]

the creatine phosphokinase was normal. The antistreptolysin O titer, the streptococcal enzyme slide agglutination test, and the heterophil titer were all negative. Hepatitis B surface antigen and core antibody were absent. Two bacterial blood cultures were sterile, and a throat culture was negative for group A β-hemolytic streptococci. Serum protein electrophoresis was normal. Roentgenograms of the chest and abdomen were normal. An electrocardiogram showed no abnormalities.

During the next 2 days in the hospital, the patient received intravenous fluids, intravenous penicillin, 6 million U/d, and naproxen sodium (Naprosyn; Syntex Laboratories, Inc., Palo Alto, California), 250 mg orally twice a day. Her temperature rapidly subsided. It was 37.6°C on the second hospital day and was normal on the third. The leukocyte count at that time was 6700/mm³ with a normal differential except for 9 eosinophils. The patient's subsequent recovery was uneventful except for a tachycardia of about 90 beats per minute that was still present at discharge on the sixth hospital day. The only other striking physical finding was the desquamation of her palms and soles.

Two weeks after hospitalization the patient developed a sore throat and unilateral conjunctivitis. On physical examination she was noted to have a pulse rate of 92. She was afebrile, and the rest of her examination was unremarkable except for injection of the pharynx and conjunctiva and continuing desquamation of palms and soles. The leukocyte count, the platelet count, and the sedimentation rate were normal. Throat culture was negative for group A β-hemolytic streptococci; bacterial culture of the conjunctiva was sterile. Heterophil, antistreptolysin O titer, and hepatitis B core-antibody titer were negative. Liver function test results were normal.

Four weeks after hospitalization the patient had an episode of shaking chills, nausea, and copious vomiting accompanied by right upper quadrant pain and diffuse myalgia. She was admitted to the University of California at Los Angeles Hospital. Physical examination revealed an acutely ill young woman. The temperature was 38°C, the pulse 116, and the respirations 16. The blood pressure was 90/60 mm Hg. The skin was clear except for a residual scaling of her feet. Conjunctivae were pink. There was no erythema of the posterior pharynx, but the tongue was bright red. Chest was clear. Heart examination was normal. There was tenderness to palpation in the right upper quadrant. Liver span was 14 cm, and the spleen tip was palpable. Results of pelvic and rectal examination were normal. The muscles were diffusely tender. There were peripheral edema of the extremities and swelling and pain of the metacarpophalangeal joints of both thumbs. Results of neurologic examination were normal. The leukocyte count was 22,200/mm³ with 71 segmented neutrophils, 24 band forms, 1 basophil, 2 lymphocytes, and 2 monocytes. The erythrocyte sedimentation rate was 27 mm/hour. The platelet count was 253,000/mm³. The urinalysis revealed 5 to 10 leukocytes/hpf.

During the first 3 days in the hospital, the patient continued to have fever spikes up to 39.5°C. On the fourth day, the patient's fever subsided. This coincided with the administration of 2 doses of naproxen, 250 mg. Along with the fever, she experienced severe myalgias. The marked palmar and plantar erythema recurred. A pericardial friction rub was heard on several occasions over a 2-day period. The patient was discharged on the tenth day of hospitalization. The leukocyte count on the day of discharge was 5900/mm³ with 49 segmented neutrophils, 14 band forms, 31 lymphocytes, and 6 monocytes. The erythrocyte sedimentation rate was 54 mm/hour.

Six blood cultures and two urine cultures had been negative for bacteria, and a throat culture revealed only normal flora. Serologic testing was negative for Toxoplasma, Epstein-Barr virus, cytomegalovirus, antistreptolysin O, cold agglutinins, and leptospirosis. The mononucleosis slide agglutination test was negative. Results of antinuclear antibody tests were later performed on a serum specimen obtained during this hospitalization. The results of both tests were negative. The bone marrow and the urine were negative for acid-fast bacilli. Skin tests were negative for coccidioidomycosis, Candida, and purified protein derivative, but positive for streptokinase-streptodornase. The patient had a normal echocardiogram; a normal ultrasound examination of the liver, gallbladder, and pelvic organs; and a normal gallium scan.

Within 2 weeks of discharge, she returned to her usual state of good health.*

Case 3

A 16-year-old woman experienced weakness, dizziness, and mild nausea 3 days before hospitalization. These symptoms persisted, and a temperature of 38.3°C was noted 2 days before admission. On the day before transfer to the University of Missouri Medical Center, her temperature rose to 40°C, and she was seen by her family physician, who transferred her to a local hospital. The WBC count there showed 14,600/cu mm, with 75% neutrophils, 15% band forms, and 10% mononuclear cells. Urinalysis showed 1+ protein and 50 to 60 WBCs per high-power field. The BUN level was elevated to 38 mg/dl, and a liver profile was normal. Throat culture, CSF examination, blood culture, and urine culture were performed and were subsequently negative. The patient was given aspirin, and 600,000 units of penicillin G procaine was given intramuscularly every 8 hours. There was no

*From Milgrom, H., et al.: Ann. Intern. Med., 92:467–470, 1980. © 1980, American College of Physicians.[16]

improvement after 24 hours, and the patient was transferred to the University of Missouri Medical Center in Columbia.

At the time of admission, she appeared acutely ill, with a pulse rate of 116 beats per minute and a temperature of 40°C. She had a diffuse macular erythematous rash, reddening of the palms and soles, and red oral mucous membranes. The tongue was red with prominent papillae. Mild conjunctival injection was present, and tender occipital lymph nodes measuring 1.5 cm in diameter were present. No other family members or friends were known to have a similar illness.

The WBC count was 12,200/cu mm, with 44% band cells, 55% neutrophils, and 1% lymphocytes. Urinalysis again showed pyuria; however, a urine culture was subsequently negative. A chest roentgenogram was normal. Blood and throat cultures were obtained and were negative. Results of a heterophil agglutination and a fluorescent antinuclear antibody test were negative.

The patient continued to receive penicillin for an additional dose, but because of lack of response and her degree of clinical illness, her therapy was changed to gentamicin sulfate and methicillin. Acute and convalescent sera for antibodies to streptococci, rubella, coxsackievirus B1–6, adenovirus, and rubeola were negative. Convalescent sera 12 days after the onset of the illness showed no antibodies to Leptospira. By the third hospital day, the rash had diminished, and desquamation of the soles of her feet was noted. Her condition gradually improved, and she was afebrile by the sixth day of illness. On the eleventh day of hospitalization, membranous desquamation of the fingertips occurred. She was well on follow-up 6 weeks after discharge from the hospital.*

SUMMARY

Kawasaki syndrome is a symptom complex having some epidemiologic features of an infectious disease to which young children of Japanese ancestry appear uniquely susceptible. Although the clinical course of the syndrome resembles that of infectious disease, no infectious agent has been isolated with regularity. The inciting agents may be multiple, but the subacute stage, which is associated with thrombocytosis, cardiac complications, and arthritis, strongly suggests an immune-mediated disease. Recommendations for definitive therapy await isolation of an etiologic agent or demonstration of pathogenesis in Kawasaki syndrome.

---

*From Everett, E.D.: JAMA, *242*:542–543, 1979. Copyright 1979, American Medical Association.[7]

REFERENCES

1. Kawasaki, T.: Acute febrile mucocutaneous syndrome with lymphoid involvement with specific desquamation of the fingers and toes in children: Clinical observations of 50 cases (in Japanese). Jpn. J. Allergol., *16*:178, 1967.
2. Kawasaki, T., et al.: A new infantile acute febrile mucocutaneous lymph node syndrome (MLNS) prevailing in Japan. Pediatrics, *54*:271, 1974.
3. Yanagawa, H., Shigematsu, I., Kusakawa, S., and Kawasaki, T.: Epidemiology of Kawasaki disease in Japan (in Japanese). Acta Paediatra Japonica, *21*:1, 1979.
4. Melish, M.E., Hicks, R.M., and Dean, A.G.: Kawasaki syndrome in Hawaii (abstract). Pediatr. Res., *13*:451, 1979.
5. Melish, M.E., Hicks, R.M., and Larson, E.J.: Mucocutaneous lymph node syndrome in the United State (abstract). Pediatr. Res., *8*:427, 1974.
6. Melish, M.E., Hicks, R.M., and Larson, E.S.: Mucocutaneous lymph node syndrome in the United State. Am. J. Dis. Child., *130*:599, 1976.
7. Everett, E.D.: Mucocutaneous lymph node syndrome (Kawasaki disease) in adults. JAMA, *242*:542, 1979.
8. Snell, G.F.: Adult Kawasaki—three occurrences in the same patient. West. J. Med., *132*:548, 1980.
9. Melish, M.E.: Kawasaki syndrome: A new infectious disease? J. Infect. Dis., *143*:317, 1981.
10. Kusakawa, S., and Asai, T.: Cardiovascular lesions. *In* Kawasaki Disease. Vascular Lesions of Collagen Diseases and Related Conditions. Edited by Y. Shiokawa. Tokyo, University of Tokyo Press, 1977.
11. Kato, H., et al.: Coronary heart disease in children with Kawasaki disease. Jpn. Circ. J., *43*:469, 1979.
12. Magilavy, D.B., et al.: Mucocutaneous lymph node syndrome: report of two cases complicated by gallbladder hydrops and diagnosed by ultrasound. Pediatrics, *61*:699, 1978.
13. Melish, M.: Kawasaki syndrome (The mucocutaneous lymph node syndrome). *In* Medical Microbiology and Infectious Diseases. Edited by A.I. Braude. Philadelphia, W.B. Saunders, 1981.
14. Bell, D.M., et al.: Kawasaki syndrome. Description of two outbreaks in the United States. N. Engl. J. Med., *304*:1568, 1981.
15. Schnaar, D.A., and Bell, D.M.: Kawasaki syndrome in two cousins with parainfluenza virus infection. Am. J. Dis. Child., *136*:554, 1982.
16. Milgrom, H., et al.: Kawasaki disease in a healthy young adult. Ann. Intern. Med., *92*:467, 1980.

CHAPTER 15 LEGIONNAIRES' DISEASE

Legionnaires' disease is an acute febrile respiratory disease that was thought to have made its first appearance following a convention of the Pennsylvania American Legion in the summer of 1976 in Philadelphia.[1] It now appears that the pulmonary infection is widespread and occurred as early as 1947.[2] The flurry of research activity that followed the outbreak in Philadelphia led to the isolation of Legionnaires' disease bacillus (LDB) in less than 6 months. Since that time, a number of organisms have been associated with the disease.[3-8]

The manifestations of Legionnaires' disease range from an asymptomatic infection to severe pneumonia. Some individuals experience only mild influenza-type illnesses.[9,10] Legionnaires' disease has aroused the curiosity of microbial sleuths around the world because the disease sometimes occurs as an opportunistic infection and at other times occurs as a primary infection.

PNEUMONIC LEGIONNAIRES' DISEASE

The pneumonic form of Legionnaires' disease qualifies for classification as an atypical pneumonia. In contrast to many bacterial pneumonias, atypical pneumonias are characterized by a paucity of physical symptoms; however, extensive roentgenographic evidence exists on chest films for the presence of an infectious process.[11] There are no clinical or x-ray markers that differentiate pneumonic Legionnaires' disease from a host of other atypical pneumonias. Atypical pneumonias may be caused by a variety of microorganisms, including viruses, bacteria, parasites, and fungi (Table 15–1). A thorough history, with emphasis on recent travel, environmental exposure to birds, arthropods, domestic or wild animals, patient contact, and use of immunosuppressive drugs, is important in making a differential diagnosis.

Extrapulmonary findings occur with sufficient consistency to make them useful in a differential diagnosis (Table 15–2).

Table 15–1. Etiologic agents of atypical pneumonia.

Bacteria	Viruses	Fungi	Parasites
Chlamydia psittaci*	Orthomyxoviruses, serotypes A, B	Aspergillus fumigatus	Pneumocystis carinii
Coxiella burnetii*		Blastomyces dermatitidis	
Mycoplasma pneumoniae*	Paramyxoviruses respiratory syncytial (RS), serotype 1 parainfluenza serotypes 1, 2, 3, 4	Candida albicans	Toxoplasma gondii
Rickettsia rickettsii*		Cryptococcus neoformans	
Bacillus anthracis		Histoplasma capsulatum	Strongyloides stercoralis
Yersinia pestis		Nocardia asteroides	
Legionella species	Adenoviruses serotypes 1, 2, 3, 4, 5, 6, 7, 14, 21	Pseudallescheria boydii	
Salmonella species			
Brucella species			
Franciscella tularensis	Herpesviruses herpes simplex cytomegalovirus		
Leptospira interrogans, sero-type icterohaemorrhagiae	Picornavirus rhinovirus, serotypes 1–90 coxsackievirus, serotypes A2, A4, A5, A6, A7, A12, A21, B2, B3, B5 Coronaviruses serotypes B814, B229E, C43		

*The pneumonias caused by those agents are most likely to mimic symptoms of the pneumonic form of Legionnaires' disease.

Table 15–2.   Clinical manifestations of pneumonic Legionnaires' disease.

Pulmonary Manifestations	Extrapulmonary Manifestations
Extensive x-ray evidence	Abnormal kidney function
Nonproductive cough	Abnormal liver function
Pneumonia	Bradycardia
	CNS involvement
	Diarrhea
	Fever
	Hyponatremia
	Hypophosphatemia
	Leukocytosis

Adapted from Lattimer, G.L., and Ormsbee, R.A.: Legionnaires' Disease. New York, Marcel Dekker, 1981.

NONPNEUMONIC LEGIONNAIRES' DISEASE

In 1968, an outbreak of an acute nonpneumonic febrile illness occurred in Pontiac, Michigan among employees and visitors who were in an air-conditioned health department building.[12] The disease was called Pontiac fever after the Michigan city. Subsequent investigation connected the illness to the air-conditioning system of the health department building and established LDB as the etiologic agent. Pontiac fever differs from the pneumonic infection because it is milder, is self-limiting, and has a shorter incubation period.

NOSOCOMIAL LEGIONNAIRES' DISEASE

Outbreaks of nosocomial Legionnaires' disease have occurred in several cities, but the best studied outbreak occurred at the Wadsworth Veterans Administration Hospital in Los Angeles between May and December of 1978.[13] Sixty patients and five employees, most of whom had underlying disease or a history of recent immunosuppressive therapy, acquired Legionnaires' disease. Only four individuals were enjoying good health before onset of the disease. Some clinical and epidemiologic features of community-acquired Legionnaires' disease, Pontiac fever, and nosocomial Legionnaires' disease are compared in Table 15–3.

ETIOLOGY

The etiologic agent of the Philadelphia outbreak of Legionnaires' disease proved to be a pleomorphic gram-negative motile bacillus, which was subsequently named Legionella pneumophila. The name is derived from the word legion and the primary anatomic site affected. At the present time, any disease caused by a Legionella species or a Legionella-like organism (LLO) is called Legionnaires' disease. Other recognized species of Legionella include L. bozemanii, L. micdadei, L. dumoffii, L. gormanii, L. longbeachae, and L. jordanis.[12–16] The term Legionnaires' disease bacillus (LDB) is a comprehensive description of any Legionella or LLO that causes the clinical entity now recognized as Legionnaires' disease.

LDB usually can be found extracellularly in alveolar spaces and intracellularly in macrophages and leukocytes (Fig. 15–1). Despite the frequent multisystem involvement in Legionnaires' disease, LDB has only been isolated from pulmonary exudate, lung tissue, and blood.[17] The exact mechanism of pathogenesis remains to be elucidated. No enterotoxin or exotoxin has been found in patients with Legionnaires' disease, but the inflammatory response initiated by LDB is consistent with a toxinogenic reaction.[11] Cell suspensions of LDB do promote gelation of a substance obtained from red blood cells of the horseshoe crab Limulus polyphemus, but no evidence of endotoxin has been demonstrated in patients with Legionnaires' disease. The Limulus test has been used to detect very small amounts of endotoxin in the peripheral blood of patients with bacteremia caused by other gram-negative bacilli.

PREDISPOSING FACTORS

Underlying disease was not found to be a significant factor in the Philadelphia epidemic of Legionnaires' disease in 1976 nor in the Pontiac fever outbreak in 1968; however, hospitalized patients with underlying disease or those who have been compromised by immunosuppressive drugs appear to be at higher risk than immunocom-

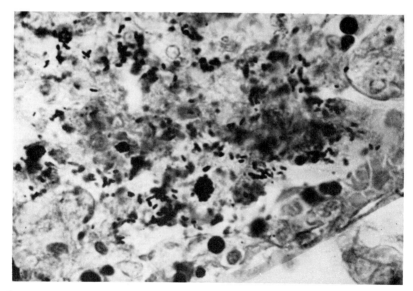

Figure 15–1. LDB in lung tissue. The bacilli appear extracellularly and in clusters of macrophages. (From Lattimer, G.L., and Ormsbee, R.A.: Legionnaires' Disease. New York, Marcel Dekker, 1981.)

petent hosts.[18] Clearly, any factor that predisposes an individual to chronic bronchitis and emphysema increases an individual's susceptibility to disease. A postmortem study of 263 sporadic cases of nosocomial pneumonia revealed that LDB was the etiologic agent in 10 cases.[19] Eight patients had a history of receiving corticosteroid therapy before onset of LDB-associated pneumonia.

The incidence of epidemic and sporadic pneumonic Legionnaires' disease is higher in men than in women. The risk of the pneumonic disease increases with age. The median age of individuals in the epidemic form of Legionnaires' disease has been between 55 and 60 years.[20] The ratio of males to females in epidemic or sporadic cases of pneumonic disease has been approximately 2 to 1.[20,21] Sex and age were not risk factors in at least 2 nonpneumonic outbreaks of Legionnaires' disease.

EPIDEMIOLOGY

No person-to-person transmission of Legionnaires' disease has been demonstrated. It is assumed that aerosols figure predominantly in transmission of LDB. It appears that excavation of soil in an immediate or adjacent area, air-conditioning equipment, and humidifying or ventilation systems may act to disperse LDB-containing aerosols.[18] LDB appears to be widely distributed in nature. Habitats include lakes, rivers, hospital showers, nebulizers, and cooling tanks. In natural aquatic habitats, LDB is often associated with cyanobacteria.[18] Sporadic and epidemic forms of disease caused by LDB occur with greater frequency during summer months. Sporadic cases have been reported from at least 43 states, Australia, Canada, Great Britain, Israel, the Netherlands, Scotland, and Switzerland.[21,22-28] The attack rate was 6% in the Philadelphia outbreak of Legionnaires' disease and 0.4% in the nosocomial outbreak of Legionnaires' disease in Los Angeles (Table 15-3). There was an attack rate of 95% in the outbreak of the nonpneumonic form of the disease that occurred in Pontiac. The fatality rate was 21% in Philadelphia and 25% in Los Angeles. No deaths occurred in Pontiac. The overall fatality rate based on larger epidemiologic data is estimated to be 20%.

LABORATORY DIAGNOSIS

Most laboratories do not attempt isolations of LDB from sputum, transtracheal aspirations, pleural fluid, bronchial washings, or lung tissue unless there is reason clinically or epidemiologically to suspect a diagnosis of Legionnaires' disease or Pontiac fever. The seriousness of the disease, particularly in immunocompromised individuals, warrants an all-out effort to recover and identify LDB as rapidly as possible. It may be necessary to rely on the services of a nearby reference laboratory for confirmation of a diagnosis of Legionnaires' disease.

Table 15–3. Epidemiologic parameters of three outbreaks of Legionnaires' disease.

	Legionnaires' Disease (Philadelphia)	Pontiac Fever (Pontiac)	Nosocomial Legionnaires' Disease (Los Angeles)
Source	Unknown	Air-conditioning system	Unknown
Incubation period	2 to 11 days	5 to 66 hours	1 to 28 days
Attack	6%	95%	0.4%
Underlying disease	61%	none	94%
Fatality rate	21%	0%	25%

Adapted from Lattimer, G.L., and Ormsbee, R.A.: Legionnaires' Disease. New York, Marcel Dekker, 1981.

Some laboratories may want to set up screening procedures for certain clinical specimens. All laboratorians should be familiar with the major characteristics of LDB.

Microscopic Examination

Legionnaires' disease bacterium (LDB) is a gram-negative bacillus, but it does not stain well when the usual gram-stain technique is employed.[29] Somewhat better results are obtained when carbolfuchsin, rather than safranin, is used as the counterstain. A so-called "half-a-Gram-stain" has been used successfully to visualize LDB in tissue sections.[30] In that procedure, the decolorizing and counterstaining steps are eliminated. The organisms appear as gram-positive bacilli, measuring approximately 0.2 μm long and 0.2 to 0.8 μm wide, but coccobacillary and filamentous forms also may be seen.[18] If the Giménez technique is used, filamentous forms as long as 50 μm can be observed in cultures incubated for prolonged periods (Fig. 15–2).[31] The Dieterle silver impregnation (DSI) stain is a reliable method available for rapid detection of LDB in tissue sections.[29] The DSI stain is not specific for LDB since other bacteria and pigments also take up the stain. Other histopathologic stains have only limited use in demonstrating LDB in tissue.

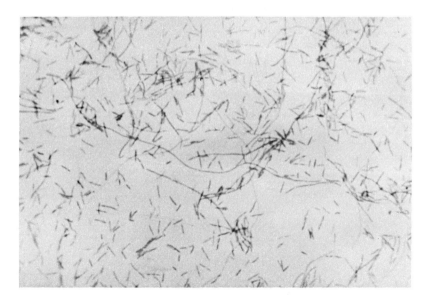

Figure 15–2. Filamentous forms of LDB stained by the Giménez method. (From Lattimer, G.L., and Ormsbee, R.A.: Legionnaires' Disease. New York, Marcel Dekker, 1981.)

Cultural Techniques

Primary in vitro isolation of LDB on enriched media is often difficult. The bacillus grows slowly, often requiring several days or more for sufficient growth to be detected. Mueller-Hinton-IsoVitaleX Hemoglobin (MH-IH) agar, modified Mueller-Hinton (MM-H) agar with L-cysteine, monosodium glutamate, hemoglobin, and a small amount of additional agar, Feeley-Gorman (FG) agar, charcoal-yeast extract (CYE) agar with L-cysteine and ferric pyrophosphate, and a yeast extract phosphate-hemin (YPH) medium have been used for primary isolation with some degree of success.[32-34] CYE agar has emerged as the medium of choice although some strains of LDB may require hemin for optimal growth.[34] The media are inoculated by placing two 0.5 ml aliquots of the specimen with a loop on the surface of each plate. One spot is left undisturbed and the other is streaked for colony isolation in the usual manner. All plates, with the exception of the FG agar plates, are incubated aerobically at 37°C. FG plates are incubated in air plus 2.5% CO_2 or in a candle extinction jar. Colonies have a ground-glass appearance on artificial culture media (Fig. 15–3). Blood cultures, if required, are taken in the usual manner,

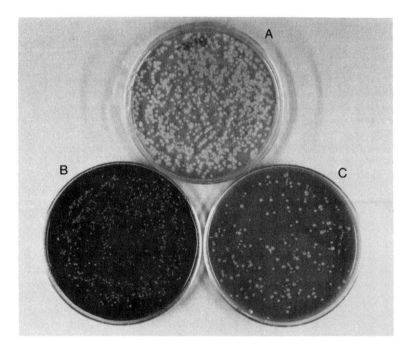

Figure 15–3. Growth of Legionella pneumophila, strain Bloomington 2, on (A) YPH, (B) CYE, and (C) MM-H agars. (From Johnson, S.R., Schalla, W.O., Wong, K.H., and Perkins, G.H.: Simple transparent medium for study of Legionellae. J. Clin. Microbiol., *15*:342, 1982. Courtesy W.O. Schalla.)

inoculated into CYE-diphasic blood culture medium, and incubated aerobically at 37°C.[35]

LDB grows abundantly in embryonated eggs and in guinea pigs. Suspensions are prepared by emulsifying 1 g of tissue in 9.0 ml of sterile distilled water in a sterile mortar with a pestle and sterile 60-mesh Alundum. Further dilution before plating may be required if antibiotic treatment has been initiated before the specimen is obtained from the patient.

A new antiserum-agar plate method for simultaneous detection and direct isolation of Legionella species has been successfully used on contaminated environmental and clinical specimens.[36] The method employs a modification of a filtered yeast extract, agarose, and antisera from rabbits immunized with formalinized Legionella vaccines. Colonies of LDB develop after 2 to 4 days of incubation at 37°C in an atmosphere of 60% relative humidity. Precipitin rings surround colonies of Legionella, but no rings are observable around colonies of contaminating organisms, such as Pseudomonas aeruginosa, Proteus vulgaris, or Escherichia coli.

Serologic Tests

By far the most specific staining technique is the direct fluorescent stain (DFS), using specific rabbit antisera. Specific conjugates have been used to demonstrate LDB in both clinical specimens and in laboratory cultures.[37] Six serogroups of Legionella pneumophila have been identified.[38] A polyvalent conjugate, which can be applied to sputum, transtracheal aspirates, or bronchial washings, is also available.[39–43] Some early preparations of direct-fluorescent antibody (DFA) conjugates also contained antibodies to mycobacteria because Freund's adjuvant was used when rabbits were inoculated with LDB. If positive LDB smears are obtained with some conjugates, some caution must be exercised. A Ziehl-Neelsen stain will differentiate mycobacteria from LDB. LDB is not acid-fast, whereas mycobacteria are acid-fast bacilli.

A variety of serologic tests is available for detection of LDB antibodies in sera. Indirect fluorescence (IF), microagglutination (MA), indirect hemagglutination (IHA), immune adherence hemagglutination (IAHA), and micro-enzyme-linked immunosorbence assay (ELISA) have all been used to measure antibody against LDB.[44–48] The IF test is the standard diagnostic test used in most laboratories, although cross reactions with other antibodies of gram-negative bacteria have been reported.[49] Paired and convalescent sera, taken at approximately 7 and 21 days, should show a fourfold or greater rise in titer to 1:128 or greater for a diagnosis of legionellosis; however, a single titer of 1:256 or greater could be significant.

A newer and promising approach for diagnosis of Legionnaires' disease has been used to detect Legionella antigenuria by reverse passive agglutination (RPA).[50] The test is based on the agglutination of antibody-sensitized protein-A bearing Staphylococcus aureus in the presence of soluble Legionella antigens. No expensive equipment is required to perform the test. More studies are required to assess the sensitivity and specificity of RPA in the rapid diagnosis of Legionnaires' disease. If additional studies confirm the results of preliminary studies using RPA, the test would be particularly valuable for small hospital laboratories.

Biochemical Characterization

The complete biochemical characterization of Legionella species and LLO has been difficult because the organisms do not grow on conventional media commonly used for species identification of other bacteria. Moreover, a single basal medium to which test substrates are added is not universally acceptable for the performance of tests.

All LDB isolated to date are catalase- and gelatinase-positive, but negative for urease activity.[7,8] All LDB produce yellow or blue-white fluorescence under ultraviolet light of 366 nm. All strains of L. pneumophila isolated to date produce β-lactamase, but some strains of LLO are β-lactamase negative.[8,51,52] Other characteristics of the Legionellaceae are listed in Table 15–4. Knowledge of other metabolic characteristics of LDB is emerging, and it can be expected that the full profiles for Legionella species will be available as more strains are isolated. With the exception of the ability to degrade starch, the legionellae do not utilize carbohydrates. Amino acids appear to be the major source of energy and carbon for the organisms. Much remains to be learned of the biochemistry of the legionellae and the as yet unclassified LLO.

Profiles of Cellular Composition

The relatively few positive biochemical reactions that can be used for identification of LDB have led to attempts to identify the organisms by fatty acid, enzyme, and carbohydrate profiles of cell contents. Chromatograms obtained by capillary gas chromatography have revealed characteristic "fingerprints" of both fatty acid and carbohydrate composition of representative strains of several species of Legionella.[53,54]

An aminopeptidase profile of four strains of L. pneumophila, using synthetic substrates and the API ZYM system (Analytab Products, Plainview, New York) appears to be of use in identifying that organism.[55] Aminopeptidase profiles could also explain conditions required for growth and even the mechanism of virulence in the host.

The special equipment and expertise required for profiling cellular components of LDB preclude use of these techniques by most hospital

Table 15–4. Biochemical characteristics of Legionella species.

	L. pneumophila	L. bozemanii	L. micdadei	L. dumoffii	L. gormanii	L. longbeachae	L. jordanis
Beta-lactamase	+	±	–	+	+	±	+
Brown pigment on FG* agar	+	+	–	+	+	+	+
Catalase	+	+	+	+	+	+	+
Gelatinase	+	+	+	+	+	+	+
Hippurate hydrolysis	+	–	–	–	–	–	–
Nitrate reduction	–	–	–	–	–	–	–
Oxidase	±	–	+	–	–	+	+
Urease	–	–	–	–	–	–	–

*FG (Feeley-Gorman)

Adapted from Cherry, W.B.: Legionella jordanis: a new species of Legionella iolated from water and sewage. J. Clin. Microbiol., 15:290, 1982.

laboratories. It is likely, however, that the procedures may become increasingly available in reference laboratories.

PROGNOSIS

The prognosis in Legionnaires' disease is not predictable, because the LDB in some hosts acts as a virulent primary pathogen, but in other hosts, as an opportunistic organism. The assessment of factors such as underlying respiratory disease and immunocompetency of the patients is necessary to understand the progressions of the disease. Emphasis on prompt diagnosis is important because data obtained to date indicate that early initiation of erythromycin and tetracycline therapy appears to be effective against LDB.[56]

CASE REPORTS

Case 1

On July 27, 1976, 2 days after returning home from the annual Pennsylvania American Legion convention, a previously healthy 39-year-old Legionnaire became ill with symptoms of shortness of breath, cough, fever, and nausea. Within 24 hours, uncontrollable shaking chills developed, the cough and shortness of breath became more severe, and he was admitted to the hospital on July 29, 1976. The only abnormalities noted on his admission physical examination were a temperature of 39.8°C (103°F), pulse 110/minute, and prominent, right-sided pulmonary rales. Chest roentgenogram revealed a right-sided, middle-lobe pneumonia. Admission laboratory data showed a hemoglobin of 12.6 g/dl, and a white blood cell count of 5900/mm^3 with 44% polymorphonuclear leukocytes, 8% band forms, and 48% lymphocytes. Arterial blood gas concentrations on room air showed a pH of 7.32, Po_2 56 mm Hg, and a Pco_2 19 mm Hg. Microscopic examination of spun urine sediment revealed 4+ protein, moderate blood, and rare casts. Serum concentration of sodium was 122 mEq/L; potassium, 3.1 mEq/L; chloride, 93 mEq/L; CO_2, 22 mEq/L; creatinine, 1.4 mg/dl; bilirubin, 1.7 mg/dl. Multiple cultures of blood and urine were negative, and sputum culture showed expected normal flora. Two days after admission, despite therapy with ampicillin, cephalothin, gentamicin, hydrocortisone, furosemide, aminophylline, and digoxin, the pneumonia progressed, and his temperature rose to over 41.1°C (> 106°F). The chest roentgenogram now revealed diffuse bilateral pneumonia. Measurements of arterial blood gases showed a progressive decrease in the Po_2 concentration to a level of 40 mm Hg, despite oxygen therapy. Because of progressive respiratory failure, mechanical ventilation was instituted. Persistent hypoxemia and cardiac arrhythmias developed, and he died on August 1, 1976, the day before LD was recognized as a clinical entity.

Autopsy revealed death was due to severe bilateral pneumonia. Histopathologic findings in lung tissue were unusual in that they demonstrated features of bacterial and nonbacterial pneumonia. Some sections showed mononuclear cell predominance as seen in pneumonias due to infection due to chlamydial, rickettsial, and zoonotic bacterial agents. Although other areas in the same section showed polymorphonuclear cellular predominance typical of bacterial pneumonia, no bacterial agent was identified. Three years later, DFA staining of formalin-fixed lung tissue confirmed the presence of LDB.*

Case 2

A 56-year-old woman with uncomplicated aortic valvular stenosis developed symptoms of fever, chills, malaise, and right-sided chest pain on May 15, 1978. During the subsequent 4 days, progressive dyspnea and cough, productive of blood-tinged sputum, were noted, and the right-sided pain increased in intensity. She was admitted to the hospital for diagnosis and treatment. On physical examination, fever 39.4°C with relative bradycardia (80/minute) was noted. Rales were heard in the posterior aspect of the thorax, and a chest roentgenogram revealed right-sided basilar pneumonia. Blood, sputum, and urine cultures were obtained, and ampicillin was administered. No pathogens were isolated from these materials, and therapy with cefazolin, gentamicin, and clindamycin was started. The pneumonic process extended to include the entire right lung and a portion of the left lung. On May 26, erythromycin was added to the regimen. Twenty-four hours later, because of progressive pulmonary infiltrates and lack of response to therapy, diagnostic lung biopsy was performed. The patient died of cardiac arrest after the biopsy procedure.

Immediately before biopsy, transtracheal aspiration was performed. Gram stain of the aspirated material was characterized by many polymorphonuclear leukocytes but did not demonstrate the etiologic agent. A portion of the aspirate was inoculated by drop technique onto Mueller-Hinton chocolate agar supplemented with IsoVitaleX. An additional Mueller-Hinton chocolate agar plate was inoculated and streaked for isolation. Expectorated sputa and lung biopsy material were cultured in the same manner. At 10 days of incubation, many small, convex, cream-colored colonies were noted on the drop-inoculated plates from the aspirate. Gram stain of the colonies revealed small, thin, gram-negative bacilli of uniform width and length. Staining of the same growth at 14 days showed filamentous, gram-negative bacilli demonstrating beaded morphology. DFA conjugate strongly stained organisms in the transtracheal aspirate and lung

---

*Reprinted from Lattimer, G.L. and Ormsbee, R.A.: Legionnaires' Disease. New York, Marcel Dekker, 1981, pp. 33–34. By courtesy of Marcel Dekker, Inc.[18]

biopsy specimen, as well as the cultured organisms. Epidemiologic and serologic surveys of family and co-workers did not show an increased incidence of seroprevalence nor were there symptoms to suggest that clinical illness occurred.

It seemed unusual that, although organisms were numerous in lung tissue examined by DFA staining, no growth occurred using undiluted lung tissue or lung tissue diluted 10^{-1}. Yet organisms were isolated from sputum obtained from transtracheal aspiration, which contained fewer organisms. Approximately 1 year later, LDB was isolated from freshly thawed lung tissue from this case by diluting the tissue suspension 10^{-2} through 10^{-3} but not with tissue diluted to a lesser degree.*

Case 3

A 59-year-old man was admitted to a Long Beach, California, hospital on 7 April, 1980, because of fever and pneumonia. His case has been followed at the hospital clinic since 1978 for rheumatoid arthritis, for which he was receiving gold therapy. Serum immunoglobulin levels had decreased during therapy; in March, 1980, IgG was 743 mg/dl; IgM, 70 mg/dl, and IgA, 175 mg/dl. During the 4 days before admission he developed a dry nonproductive cough, myalagia, fever, and anorexia. The patient was alert and cooperative but appeared to be in a mildly toxic state. A chest roentgenogram taken on 7 April revealed a right lower lobe alveolar infiltrate, and he was admitted.

Physical examination of the chest showed dullness to percussion, egobronchophony, and rales at the right base. The leukocyte count was $19,200/mm^3$ with a left shift. Arterial blood gases measured while the patient breathed room air were Po_2, 60 mm Hg; Pco_2, 34 mm Hg; and pH 7.46. A transtracheal aspirate was obtained before antimicrobial therapy; occasional neutrophils without bacteria were seen on a Gram smear.

Penicillin G, 2.4 million U/d, was given intravenously. He became afebrile over 2 days, but experienced respiratory failure; arterial blood gases taken while he was on 28% fraction of inspired oxygen were Po_2, 48 mm Hg; Pco_2, 40 mm Hg; and pH, 7.36. Ampicillin, 6 g/d intravenously, was substituted on hospital day 2 for the penicillin, when Haemophilus influenzae was grown in moderate numbers from the transtracheal aspirate culture. An exudative right pleural effusion was detected and tapped the same day; aerobic and anaerobic cultures on routine media yielded no growth. On hospital day 3 he needed cardiopulmonary resuscitation and intubation for a respiratory arrest. Coma and seizures occurred after resuscitation and persisted until

---

*From Lattimer, G.L., McCrone, C., and Galgon, J.: N. Engl. J. Med., *299*:1172–1173, 1978. Reprinted by permission of the New England Journal of Medicine.[41]

death. Renal failure developed, requiring peritoneal dialysis. Erythromycin, 2 g/d intravenously, was started on day 4. Arterial blood gases improved slowly over the next 5 days, but upper gastrointestinal bleeding on day 10 resulted in death.

A Legionella-like organism was isolated from the transtracheal aspirates after 3 days' incubation on CYE medium (strain Long Beach 4). The blood cultures were negative. A postmortem examination of the chest showed a consolidated right lower lobe with multiple abscesses and hemorrhage with penumonitis in the remainder of both lungs.*

SUMMARY

Since Legionnaires' disease emerged as an acute febrile pneumonic disease in 1976, both sporadic and epidemic forms of the disease have been recognized with increasing frequency. Although nonpneumonic and nosocomial infections have been reported, most primary infections are aptly described as atypical pneumonias. The seven species of Legionella, which are collectively called Legionnaires' disease bacillus (LDB), appear to be widely distributed in nature. No person-to-person transmission of LDB has been demonstrated. It is assumed that aerosols are the major vehicles of transmission. Several serologic techniques are available for screening clinical specimens for the presence of Legionella organisms. Rapid identification of LDB is important in selecting appropriate antimicrobial therapy.

REFERENCES

1. Center for Disease Control: Respiratory infection—Pennsylvania. Morbid. Mortal. Weekly Rept., *25*:244, 1976.
2. McDade, J.E., Brenner, D.J., and Bozeman, F.M.: Legionnaires' disease bacterium isolated in 1947. Ann. Intern. Med., *90*:659, 1979.
3. Brenner, D.J., et al.: Legionella bozemanii sp. nov. and Legionella dumoffii sp. nov: Classification of two additional species of Legionella associated with human pneumonia. Curr. Microbiol., *4*:111, 1980.
4. Garrity, G.M., Brown, A., and Vickers, R.M.: Tatlockia and Fluoribacter. Two new genera of organisms resembling Legionella pneumophila. Int. J. Syst. Bacteriol., *30*:609, 1980.
5. Hébert, G.A., Steigerwalt, A.G., and Brenner, D.J.: Legionella micdadei species nova: Classification of a third species of Legionella associated with human pneumonia. Curr. Microbiol., *3*:255, 1980.
6. Morris, G.K., et al.: Legionella gormanii sp. nova. J. Clin. Microbiol., *12*:718, 1980.
7. McKinney, R.M., et al.: Legionella longbeachae species novum, another etiologic agent of human pneumonia. Ann. Intern. Med., *94*:739, 1981.
8. Cherry, W.B., et al.: Legionella jordanis: a new species of Legionella isolated from water and sewage. J. Clin. Microbiol., *15*:290, 1982.
9. Sanford, J.P.: Legionnaires' disease—The first thousand days. N. Engl. J. Med., *300*:654, 1979.

---

*From McKinney, R.M., et al.: Ann. Intern. Med., *94*:739–743, 1981. © 1981 American College of Physicians.[7]

10. Swartz, M.N.: Clinical aspects of Legionnaires' disease. Ann. Intern. Med., *90*:492, 1979.

11. Tsai, T.F., et al.: Legionnaires' disease. Clinical features of the epidemic in Philadelphia. Ann. Intern. Med., *90*:509, 1979.

12. Glick, T.H., et al.: Pontiac fever: An epidemic of unknown etiology in a health department. I. Clinical and epidemiologic aspects. Am. J. Epidemiol., *107*:149, 1978.

13. Kirby, B.D., Snyder, K.M., Meyer, R.D., and Finegold, S.M.: Legionnaires' disease: Report of sixty-five nosocomially-acquired cases and review of the literature. Medicine, *59*:188, 1980.

14. Williams, D.M., Krick, J.A., and Remington, J.S.: Pulmonary infection in the compromised host. Am. Rev. Resp. Dis., *114*:359, 1976.

15. Valdivieso, M., et al.: Gram-negative bacillary pneumonia in the compromised host. Medicine, *56*:251, 1977.

16. Ramsey, P.G., et al.: The renal transplant patient with fever and pulmonary infiltrates: Etiology, clinical manifestations, and management. Medicine, *59*:206, 1980.

17. Ormsbee, R.A., et al.: Legionnaires' disease: Antigenic peculiarities, strain differences, and antibiotic sensitivities of the agent. J. Infect. Dis., *138*:260, 1978.

18. Lattimer, G.L., and Ormsbee, R.A.: Legionnaires' Disease. New York, Marcel Dekker, 1981.

19. Cohen, M.L., et al.: Fatal nosocomial Legionnaires' disease: Clinical and epidemiologic characteristics. Ann. Intern. Med., *90*:611, 1979.

20. Broome, C.V., and Fraser, D.W.: Epidemiologic aspects of legionellosis. Epidemiol. Rev., *1*:1, 1979.

21. Center for Disease Control: Legionnaires' disease. Morbid. Mortal. Weekly Rept., *27*:439, 1978.

22. Harkness, J., et al.: Legionnaires' disease. Med. J. Aust., *2*:266, 1978.

23. Bennett, J.S.: Legionnaires' disease in Canada. Can. Med. Assoc. J., *118*:1031, 1978.

24. Bartlett, C.L.R.: Sporadic cases of Legionnaires' disease in Great Britain. Ann. Intern. Med., *90*:592, 1979.

25. Berman, J., Loon, G., and Rubenstein, E.: Legionnaires' disease. Isr. J. Med. Sci., *15*:227, 1979.

26. Meenhorst, P.L., Van der Meer, J.W.M., and Borst, J.: Sporadic cases of Legionnaires' disease in the Netherlands. Ann. Intern. Med., *90*:529, 1979.

27. Fallon, R.J., and Abraham, W.H.: Scottish experience with the serologic diagnosis of Legionnaires' disease. Ann. Intern. Med., *90*:684, 1979.

28. Krech, U., Kohli, P., and Pagon, S.: "Legionnaires' disease" in der Schweiz. Schweiz. Med. Wochenschr., *108*:1653, 1978.

29. Chandler, F.W., Hicklin, M.D., and Blackmon, J.A.: Demonstration of the agent of Legionnaires' disease in tissue. N. Engl. J. Med., *297*:1218, 1977.

30. de Freitas, J.L., Borst, J., and Meenhorst, P.L.: Easy visualization of Legionella pneumophila by "half-a-gram" stain procedure. Lancet, *1*:270, 1979.

31. Giménez, D.F.: Staining rickettsiae in yolk-sac cultures. Stain Technol., *39*:135, 1964.

32. Feeley, J.C., et al.: Primary isolation media for the Legionnaires' disease bacterium. J. Clin. Microbiol., *8*:320, 1978.

33. Feeley, J.C., et al.: Charcoal-yeast extract agar: primary isolation medium for Legionella pneumophila. J. Clin. Microbiol., *10*:437, 1979.

34. Johnson, S.R., Schalla, W.O., Wong, K.H., and Perkins, G.H.: Simple transparent medium for study of Legionellae. J. Clin. Microbiol., *15*:342, 1982.

35. Feeley, J.C., and Gorman, G.W.: Legionella. *In* Manual of Clinical Microbiology, 3rd Ed. Edited by E.H. Lennette. Washington, D.C., American Society for Microbiology, 1980.

36. Janssen, W.A., and Hedlund, K.W.: Antiserum-agar plate method for simultaneous detection and direct isolation of Legionella species in clinical and environmental specimens. J. Clin. Microbiol., *15*:1176, 1982.

37. Cherry, W.B., et al.: Detection of Legionnaires' disease bacterium by direct immunofluorescent staining. J. Clin. Microbiol., *8*:329, 1978.

38. McKinney, R.M., et al.: Legionella pneumophila serogroup six: Isolation from cases of legionellosis, identification by immunofluorescence staining and immunologic response to infection. J. Clin. Microbiol., *12*:395, 1980.
39. Katz, S.: Examination of sputum in Legionnaires' disease. Lancet, *2*:987, 1978.
40. Edelstein, P.H., and Finegold, S.M.: Isolation of Legionella pneumophila from a transtracheal aspirate. J. Clin. Microbiol., *9*:457, 1979.
41. Lattimer, G.L., McCrone, C., and Galgon, J.: Diagnosis of Legionnaires' disease from transtracheal aspirate by direct fluorescent-antibody staining and isolation of the bacterium. N. Engl. J. Med., *299*:1172, 1978.
42. Winn, W.C., et al.: V. Direct immunofluorescent detection of Legionella pneumophila in respiratory specimens. J. Clin. Microbiol., *11*:59, 1980.
43. Broome, C.V., Cherry, W.B., Winn, W.C., Jr., and MacPherson, B.R.: Rapid diagnosis of Legionnaires' disease by direct immunofluorescent staining. Ann. Intern. Med., *90*:1, 1979.
44. Wilkinson, H.W., Fikes, B.J., and Cruce, D.D.: Indirect immunofluorescence test for serodiagnois of Legionnaires' disease: Evidence of serogroup diversity of Legionnaires' disease bacterial antigens and for multiple specificity of human antibodies. J. Clin. Microbiol., *9*:379, 1979.
45. Farshy, C.E., Klein, G.G., and Feeley, J.C.: Detection of antibodies to Legionnaires' disease organism by microagglutination and microenzyme-linked immunosorbent assay tests. J. Clin. Microbiol., *7*:327, 1978.
46. Edson, D.C., Stiefel, H.E., Wentworth, B.B., and Wilson, D.L.: Prevalence of antibodies to Legionnaires' disease. A seroepidemiologic survey of Michigan residents using the hemagglutination test. Ann. Intern. Med., *90*:691, 1979.
47. Lennette, D.A., et al.: Comparison of indirect fluorescent antibody, immune adherence hemagglutination, and indirect hemagglutination tests. J. Clin. Microbiol., *10*:876, 1979.
48. Tilton, R.C.: Legionnaires' disease antigens detected by enzyme-linked immunosorbent assay. Ann. Intern. Med., *90*:697, 1969.
49. Wilkinson, H.W., et al.: Measure of immunoglobulin G-, M-, and A-specific titers against Legionella pneumophila and inhibition of titers against nonspecific gram-negative bacterial antigens in the indirect immunofluorescence test for legionellosis. J. Clin. Microbiol., *10*:685, 1979.
50. Tang, P.W., de Savigny, D., and Toma, S.: Detection of Legionella antigenuria by reverse passive agglutination. J. Clin. Microbiol., *15*:998, 1982.
51. Thornsberry, C., and Kirven, L.A.: B-lactamase of the Legionnaires' bacterium. Curr. Microbiol., *1*:51, 1978.
52. Hébert, G.A., et al.: The Rickettsia-like organisms TATLOCK (1943) and HEBA (1959) bacteria phenotypically similar but genetically distinct from Legionella pneumophila and the WIGA bacterium. Ann. Intern. Med., *92*:45, 1980.
53. Moss, C.W., Weaver, R.E., Dees, S.B., and Cherry, W.B.: Cellular fatty acid composition of isolates from Legionnaires' disease. J. Clin. Microbiol., *6*:140, 1977.
54. Fox, A., et al.: Capillary gas chromatographic analysis of carbohydrates of Legionella pneumophila and other members of the family Legionellaceae. J. Clin. Microbiol., *19*:326, 1984.
55. Müller, H.E.: Enzymatic profile of Legionella pneumophila. J. Clin. Microbiol., *13*:423, 1981.
56. Broome, C.V., et al.: The Vermont epidemic of Legionnaires' disease. Ann. Intern. Med., *90*:573, 1979.

CHAPTER 16 NONTUBERCULOUS MYCOBACTERIA INFECTIONS

More than 100 years have elapsed since Robert Koch announced to the Berlin Physiological Society that he had discovered the cause of tuberculosis.[1] Although there has been an overall continuing decline in cases of tuberculosis in developed countries, disease caused by nontuberculous mycobacteria is being recognized with increasing frequency[2] (Fig. 16–1). At one time acid-fast bacilli, other than Mycobacterium tuberculosis, M. bovis, or M. africanum, were referred to as "atypical acid-fast" bacilli. The organisms are probably more

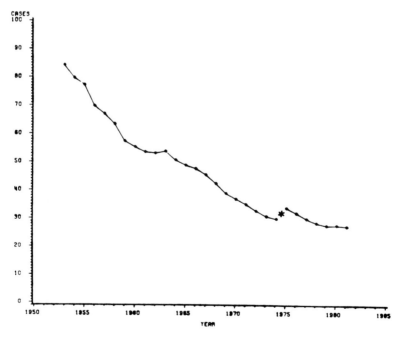

Figure 16–1. Reported cases of tuberculosis by year in thousands for the United States, 1953 to 1981. (From Reported Morbidity and Mortality in the United States, Annual Summary, 1981. Atlanta, Georgia, Centers for Disease Control, 1981.)

properly called nontuberculous mycobacteria or mycobacteria other than the tubercle bacilli (MOTT) or bacillus of Hansen's disease (leprosy).

Pulmonary disease caused by nontuberculous mycobacteria in adults is indistinguishable from classic tuberculosis. In the early stages of the infection, individuals may be asymptomatic or demonstrate only low-grade fever. Later symptoms may include temperatures up to 103° or 104°F, fatigue, anorexia, night sweats, weight loss, a cough, and hemoptysis.[3] Systemic dissemination is rare except in immunocompromised hosts. Pulmonary disease caused by nontuberculous mycobacteria in children is rarely encountered. When it does occur, children may be asymptomatic or the symptoms may span a wide clinical spectrum. The infection may manifest itself as an acute pneumonia, progressive pulmonary disease, mediastinal masses, peritonitis, septicemia, endocarditis, abscesses at sites of trauma, osteomyelitis, or unremitting disseminated disease with lung involvement.[4-13]

The most common manifestation of nontuberculous mycobacterial infection in children, however, is not lung-associated. Most cases consist of local unilateral infections of the superficial lymph nodes.[14,15] The submaxillary or submandibular lymph nodes are the ones most frequently affected. Surgical excision is the treatment of choice, but some infections respond to antituberculous drugs. Granulomatous nodules of the skin and subcutaneous tissue caused by nontuberculous mycobacteria can occur in adults and children following relatively minor trauma. The lesions, for the most part, are benign and self-limiting (Fig. 16–2). Nontuberculous myobacteria are being isolated with increasing frequency as causes of nosocomial infections in immunocompromised hosts.[16-20] Individual and clustered outbreaks in patients with infections of postsurgical wounds, artificial heart valves, and mammary implants have been reported.[18,21,22]

The cavitary lesions of the lung caused by nontuberculous mycobacteria are not always distinguishable from those associated with tubercle bacilli on roentgenograms, but most patients with cavitary lesions associated with nontuberculous mycobacteria have a history of prior or coexisting lung disease. Tsukamura describes a "primary" nontuberculous mycobacterial infection in which cavities are thin-walled and a "secondary" nontuberculous mycobacterial infection in which the disease produces thick-walled residual cavities similar to those of tuberculosis.[23] Others feel that the distinction is somewhat arbitrary and that pre-existing focal disease may remain undetected. Infiltrates are usually modest.[24]

The cross-reactivity exhibited by tubercle bacilli and the nontuberculous mycobacteria have created a new challenge in interpreting results of tuberculin skin tests.[25] The cross-reactivity accounts for most false-positive tuberculin reactions. Although a zone of induration of 10 mm or more has been adopted as the standard for a positive test,

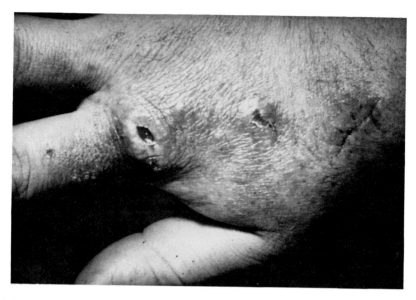

Figure 16–2. A granulomatous nodule caused by Mycobacterium marinum. The condition is so often associated with trauma incurred while cleaning tropical fish tanks that it is often called "fish fancier's finger." (Courtesy of T.B. Hugh, St. Vincent's Hospital, Sydney, Australia.)

using 5 units of purified protein derivative (PPD), many equivocal tuberculin reactions do occur in which the border of induration is not clearly defined. Comparative skin testing using homologous and heterologous antigens have some value in distinguishing nontuberculous mycobacterial infections from tuberculosis, but the antigens are no longer available in the United States.

A diagnosis of disease caused by nontuberculous mycobacteria may be complicated by the presence of transient colonization of body sites by acid-fast bacilli.[26] A distinction must also be made between an infection and actual disease. Mere colonization without evidence of disease does not appear to be a public health problem.

The criteria needed to establish the presence of a nontuberculous mycobacterial infection have been established by the American Thoracic Society.[27]

A definite diagnosis requires (1) evidence, such as an infiltrate visible on a chest roentgenogram, of disease, the cause of which has not been determined by careful clinical and laboratory studies; and (2) either (a) isolation of the same strain of mycobacteria repeatedly, usually in the absence of other pathogens, or (b) isolation of the mycobacteria from a closed lesion from which the specimen has been collected and handled under sterile conditions, for example, an abscess or biopsy tissue. Occasional isolation of these organisms from sputum, throat washings, and gastric aspirates in the absence of related disease may occur. A careful assessment of quantity of growth, repeated isolation, site of origin, species identification, and symptoms of the patient should be made before embarking on a course of therapy.

ETIOLOGY

There are 15 species of nontuberculous Mycobacterium that are potential human pathogens and at least 17 saprophytes that can be isolated from the environment, but that are rarely pathogenic (Table 16–1). The organisms that cause human disease are often classified on the basis of growth rate and pigment production. Some species are slow growing, requiring 6 to 8 weeks for observable colonies, or will not grow on artificial culture media. Other species grow in 5 to 7 days. Still other species can be differentiated on the basis of their ability either to produce yellow-orange pigments in the light or in the dark. The photochromogens produce characteristic pigments in the light, whereas the scotochromogens synthesize pigments only in the

Table 16–1. Nontuberculous Mycobacterium species.

Group	Strict or Potential Pathogen	Rarely or Never a Pathogen
Slowly growing or "nonculturable" strict pathogens	M. ulcerans M. leprae	
Photochromogens	M. kansasii M. marinum M. simiae M. asiaticum	
Scotochromogens	M. scrofulaceum M. szulgai M. xenopi	M. gordonae M. flavescens
Nonphotochromogens	M. avium M. intracellulare M. malmoense M. haemo- philum	M. terrae M. triviale M. nonchromogenicum M. gastri
Rapidly growing	M. fortuitum M. chelonei	M. vaccae M. smegmatis M. phlei M. parafortuitum M. neoaurum M. thermoresistible M. chitae M. gadium M. gilvum M. duvalii M. aurum

absence of light. Nonphotochromogens lack the ability to synthesize pigments under either environmental condition.

Most human disease caused by nontuberculous mycobacteria is attributable to Mycobacterium kansasii, the M. avian-intracellulare complex, or M. scrofulaceum. In recent years, M. xenopi has received increasing attention as a cause of pulmonary mycobacteriosis. M. ulcerans and M. marinum both grow optimally at 30 to 33°C and, therefore, are associated with cutaneous lesions where temperatures are lower than 37°C.

The lack of a suitable animal model for nontuberculous mycobacteria has hampered studies on the pathogenesis of the organisms. Some nontuberculous mycobacteria, unlike M. tuberculosis, produce soluble toxins that contribute to histologic changes observed in pulmonary disease.[28] Mycobacteria appear to resist destruction by macrophages and, ultimately, kill the scavenger cells. It is likely that the activity of lysosomal hydrolases released from the degenerating macrophages contributes to the inflammatory process. Cell-mediated immune responses initiated by the presence of the acid-fast bacilli play a major role in the production of granulomatous lesions.

The gross and microscopic lesions of nontuberculous disease, other than Hansen's disease (leprosy), in guinea pig lymph nodes are identical to those of tuberculous disease. The amount of fibrosis and caseous necrosis depends on the duration of the lesion.[29] In disseminated cases of nontuberculous mycobacterial disease, it is likely that there is insufficient time for typical granulomas to form.

PREDISPOSING FACTORS

The presence or history of underlying lung disease appears to be important in predisposing adults to infections of the lung caused by nontuberculous mycobacteria. Some of the predisposing conditions are as follows:*

Pneumoconiosis (e.g., silicosis and coal miner's pneumoconiosis; also arc welder's lung)
Healed tuberculosis or mycosis
Chronic bronchitis or emphysema
Bronchiectasis
Esophageal disease
Malignant disease

Approximately half of individuals with pulmonary disease caused by Mycobacterium kansasii or M. avian-intracellulare complex have coexisting obstructive pulmonary disease.[28] Some persons with hema-

---

*From Wolinsky, E.: When is an infection disease? Rev. Infect. Dis., 3:1025, 1981.

tologic diseases, particularly those with hair cell leukemia, are prone to infections caused by nontuberculous mycobacteria.[10] In some instances, the infection may precede the development of neoplastic disease. The use of steroids in systemic lupus erythematosus appears to be an additional predisposing factor in the development of nontuberculous mycobacterial infections.[11] Diagnosis of nontuberculous mycobacterial disease in patients with arthritis and arthralgia is often difficult because changes on radiographs are often attributed to primary disease. Persons who swim consistently in hot springs or who clean fish tanks are at risk of developing localized granulomas.[10]

EPIDEMIOLOGY

Nontuberculous mycobacteria are ubiquitous in nature. The acid-fast bacilli have been isolated from soil, air, dust, water, and food, including eggs, milk, and vegetables.[30,31] It is believed that mycobacteria are washed into river and lake waters from the soil. Droplets formed by bursting bubbles and winds transport the organisms long distances.

M. chelonei subsp. abscessus is sometimes found as a commensal on human skin.[32] Little is known about the distribution of M. malmoense, which has been described in Sweden, England, and Australia, and M. haemophilum, a hemin-requiring organism isolated in Israel.[33,34]

The exact source of nontuberculous mycobacteria in infections is often unknown, but peron-to-person transmission is probably limited. The nontuberculous mycobacteria are known to be transmitted by aerosols, mucosal penetration, or cutaneous inoculation.[35] Pulmonary infections have been associated with droplets measuring less than 10 μm in diameter. The possible contamination of operating room components of methylmethacrylate cement or of a metallic prosthesis was not eliminated in an infection caused by M. fortuitum after a total hip replacement.[36]

At least two thirds of pulmonary disease caused by Mycobacterium kansasii or M. avian-intracellulare complex occurs in males over 45 years of age.[24] The sex distribution is similar to that seen in pulmonary tuberculosis. Chronic bronchitis and emphysema represent the most common predisposing factors. M. kansasii is a more frequent cause of disease in cities. Infections associated with the M. avian-intracellulare complex are found more often in rural areas.

It is difficult to attach much significance to geographic variations in incidence of nontuberculous mycobacterial infections because it is almost certain that large numbers of infections remain undiagnosed in many countries. Mycobacterial infections in immunocompromised hosts are often masked by the presence of other opportunistic pathogens. Only with more aggressive attempts at isolation of nontuberculous mycobacteria will the actual geographic distribution of the acid-fast bacilli be known.

LABORATORY DIAGNOSIS

The potential hazard of clinical specimens possibly contaminatd with pathogenic mycobacteria deserve special consideration to protect laboratory workers. An air flow of at least 70 ft (21 m)/minute should be maintained. Ultraviolet irradiation is useful as a surface decontaminant. Laminar air-flow hoods, equipped with HEPA filters, are recommended for handling centrifuged specimens. Masks, gowns, caps, and disposable gloves should be worn at all times during processing of specimens. Only manual pipetting should be performed. Electric induction incinerators are preferable for sterilizing bacteriologic loops or wires. A more complete discussion of safety may be found in DHEW publication No. (CDC) 75-8230, entitled Procedures for the Isolation and Identification of Mycobacteria.

Microscopic examination, cultural techniques, and biochemical reactions are all of value in the diagnosis of disease caused by the nontuberculous mycobacteria. The mere presence of the organisms on a smear may not indicate disease, however, because some mycobacteria colonize the oral cavity and are likely to contaminate sputum specimens. Some species of mycobacteria grow slowly, requiring 6 to 8 weeks in order to obtain sufficient growth for descriptive colony morphology and biochemical tests.

Concentration and Decontamination

Some specimens, such as sputum and gastric washings, must be liquified and decontaminated prior to processing. The combined digestant and decontaminant N-acetyl-L-cysteine-sodium hydroxide (NALC) or trisodium phosphate-benzalkonium chloride (Zephiran) may be used.[37,38] A 5.0% solution of oxalic acid is recommended for digestion and decontamination of specimens from patients from whom Pseudomonas organisms have been consistently isolated.[39] Equal volumes of combined digestant and decontaminant reagents or 5.0% oxalic acid are added to 10-ml aliquots of specimens in 50-ml centrifugation tubes.[40] Liquifaction is facilitated by mixing on a Vortex-type mixer for 5 to 20 minutes. Mixtures should be allowed to stand 15 minutes to allow settling of aerosols before the addition of 10 ml of sterile buffer (pH 6.8) or sterile distilled water. Centrifugation of mixtures at 3000 rpm (1800 to 2400 $\times$ G) for 15 minutes concentrates any acid-fast bacilli.

Tissue should be ground in sterile 0.85% saline or 0.2% bovine albumin. A pinch of N-acetyl-L-cysteine can be added to liquify mucus. Fluid specimens may be centrifuged and inoculated directly onto culture media. Swabs can be placed in 2 ml of sterile distilled water or saline and an equal quantity of N-acetyl-L-cysteine-sodium hydroxide, mixed on a Vortex-type mixer, and allowed to stand for 15 minutes to permit decontamination.

Microscopic Examination

Acid-fast bacilli may be detected on smears prepared directly from clinical specimens or from concentrated material by brightfield or fluorescent microscopy. For observation under a brightfield microscope, fixed smears may be stained by the Ziehl-Neelsen method or Kinyoun's acid-fast stain.[41] Mycobacteria appear as red bacilli 0.5 to 5.0 μm long by 0.2 to 0.6 μm wide against a blue or green background. Auramine-rhodamine may be used to stain fixed smears if a fluorescent microscope with an ultraviolet light source is available. Acid-fast bacilli emit a bright yellow fluorescence. Fluorescent microscopy has several advantages over brightfield microscopy. Scanning can be done with a 25× objective lens with minimum eye strain. Reporting of smears should be done in accordance with the recommendations of the American Lung Association (Table 16–2).

Cultural Techniques

Culture media used for isolation of nontuberculous mycobacteria should include a primary, nonselective, inspissated egg medium (Lowenstein-Jensen or Petragnani medium), a nonselective agar medium (Middlebrook 7H10 or 7H11 medium), and one selective medium (selective Middlebrook 7H11 medium). Malachite green is used as an inhibitory agent in primary nonselective media. Selective media contain additional antifungal or antibacterial agents. Duplicate and sometimes triplicate cultures should be set up on each medium for incubation at 24°, 32°, 37°, and 42°C. Those organisms obtained from external surfaces of the body tend to grow well at the lower temperatures. Most of the organisms produce more luxuriant growth in a CO_2 incubator. Tube, bottle, or plate cultures should be examined 5 to 7 days after inoculation and once a week thereafter for 6 to 8 weeks.

Table 16–2. Recommendations for reporting smears of mycobacteria.*

Number of Bacilli	Report
0	No acid-fast bacilli found
1–2 in entire smear	Report number found and request repeat specimen
3–9 in entire smear	Rare or +
10 or more in entire smear	Few or + +
1 or more per field	Numerous or + + +†

*American Lung Association, Diagnostic Standards and Classification of Tuberculosis, 1973.
†When fluorochrome stains are used, report "numerous" if 2 or more bacilli are found per high-power field.

It is necessary to place plates in individual CO_2 polyethylene bags to prevent dehydration.

The importance of the rate of growth and of colony characteristics of mycobacteria is often overlooked. The use of symbols is of value in recording colony morphology. The symbols commonly used for describing colony characteristics of mycobacteria are as follows:*

Rg or R = rough
Sm = smooth
D = domed (hemispherical)
S = spreading, serrated edge
T = transparent, thin
X = xenopi
K = kansasii
"D" = resembles kansasii
f = filamentous
w = wrinkled (not rough)
I = interconvertible (a subculture of a single colony of mixed types, reproduces like mixed types)
Ch = chromogenic
NC = nonchromogenic
y = yellow
o = orange
s = spot in center
a = apron (thin growth at the base of the colony)

The nontuberculous mycobacteria can be divided into two groups, based on rate of growth. Those which grow at 24°C and 37°C, or at 42°C in less than 1 week are classified as rapid growers. If 2 or more weeks are required for detection of growth, the mycobacteria are designated as slow growers. The temperature–growth-rate relationships are especially important in identifying Mycobacterium ulcerans, M. marinum, M. xenopi, and M. haemophilum. All tubes, bottles, or plates of rapidly growing mycobacteria should be exposed to light for 1 hour, reincubated, and examined in 24 hours for evidence of pigment. M. fortuitum and M. chelonei are nonchromogenic. Other rapid growers may produce yellow, orange, or pink pigments. Slow growing mycobacteria may be classified as nonchromogens, photochromogens, which produce pigments after exposure to light, or scotochromogens, which produce pigment in the dark (Table 16–1).

---

*From Vestal, A.L.: Procedures for the isolation and identification of mycobacteria. Atlanta, Georgia, Center for Disease Control, 1975.

Biochemical Characterization

The number of biochemical tests needed to identify mycobacteria depends on rate of growth. Only the nonchromogens M. fortuitum and M. chelonei grow on MacConkey agar without crystal violet in 5 days. Those 2 pathogens can be differentiated from one another on the basis of nitrate reduction. Other valuable tests for rapidly growing mycobacteria are listed in Table 16–3. A number of additional tests must be performed to identify mycobacteria classified as slow growers (Table 16–4). Positive and negative controls must be used for each test for reliable results. Standard cultures of Mycobacteria species may be obtained from Dr. Maurice Lefford of the Trudeau Institute, P.O. Box 59, Saranac Lake, New York 12983. Attempts to speciate tuberculous or nontuberculous mycobacteria should be made only by those thoroughly experienced with the biochemical tests. For many laboratories, patients are better served if cultures are sent to a proficient reference or public health laboratory.

Serologic Tests

Serologic techniques have had only limited application in identifying mycobacteria, but have been of great value in epidemiologic studies.[42,43] Agglutination tests have been used to differentiate some strains of M. kansasii, M. marinum, M. simiae, M. avium, M. intracellulare, M. scrofulaceum, M. szulgai, M. gordonae, M. fortuitum, and M. chelonei.[44] Fluorescent-antibody, complement-fixation, and double diffusion in gel have also been used to differentiate Mycobacteria species, but the procedures have not been standardized for use in clinical laboratories.

Animal Inoculation

The guinea pig has been used since the time of Koch to confirm a diagnosis of tuberculous disease, because of the susceptibility of the animals to tubercle bacilli and a concomitant tolerance for contaminating commensals. Guinea pigs have been used only infrequently since the development of sensitive cultural techniques for isolation and biochemical characterization of mycobacteria. Guinea pigs are not universally susceptible to nontuberculous mycobacteria. Mice can be used to differentiate M. kansasii, M. marinum, and M. ulcerans, but are usually not necessary.[41] M. marinum and M. ulcerans produce disease in cooler parts of a mouse, such as the tail or the footpad. M. kansasii produces internal disease.

PROGNOSIS

Pulmonary disease caused by nontuberculous mycobacteria can be progressive and fatal. More often, it is merely one factor contributing

Table 6–3. Biochemical characteristics of rapidly growing mycobacteria.

Species	Pigment	Growth on MacConkey Agar	Nitrate Reduction	NaCl Tolerance	Iron Uptake	Arylsul- fatase 3 Days	Tween Hydrolysis 5 Days	Catalase >45mm	Catalase 68°C
M. fortuitum	None	+	+	+	+	+	+/–†	+	+
M. chelonei	None	+	–	Variable*	–	+	–/+‡	+	+
M. smegmatis	None	–	+	+	+	–	+	+	+
M. phlei	Orange/Yellow	–	+	+	+	–	+	+	+
Other Rapid Growers	Variable	–	+	Variable	Variable	–	+	+	+

*M. chelonei subspecies abscessus are positive; M. chelonei subspecies chelonei are negative.
†55% of strains positive.
‡30% of M. chelonei subspecies abscessus are positive; M. chelonei subspecies chelonei are negative.

Reprinted by permission of the publisher from Good, R.C.: Nontuberculous mycobacteria. Clin. Microbiol. Newsl., 1(20):1–4, 1979. Copyright 1979 by Elsevier Science Publishing Co., Inc.

Table 16–4. Biochemical characteristics of slowly growing nontuberculous mycobacteria.

Species	Colony Morphology*	Pigment†	Niacin	Growth on TCH	Nitrate Reduction	Catalase >45mm	Catalase 68°C	Tween Hydrolysis 10 Days	Tellurite Reduction 3 Days	Pyrazinamidase 4 Days	Pyrazinamidase 7 Days	Urease	NaCl (5%) Tolerance	Arylsulfatase 2 Weeks
M. ulcerans	Rg	N	-	+	-	+	+	-	-(?)	-	Unk	+	-	-
M. kansasii	Sm/Rg	P	-	+	+	+	+	+	-	+/-	+/-	+	-	+/-
M. simiae	Sm	P	+	+	-	+	+	+	-	-	-	+	-	-
M. marinum§	Sm	P	-/+	+	-	-	+	+	-	+	+	+	-	++
M. scrofulaceum	Sm	S	-	+	-	+	+	+/-	-	+/-	+	+	-	-
M. szulgai	Sm/Rg	S/P‖	-	+	+	+	+	+	-	-/+	+/-	-	-	+
M. gordonae	Sm	S	-	+	-	+	+	+	-	+/-	+/-	-	-	±
M. xenopi	Sm/Rg	S	-	+	-	-	+	-	-	+/-	+/-	-	-	-
M. avium complex	Sm/Rg	N	-	+	-	-	+/-**	-	+	+	-/+	+	-	++
M. gastri	Sm	N	-	+	-	-	-	+	-	+	+/-	+	-	-/+
M. terrae complex	Sm/Rg	N	-	+	+/-	+	+	+	-	-/+	-	+	-#	++
M. flavescens	Sm/Rg	S	-	+	+/-	+	+	+	-	+	+	+	+/-	Variable +/++

*Rg = rough; Sm = smooth.
†N = none; P = photoinducible; S = scotochromogenic.
-/+ indicates majority of strains negative.
+/- indicates majority of strains positive.
+ indicates weak reaction; Unk indicates unknown.

§If grown at 28°C–33°C, M. marinum colonies develop in 7 days.
‖M. szulgai is photochromogenic at 25°C and scotochromogenic at 35°C.

#M. triviale in the M. terrae complex will grow in the presence of 5% NaCl.
**Negative 68°C catalase may be seen with poorly growing strains.

Reprinted by permission of the publisher from Good, R.G.: Nontuberculous mycobacteria. Clin. Microbiol. Newsl., 1(20):1–4, 1979. Copyright 1979 by Elsevier Science Publishing Co., Inc.

to morbidity and mortality. In a review of 100 cases of mycobacterial infections caused by Mycobacterium avian-intracellulare complex, more than half of the cases were reported to be stable after treatment.[24] Eight patients died of their mycobacterial disease.

The outcome of cervical lymphadenitis or cutaneous disease caused by nontuberculous mycobacteria, uncomplicated by constitutional symptoms, is usually favorable. However, both M. scrofulaceum and the Mycobacterium avian-intracellulare complex are relatively resistant to antituberculous drugs.

Nontuberculous mycobacterial disease in immunocompromised hosts has a less favorable prognosis. Although the nontuberculous mycobacteria do not appear to be major causes of nosocomial infections, their contribution to persistent morbidity needs continuing surveillance.

CASE REPORTS

Case 1

This 6-month-old white male infant was admitted to a local hospital with a 1-week history of an afebrile illness characterized by wheezing and progressive respiratory symptoms. On admission, a roentgenogram of the chest revealed hyperinflation of the right lung, and fluoroscopy revealed paradoxical motion. Bronchoscopy revealed an intraluminal mass in the right main-stem bronchus. Immediately after the procedure, the child developed cyanosis and bradycardia. He was transferred to North Carolina Baptist Hospital with an endotracheal tube in place; he required mechanical ventilatory assistance.

On physical examination, he was afebrile and normotensive. Pulse rate was 160/minute. There were generalized wheezes on auscultation of the chest. No other abnormalities were observed. The peripheral blood count, urinalysis, and serum electrolyte values were within normal limits. A chest roentgenogram revealed peristent hyperinflation of the right lung and some compression of the left upper lobe. A right thoracotomy was performed; a large, rubbery, gray-white mass involving the anterior portion of the trachea extended across the bifurcation of the trachea and both main-stem bronchi, and compressed the anterior portion of the trachea and right main-stem bronchus. An area of central necrosis was present in the mass. A portion of the capsule of the extraluminal mass could not be removed without perforation of the tracheal wall, and was left attached.

Postoperatively, the child had complete relief from respiratory distress. Histologic examination of the surgical specimen was interpreted as lymph nodes with a necrotizing granulomatous inflammatory process. Cultures for bacterial pathogens were negative, but acid-fast cultures were positive for Mycobacterium intracellulare avium complex.

These cultures were subsequently confirmed by the North Carolina State Health Department Laboratory. Drug sensitivities performed by the Center for Disease Control in Atlanta showed a multiple resistance pattern to all the commonly used antituberculous agents, including isoniazid, streptomycin, kanamycin, ethambutol, pyrazinamide, and rifampin.

There was no family history of tuberculosis or nontuberculous mycobacterial infection, although the family resides in a rural area with many domestic farm animals in the vicinity.

Six weeks after surgery, the child was thriving. Except for the well-healed thoracotomy scar and an occasional wheeze on auscultation of the chest, no abnormalities were detected. At this time, the nontuberculous mycobacterial skin tests for Groups I, II, and III were applied; the result of the Group II test was strongly positive, with 16 mm induration. There was minimal reactivity to the other groups and to an intermediate strength PPD. Chest radiograph revealed a normal cardiac silhouette and mediastinal structures, but there were prominent bilateral interstitial markings. Fluoroscopic examination revealed normal diaphragmatic excursion. In consideration of the infant's clinical well being and the multiple drug resistant pattern of the etiologic agent, it was decided to continue close clinical observation without specific drug therapy. The child is now 2½ years of age, is in the seventy-fifth percentile for height and weight, and is active and playful, with a normal physical examination. He has no manifestation of residual illness, and his chest radiograph is normal.*

Case 2

A 70-year-old plumber was first seen at our institution on October 10, 1979, because of an exacerbation of chronic obstructive pulmonary disease. He had suffered from recurring bouts of bronchitis and shortness of breath for 10 years. In 1973 he had received ethambutol and isoniazid for 1 year as a treatment for pulmonary tuberculosis: a chest roentgenogram from this period featured a small cavity surrounded by some flocky infiltration in the left upper lobe, and a sputum culture had yielded M. tuberculosis. No details of this bacteriologic investigation could be traced. Furthermore, the patient admitted a moderate alcohol abuse.

The clinical examination showed prominent signs of emphysema. There was cyanosis and pitting oedema of both legs. The pulmonary function tests revealed severe bronchial obstruction. The chest roentgenogram was consistent with widespread emphysema, and the left hilum was displaced cranially as a result of extensive fibrosis covering

---

*From Kelsey, D.S., Chambers, R.T., and Hudspeth, A.S.: J. Pediatr., *98*:431, 1981.[6]

the whole left upper zone. Interspersed between the fibrotic lesions were irregular translucent areas. Tomographic examination could not establish whether these were of an emphysematous or infectious nature. The apex of the right lung showed fibrosis only. The Ziehl-Neelsen stain of 3 consecutive sputum specimens was negative, but M. xenopi was cultured from all 3. The isolate was susceptible to 20 μg/ml rifampicin, 5 μg/ml ethionamide, and 10 μg/ml PAS but resistant to 5 μg/ml ethambutol, 1 μg/ml isoniazid, and 10 μg/ml streptomycin (Löwenstein medium). Before these results became available, the patient had been discharged, not to be seen again until April 21, 1980, when he was readmitted because of a new exacerbation of dyspnoea. In the right upper zone a new poorly delineated infiltrate was seen. In 3 or 4 new sputum smears, acid-fast bacilli were identified and again all cultures yielded M. xenopi. Treatment was instituted with a regimen of 600 mg rifampicin, 300 mg isoniazid and 1000 mg pyrazinamide daily, and the patient was discharged.

On July 16, 1980, he had to enter the hospital once again. He was very dyspnoeic and produced copious yellow sputa. Four sputum specimens were examined for mycobacteria; microscopy was negative in all and M. xenopi could be cultured from only one. While the patient was in hospital, he developed hectic fever and extensive pneumonic infiltrates appeared throughout the right lung. Staphylococcus aureus was cultured from a transtracheal aspirate and in spite of intensive antibiotic treatment the patient died on August 17, 1980.

At autopsy the lungs showed severe emphysema and large cavities were found in the right middle and both upper lobes. Microscopically, multiple caseating granulomas were seen but no acid-fast bacilli or fungi could be identified. A tissue culture was not attempted.*

Case 3

A 21-year-old soldier, who has been well prior to October, 1977, initially presented with a history of ill-defined abdominal discomfort in the left upper quadrant followed by progressive weight loss. In April, 1978, he developed a generalized lymphadenopathy, accompanied by fever, malaise, and diarrhoea. He was admitted to a military hospital, where a bone marrow aspirate and a cervical lymph node biopsy were performed and found to contain many foam cells filled with acid-fast bacteria. Cultures of lymph node, urine, faeces, and pleural effusions grew M. fortuitum. The subsequent treatment with isoniazid, cycloserine, rifampicine, and ethambutol did not result in any clinical improvement. Four months later, in October, 1978, the patient was found to have a rapidly enlarging inflammatory abdominal

*From Bogaerts, Y. et al.: Eur. J. Respir. Dis., *63*:298, 1982. © 1982 Munksgaard International Publishers, Copenhagen, Denmark.[15]

pseudotumor with abscess cavities from which the same mycobacterium was isolated. Testing of antibiotic sensitivities led to therapy with capriomycine, protionamide and cycloserine. A presumed immune deficiency and granulocyte dysfunction were treated with leucocyte transfusions and transfer factor. These changes in therapy resulted in a transient improvement.

When the patient was transferred to the Department of Medicine of the University Hospital, Ulm, on December 4, 1978, he appeared cachectic, having lost 20 kg body weight, and he had a generalized lymphadenopathy, hepatosplenomegaly, and tender, palpable masses in the abdominal cavity and the abdominal wall. Small bilateral effusions were seen on chest films but the lung parenchyma was unremarkable. Contrast studies of the gut disclosed an extrinsic compression of both stomach and duodenum and a coarse mucosal pattern of small and large bowel. A lymphangiogramm showed enlarged para-aortic nodes with a coarse storage pattern. There was a moderate anaemia (Hgb 10, 1 g/dl; Hct 31%), a hyperalbuminaemia of 3.5 g/dl and a marked hypergammaglobulinaemia of 28.8 g/dl. The white cell count was 8500 mm^3 with 73% neutrophils, 1% band forms, 20% lymphocytes, and 6% monocytes. The moderately hypercellular bone marrow contained normal haematopoietic elements and many foamy macrophages with masses of mycobacteria, some haemosiderin pigment and occasionally showed erythrophagocytosis.

Karyotyping of bone marrow cells failed to detect any abnormality except for a "clonal instability" (Prof. Dr. Fliedner, Department of Clinical Physiology, University of Ulm). This change was not observed in peripheral blood lymphocytes. Granulocyte function tests for chemotactic reactivity, phagocytosis, increase in oxidative metabolism during particle uptake, and intracellular killing of Staph. aureus were all within normal range.

Quantitative determinations of immunoglobulins indicated a marked increase of IgG (5104 mg/dl), IgA (707 mg/dl), and IgM (655 mg/dl) in patient's serum. Skin reactions for testing delayed hypersensitivity were negative with Candida albicans, trichophytin, tuberculin, and streptococcal antigens. The proliferative responses of the patient's blood lymphocytes (total lymphocyte count: 1700/mm^3) to phytohaemagglutinin, concanavalin A, pokeweed mitogen, and to a pool of allogeneic, irradiated, frozen-thawed cells in mixed lymphocyte reaction were regular. Lymphocyte subpopulations in the peripheral blood were quantitated using routine techniques: the percentage of lymphocytes reacting with 5-2 aminoethyl-isothiuronium-bromidxHBr (AET)-treated sheep erythrocytes was 80% and thus in normal range. T-lymphocytes, expressing receptors with high avidity for sheep erythrocytes, were found to be 30% (normal range: 25 to 35%). Lymphocytes with receptors for human C3 were found to be

29%, those with receptors for mouse C3 (predominantly C3d) were 21%. The percentage of lymphocytes bearing surface immunoglobulins was 3% (normal range: 8 to 18%).

To investigate differentiation of B-cells into plasma cells in vitro, various cell combinations of mononuclear cells of the patient and a control person were stimulated in vitro by pokeweed mitogen. After 7 days in culture, cytocentrifuge smears were performed and the number of cells with intracellular immunoglobulins (= plasma cells) was determined by means of immunofluorescence; 500 cells were scored in each preparation. The mononuclear cells (MNC) of the patient did not differentiate into plasma cells. When the MNC of the patient were cocultured with T-lymphocytes (isolated by rosette formation with AET-treated sheep erythrocytes) of the control person, some plasma cell differentiation was obtained. The patient's T-lymphocytes did not suppress the plasma cell differentiation of the normal donor, but they also did not cooperate with the non-T-cells of the normal donor. These data suggested that the patient's T-lymphocytes were incapable of providing help for autologous and allogeneic non-T-cell in the pokeweed mitogen driven B-cell differentiation system (helper T-lymphocyte defect).

The patient's status during this last hospitalization did not improve, and he expired about 15 months after onset of his disease in sudden right heart failure from thrombosis of both main trunks of the pulmonary artery.*

Case 4

In October, 1973, a 78-year-old woman had bilateral total hip replacements with Aufranc-Turner prostheses because of severe degenerative joint disease. She did well until August, 1979, when a fall resulted in a subtrochanteric fracture of the left femur. Because of loosening of the femoral prosthesis, it was replaced with a long-stem Aufranc-Turner femoral prosthesis; the acetabular component was stable. Three weeks later, dark, bloody fluid was draining from the incision. Physical examination was otherwise unremarkable. The patient's peripheral white blood cell count was 7200/cu mm with a normal differential. The erythrocyte sedimentation rate was 82 mm/hour; the hematocrit was 37%. Serum electrolytes and creatinine were normal. The alkaline phosphatase was 165 mU/ml (normal, 30 to 85).

Small numbers of Staphylococcus epidermidis and S. aureus were isolated from drainage from the incision site. In addition, there was a moderate growth of gram-variable, acid-fast, coccobacilli after 48 to 72 hours of incubation. The patient was initially treated with par-

---

*From Bültmann, B.D., et al.: Virchows Arch., *395*:217, 1982. © 1982, Springer-Verlag, New York.[20]

enteral cephalosporins; sulfonamides were then added because of the possibility of nocardiosis.

Because of increasing drainage, the wound was debrided. Pus was found within the neocapsule but there was no loosening of the components. Suction irrigation was instituted and the wound was closed. Irrigation was discontinued after 4 days.

The patient did well for 10 days postoperatively, but purulent drainage from the proximal wound necessitated surgical reexploration on the twenty-second hospital day. Because loosening of the components was found, a Girdlestone resection arthroplasty with removal of the prosthesis and extensive debridement of necrotic bone and soft tissue was performed and the operative wound left open.

Histopathologic examination of a fragment of resected bone disclosed acute and chronic osteomyelitis and a clump of acid-fast bacilli. Gram-variable, acid-fast bacilli, identical to those isolated earlier, were isolated from cultures of material obtained deep within the surgical wound, as well as from the hip joint capsule, cortical and intramedullary bone of the femur, and the acetabulum. The microorganism was tentatively identified as an atypical mycobacterium and subsequently as M. fortuitum. The organism was susceptible to erythromycin 8 μg/ml, kanamycin 8 μg/ml, tetracycline 2 μg/ml, amikacin 2 μg/ml, and ethionamide 5 μg/ml. It was considered intermediately susceptible to cefoxitin 16 μg/ml, gentamicin 8 μg/ml, and trimethoprim-sulfamethoxazole 0.5 μg/ml to 10 μg/ml. It was resistant to ampicillin, carbenicillin, methicillin, penicillin G, cefamandole, cephalothin, colistimethate, clindamycin, streptomycin, isoniazid, PAD, ethambutol, and rifampin. Pseudomonas aeruginosa was also recovered from several of the operative specimens.

After removal of the prosthesis, gentamicin, and subsequently, tobramycin were prescribed. When the M. fortuitum was identified, amikacin was administered for 12 days. It was discontinued when renal failure due to obstructive uropathy developed. No antibiotics were prescribed thereafter.

Two and 3 weeks later, no mycobacteria could be recovered from the open wound with either routine or selective media. Although the wound appeared to heal during this period, the patient's condition slowly deteriorated and she died. No autopsy was done.

Cultures of bone cement from the same lot number as that used in the insertion of the second prosthesis were negative.*

---

*Reprinted by permission from Horadam, V.W., Smilack, J.D., and Smith, E.C.: Southern Medical Journal, 75(2):244–246, 1982. Copyright © by Southern Medical Association, Birmingham, Alabama.[36]

SUMMARY

Pulmonary disease is the most common manifestation of nontuberculous mycobacterial infections, but the acid-fast bacilli are being isolated with increasing frequency from a variety of clinical sites. It is important, but sometimes difficult, to distinguish whether colonization, infection, or actual disease is present. The quantity of growth, frequency of isolation, site of origin, species identification, presence of underlying disease, state of immunocompetence, and clinical manifestations must be carefully assessed in making a diagnosis.

Microscopic demonstration of acid-fast bacilli, growth rate, colony characteristics, and biochemical tests are important in speciation of nontuberculous mycobacteria. The bulk of human nontuberculous mycobacterial disease is caused by Mycobacterium kansasii and the M. avian-intracellulare complex.

Environmental sources of the organism are believed to be responsible for the majority of infections. Nontuberculous mycobacterial disease can be progressive and fatal because drug treatment is often less effective than in tuberculosis. Eradication of the nontuberculous mycobacterial infections awaits development of more effective drugs.

REFERENCES

1. Centers for Disease Control: Centennial: Koch's discovery of the tubercle bacillus. Morbid. Mortal. Weekly Rept., *31*:121, 1982.
2. Good, R.C.: Nontuberculous mycobacteria. Clin. Microbiol. Newsl., *1*:1, 1979.
3. Harris, H.W., and McClement, J.: Pulmonary tuberculosis. *In* Infectious Diseases, 3rd Ed. Edited by P.D. Hoeprich. Hagerstown, Maryland, Harper & Row, 1983.
4. Dornetzhuber, V., et al.: Pulmonary mycobacteriosis caused by Mycobacterium xenopi. Eur. J. Respir. Dis., *63*:293, 1982.
5. Bevelaqua, F.A., Kamelhar, D.A., Campion, J., and Christianson, L.C.: Mycobacterium fortuitum-chelonei—Two patients with fatal pulmonary infection. N.Y. State J. Med., *11*:1621, 1981.
6. Kelsey, D.S., Chambers, R.T., and Hudspeth, A.S.: Nontuberculous mycobacterial infection presenting as a mediastinal mass. J. Pediatr., *98*:431, 1981.
7. Gilligan, P.H., and McCarthy, L.R.: Peritonitis caused by Mycobacterium chelonei. Clin. Microbiol. Newsl., *1*:8, 1979.
8. Katz, M.A., and Hull, A.R.: Probable Mycobacterium fortuitum septicemia: Complication of home dialysis. Lancet, *1*:499, 1971.
9. Repath, F., Seaburg, J.N., and Saunders, C.V.: Prosthetic valve endocarditis due to Mycobacterium chelonei. South. Med. J., *69*:1244, 1976.
10. Beck, A.: Mycobacterium fortuitum in abscesses of man. J. Clin. Microbiol., *18*:307, 1965.
11. Borghas, J.G.L., and Stanford, J.L.: Mycobacterium chelonei in abscesses after injection of diphtheria-pertussis-tetanus polio vaccine. Am. Rev. Respir. Dis., *107*:1, 1973.
12. Hoffman, G.S., Myers, R.L., Stark, F.R., and Thoen, C.O.: Septic arthritis associated with Mycobacterium avium: A case report and literature review. J. Rheumatol., *5*:199, 1978.
13. Fainstein, V., Bolivar, R., and Mavlight, G.: Disseminated infection due to Mycobacterium avium-intracellulare in a homosexual man with Kaposi's sarcoma. J. Infect. Dis., *145*:586, 1982.
14. Lincoln, E.M., and Gilbert, L.A.: Disease in children due to mycobacteria other than Mycobacterium tuberculosis. Am. Rev. Respir. Dis., *105*:683, 1972.

15. Schaad, U.B., Votteler, T.P., McCracken, G.H., and Nelson, J.D.: Management of atypical mycobacterial lymphadenitis in childhood. J. Pediatr., 95:356, 1979.
16. Beck, A., Stanford, J.L., Inman, P.M., and Brown, A.E.: Mycobacteria, skins, and needles. Lancet, 2:801, 1962.
17. Foz, A., et al.: Mycobacterium chelonei iatrogenic infections. J. Clin. Microbiol., 7:319, 1978.
18. Center for Disease Control: Atypical mycobacterial wound infection. Morbid. Mortal. Weekly Rept., 25:233, 1976.
19. Wolinsky, E.: Nontuberculous mycobacteria and associated diseases, state of the art. Am. Rev. Respir. Dis., 119:107, 1979.
20. Bültmann, B.D., et al.: Disseminated mycobacterial histiocytois due to M. fortuitum associated with helper T-lymphocyte immune deficiency. Virchows Arch., 395:217, 1982.
21. Center for Disease Control: Follow-up on mycobacterial contamination of porcine heart valve prostheses. Morbid. Mortal. Weekly Rept., 27:92, 1978.
22. Center for Disease Control: Mycobacterial infections associated with augmentation mammoplasty. Morbid. Mortal. Weekly Rept., 27:513, 1978.
23. Tsukamura, M., et al.: Epidemiologic studies of lung disease due to mycobacteria other than Mycobacterium tuberculosis in Japan. Rev. Infect. Dis., 3:997, 1981.
24. Rosenzweig, D.Y., and Schleuter, D.P.: Spectrum of clinical disease in pulmonary infection with Mycobacterium avium-intracellulare. Rev. Infect. Dis., 3:1046, 1981.
25. Hsu, K.H.K.: Atypical mycobacterial infections in children. Rev. Infect. Dis., 3:1075, 1981.
26. Wolinsky, E.: When is an infection disease? Rev. Infect. Dis., 3:1025, 1981.
27. American Thoracic Society, Committee on Diagnostic Skin Testing: Tuberculin skin testing techniques: current status. Am. Rev. Respir. Dis., 87:607, 1963.
28. Mims, C.A.: The Pathogenesis of Infectious Disease, 2nd Ed. New York, Academic Press, 1982.
29. Narayanan, R.B., Jones, B.P., and Turk, J.L.: Experimental mycobacterial granulomas in guinea pig lymph nodes: ultrastructure observations. J. Pathol., 134:253, 1981.
30. Wolinsky, E., and Rynearson, T.K.: Mycobacteria in soil and their relation to disease-associated strains. Am. Rev. Respir. Dis., 97:1032, 1968.
31. Hatch, T.F.: Distribution and disposition of inhaled particles in respiratory tract. Bacteriol. Rev., 25:237, 1961.
32. Runyon, E.H.: Whence mycobacteria and mycobacterioses? Ann. Intern. Med., 75:467, 1971.
33. Schroder, K.H., and Juhlin, I.: Mycobacterium malmoense sp. nov. Int. J. Syst. Bacteriol., 27:241, 1977.
34. Sompolinsky, D.A., Lagziel, D.N., and Yankilevitz, T.: Mycobacterium haemophilum. sp. nov. a new pathogen of humans. Int. J. Syst. Bacteriol., 28:67, 1978.
35. Lester, W.: Nontuberculous mycobacterial infections. In Medical Microbiology and Infectious Diseases. Edited by A.I. Braude. Philadelphia, W.B. Saunders, 1981.
36. Horadam, V.W., Smilack, J.D., and Smith, E.C.: Mycobacterium fortuitum infection after total hip replacement. South. Med. J., 75:244, 1982.
37. Kubica, G.P., Dye, W.E., Cohn, M.L., and Middlebrook, G.: Sputum digestion and decontamination with N-acetyl-L-cysteine-sodium hydroxide for culture of mycobacteria. Am. Rev. Respir. Dis., 87:775, 1963.
38. Wayne, L.G., Krasnow, I., and Kidd, G.C.: Finding the "hidden positive" in tuberculosis eradication programs. The role of sensitive trisodium phosphate-benzalkonium (Zephiran) culture technique. Am. Rev. Respir. Dis., 86:537, 1962.
39. Corper, H.J., and Uyei, N.: Oxalic acid as a reagent for isolating tubercle bacilli and a study of the growth of acid fast non-pathogens on different mediums with their reactions to chemical reagents. J. Lab. Clin. Med., 15:348, 1930.
40. Vestal, A.L.: Procedures for the isolation and identification of mycobacteria. Atlanta, Georgia, U.S. Department of Health, Education, and Welfare, 1975.
41. Runyon, E.H., et al.: Mycobacterium. In Manual of Clinical Microbiology, 3rd Ed. Edited by E.H. Lennette. Washington, D.C., American Society for Microbiology, 1980.
42. Goslee, S., Rynearson, T.K., and Wolinsky, E.: Additional serotypes of Mycobac-

terium scrofulaceum, Mycobacterium gordonae, Mycobacterium marinum, and Mycobacterium xenopi determined by agglutination. Int. J. Syst. Bacteriol., *26*:136, 1976.

43. Wolinsky, E., and Schaefer, W.B.: Proposed numbering scheme for mycobacterial serotypes by agglutination. Int. J. Syst. Bacteriol., *23*:182, 1973.
44. Wolinsky, E.: Nontuberculous mycobacteria and associated diseases. Am. Rev. Respir. Dis., *119*:107, 1979.
45. Bogaerts, Y., et al.: Pulmonary disease due to Mycobacterium xenopi: Report of two cases. Eur. J. Respir. Dis., *63*:298, 1982.

CHAPTER 17 PNEUMOCYSTIS INFECTION

Pneumocystis infection was first recognized during World War II as a cause of interstitial pneumonia in premature infants, foundlings, and orphans in central Europe and Asia.[1] The syndrome has also been described in infants 3 to 5 months of age in Canada, Iran, Korea, and Spain.[2-5] In most instances, the children were suffering from malnutrition and were unable to mount effective immune responses in the presence of the infectious agent. For the past several decades, the organism Pneumocystis carinii has been also associated with pneumonia in immunocompromised individuals.[6-8] More recently, Pneumocystis carinii pneumonia (PCP) has occurred in previously healthy homosexual men and in children under 2 years of age who had unexplained immunodeficiency.[9-11] In 1981, an unexpected outbreak of PCP and Kaposi's sarcoma (KS) occurred in the United States among homosexual men.[9,12]

The enigmatic relationship between PCP or other opportunistic infections and KS has piqued the curiosity of public health officials and intensified the quest for the underlying mechanisms that cause the proliferation of both an infectious agent and neoplastic cells.

It is likely that most human infections caused by P. carinii are asymptomatic. Symptomatic pneumocystosis has been associated with a defect in cellular immunity.[13] The acquired cellular immunodeficiency is characterized by lymphopenia, T-lymphocyte depletion, defective natural killer-cell activity, anergy to cutaneous antigens, and an inability of the lymphocytes to proliferate.[13-15]

Interstitial plasma-cell pneumonia in premature, institutionalized, and malnourished children is characterized by dyspnea, tachypnea, coughing, the inability to gain weight, cyanosis, and sometimes, fever.[16] The onset is typically slow and insidious. Fine crepitant rales may be present on deep breathing, but other auscultatory findings are usually absent.[17] In older children and adults, the onset of pneumocystosis may be more abrupt.

Chest roentgenograms reveal a uniform density that may be more marked in the hilar areas (Fig. 17–1). The alveolar infiltration with Pneumocystis leads to progressive dyspnea. The term interstitial

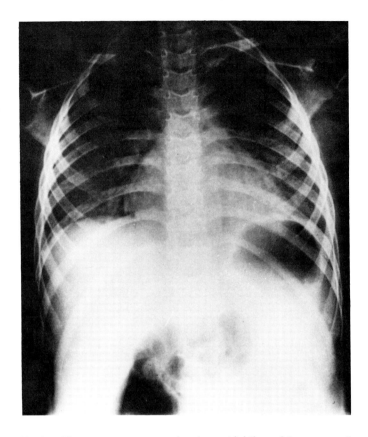

Figure 17–1. Chest roentgenogram of patient with bilateral Pneumocystis carinii pneumonia (PCP). (From Cohen, S.N.: Infection with Pneumocystis carinii. *In* Medical Microbiology and Infectious Diseases. Edited by A.I. Braude. Philadelphia, W.B. Saunders, 1981.)

plasma cell pneumonia is descriptive for the plasma cell infiltration of the interalveolar septa seen in newborns.

PCP may have a rapidly fulminating course both in infants and immunocompromised adults. The contribution of P. carinii to either the course of the disease or the death of patients is difficult to assess because underlying diseases or infections are often multiple. The fatality rate of untreated PCP is approximately 95%.

ETIOLOGY

The organism Pneumocystis carinii was first described in the lungs of guinea pigs and rats in Brazil in 1909 and 1910, and was at first thought to be a variant of a trypanosome.[18,19] Like Toxoplasma gondii, P. carinii has also been considered a coccidian, although only a probable life cycle for the organism has been described.[20] The trophozoite is believed to be motile and probably reproduces by binary fission before invading the parenchyma of the lung.[21]

P. carinii has a cell wall that contains chitin and, therefore, is considered to be closely related to fungi. The taxonomic position of P. carinii remains uncertain, however, because the organism appears also to have characteristics classically associated with protozoa. Intra-alveolar material in the infected lungs of animals and humans consists largely of masses of P. carinii. In terminal cases, alveoli contain fat-laden cells, exudate, and the parasites. It is presumed that organisms can persist in a host because they are able to encyst and escape destruction by host defenses or drugs.

The rat has been used as a model to study induction of latent infections of P. carinii.[22] In most colonies of rats, the animals are infected subclinically. After a 4- to 6-week period of hypercorticism or administration of cyclophosphamide, the disease becomes apparent. Despite certain similarities between PCP in rats and humans, much needs to be learned of the host-parasite relationship that exists between humans and P. carinii.

PREDISPOSING FACTORS

Pneumocystis infection gives rise to overt disease in immunodeficient hosts. Prematurity, low birth weight, use of intravenous drugs by the mother, malnutrition, and unexplained immune deficiencies predispose neonates to interstitial plasma-cell pneumonia caused by Pneumocystis carinii. Institutionalization of infants appears to provide a unique opportunity for the organism to spread. Severe combined immunodeficiency (SCID) or any form of chemotherapy that depresses cellular immune responses predisposes older children and adults to pneumocystosis. One study of over 100 cases of SCID from 19 geographically distinct areas of the United States reported that 27% of the individuals had infections caused by P. carinii.[23] Persons with chronic granulomatous disease (CGD) may also be particularly prone to develop Pneumocystis infection.[24,25] CGD is characterized by recurrent purulent infections of the skin, lungs, and organs of the reticuloendothelial systems. In CGD, phagocytes lack the ability to form the high-energy metabolites necessary for the destruction of microorganisms.

Male homosexuals with acquired immune deficiency syndrome (AIDS) constitute a high-risk group for the development of a variety of opportunistic viral infections, including those caused by cytomegalovirus (CMV), Epstein-Barr virus (EBV), and hepatitis B virus (HBV). CMV causes immunosuppression in both mice and humans.[26,27] Since homosexuality is not a new life style and CMV is not a new pathogen, it is unlikely that CMV infection can be entirely responsible for the circumstances that permit proliferation of P. carinii.[12] So-called "recreational drugs," such as amyl nitrite, may represent a risk factor.[28] A subgroup of homosexuals living in Los Angeles and New York, where PCP was first reported, are known to inhale amyl nitrite to intensify orgasm. Whether susceptibility to PCP is related to a synergistic effect occurring with drug use in the presence of an opportunistic agent or of another infectious agent remains speculative. In 1982, three cases of PCP were reported in heterosexual males with hemophilia A in the United States. None had a history of drug abuse, other underlying disease, or therapy that could induce immunosuppression.[29]

Familial pneumocystosis has been reported in siblings and in a three-member family that included a husband and wife.[30-32] Contagion is usually not believed to be responsible for familial outbreaks. Siblings and other family members probably share an inherited susceptibility. The husband of the three-member family involved in familial pneumocystosis had been treated with corticosteroids.

EPIDEMIOLOGY

Pneumocystis carinii is believed to be ubiquitous in nature, but the prevalence of latent infections or carrier states is impossible to determine. Until recently, the largest number of PCP cases occurred in infants and children between the ages of 1 and 4 years. Clustering of overt pneumocystosis has been recognized in cancer patients receiving aggressive chemotherapy, in organ-transplant patients receiving corticosteroids, and in homosexual males. It is almost impossible to document how PCP is spread, but intimate sexual contact in homosexual males could provide an opportunistic mode of transmission. Person-to-person transmission was believed to be responsible for the spread of P. carinii in European institutions for children where health-care personnel may have acted as healthy carriers. Blood products are suspected as vehicles of transmission in hemophiliacs who require multiple units of Factor VIII.[29] Factor VIII is available as a cryoprecipitate made from single units of fresh-frozen plasma or as lyophilized Factor VIII-concentrate obtained from plasma pools collected from 1000 or more donors.

Direct transmission of P. carinii has been demonstrated in immunosuppressed rats. A unique susceptibility caused by underlying disease or immune deficiencies appears to be the common thread in human PCP. For that reason, persons developing PCP should be isolated from other immunocompromised patients in a hospital setting.

LABORATORY DIAGNOSIS

Chest roentgenograms showing interstitial or alveolar infiltrates, arterial hypoxemia, and hypocapnia are consistent findings in Pneumocystis carinii pneumonia (PCP). Those findings, however, are not definitive for the presence of the organism in lung tissue.[7] It is imperative, therefore, that immediate steps be taken to identify the etiologic agent.

Microscopic Examination

The most reliable technique for a definitive diagnosis of PCP has been microscopic examination of stained smears obtained from transtracheal aspirates, from endobronchial brush biopsies, or from histopathologic sections from biopsy or autopsy material. The application of hematoxylin-eosin or Gomori's methenamine silver nitrate to slides prepared from lung sections has been of value in detecting the presence of P. carinii.[33] The Giemsa, toluidine blue O, or methenamine-silver stains may be used to stain impression smears. A 10-minute methenamine-silver stain which employs metabisulfite, a 10:1 mixture of methenamine-silver nitrate, direct heating of the working solution to 90° to 95°C, and gold chloride toning after silver staining provides both rapid and consistent results.[34] It is recommended that duplicate slides be stained by the various techniques and that a positive control be included for each stain.[35] A variety of morphologic forms has been described.[36] Trophozoites are highly pleomorphic and may be as large as 2.0 to 12.0 μm in length.[37] Cysts are usually spherical and measure 3.5 to 4.0 μm in diameter (Fig. 17–2).

Detailed morphology of trophozoites and cysts of P. carinii in the lung is best observed by electron microscopy of tissue obtained by biopsy. Trophozoites often contain fine projections measuring 0.1 μm in diameter. Four forms of cysts have been described: a precyst, a mature cyst, a cyst liberating trophozoites, and an empty collapsed cyst. Mature cysts contain distinct intracystic bodies (Fig. 17–3).

Cultural Techniques

P. carinii has been successfully cultured in embryonic chicken epithelial cells, MRC-5 cells, and WI-38 human embryonic lung fibroblasts.[38–40] The cultural techniques are applicable to studies of pathogenesis and immunology but are not used as diagnostic procedures.

Serologic Tests

Serologic techniques for diagnosing PCP have been largely unrewarding.[41,42] It appears unlikely that patients with the severe immune deficiencies found in PCP can produce detectable levels of antibody. Measurement of P. carinii antigens by enzyme immunoassay may hold some promise for the eventual testing of clinical specimens.[43]

PROGNOSIS

Interstitial plasma-cell pneumonia in the neonate is usually fatal. Prompt recognition and treatment with trimethoprim-sulfamethox-

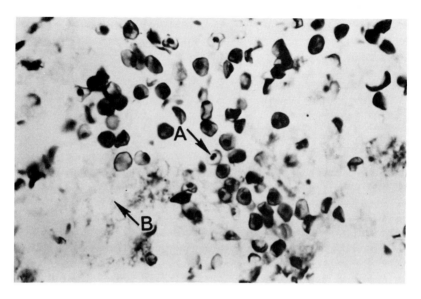

Figure 17–2. Cysts of Pneumocystis carinii in alveolar spaces as demonstrated by Gomori's methenamine silver-nitrate stain. Several of the cysts contain small intracystic bodies (A →). These cysts correspond to the thick-walled cysts in electron microscopic preparations. The thin-walled cysts do not stain readily and appear only as amorphous or finely reticulated background (B →). (Courtesy H. Sepp, Toronto.)

azole or pentamidine isethionate has reduced mortality rates to 20 to 30% in older children and adults.[44] Children who recover from acute pneumocystosis may have persistent lung dysfunction.[45] Previously healthy adults who recover from Pneumocystis carinii pneumonia have little or no permanent lung damage, but relapses are not uncommon in immunosuppressed patients. The severity of underlying disease and presence of multiple opportunistic infections in patients with PCP may mask sequelae. Survival rates appear to be dependent on the severity of the immune impairment, the age of the patient, and appropriate therapy.

CASE REPORTS

Case 1

This 2948-g full-term female infant did well until 5 months of age, when she was admitted to the Bethesda Naval Hospital because of congestive heart failure. Cardiac catheterization revealed a small atrial septal defect with elevated pulmonary arterial pressures. Despite vigorous treatment with digoxin and diuretics, she showed no clinical improvement and was transferred to the Johns Hopkins Hospital for further evaluation.

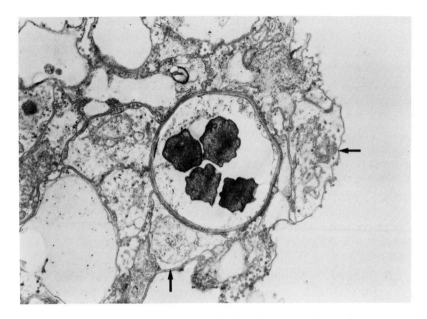

Figure 17–3. Electron micrograph of a thick-walled cyst of Pneumocystis carinii containing dense intracystic bodies from biopsy material. (From Sepp, H.: Ann. Eston. Med. Assoc., p. 49, 1975.)

The family history was remarkable for death in a maternal great uncle at 1 year of age from an unknown pulmonary disease. Another maternal great uncle was found to have desquamative interstitial pneumonia (DIP) at Jefferson Medical College in 1966 and required long-term steroid administration for clinical management. This case was previously published by Patchefsky et al.

Physical examination on admission at 7 months of age showed this infant to be pale and malnourished, with intercostal retractions and a respiratory rate of 75. Diffuse coarse crackling rales were present, and there was a grade 2–3/6 systolic ejection murmur at the left sternal border with fixed splitting of S_2 and accentuation of P_2. The liver was 2.5 cm below the right costal margin, and the spleen tip was palpable. Arterial blood gas in room air revealed a PO_2 of 58 mm Hg, PCO_2 of 31 mm Hg, and a pH of 7.48. Chest roentgenograms showed diffuse interstitial and intra-alveolar infiltrates. Subsequent evaluation of her pulmonary disease included the following negative findings: non-reactive PPD, normal sweat chloride, normal esophagram with no reflux or tracheo-esophageal fistula, normal α_1-antitrypsin with Pi type MM, normal quantitative immunoglobulins, C_3 and C_4, normal T cell functions as assessed by response to mixed lymphocyte culture and phytohemagglutinins, and negative antinuclear antibody and rheumatoid factor. An open lung biopsy showed an interstitial pneumonitis with a desquamative component and the presence of scattered Pneumocystis carinii cysts. Bacterial, viral, mycobacterial, and chlamydial cultures of the biopsy specimen were sterile. Despite a 3-week course of Bactrim (combination of 20 mg/kg of trimethoprim and 100 mg/kg of sulfamethoxazole), no significant clinical change was noted. Prednisone therapy at 2.0 mg/kg was started, and within 72 hours marked clinical improvement was observed. The patient did relatively well over the next 12 months, and the prednisone dosage was gradually reduced to 1.0 mg/kg every other day. However, she received maintenance prophylactic therapy with Bactrim, since several attempts to discontinue giving the antibiotic resulted in fever and respiratory distress.

Fifteen months after the initial diagnosis, the patient became ill with tachypnea, fever, and weight loss and was admitted to Wilford Hall USAF Medical Center. At that time, her steroid dosage had been reduced to 0.5 mg/kg. She had a prolonged and complicated hospital course marked by spiking temperatures, hypoxia, and requirement for mechanical ventilation. A chest roentgenogram showed diffuse bilateral interstitial infiltrates. Repeated open lung biopsy showed usual interstitial pneumonitis with mild interstitial fibrosis and no evidence of Pneumocystis. All bacterial and viral cultures were sterile. The patient gradually responded to reinstitution of high-dose corticosteroid and Bactrim. Since then she has remained well with alternate-day therapy of low-dose prednisone and Bactrim.

The first lung biopsy obtained at 7 months of age showed active interstitial inflammation with lymphocytes, plasma cells, and scattered polymorphonuclear leukocytes diffusely infiltrating the alveolar walls. Marked alveolar hyperplasia, desquamation, and focal epithelial necrosis were present. The alveoli contained numerous macrophages and a few foci of polymorphonuclear leukocytes. A few scattered P. carinii cysts were demonstrated in the alveoli by the Gram-Weigert stain. These changes were consistent with an active phase of usual interstitial pneumonitis.

Results of the second lung biopsy, at 22 months of age, showed considerably less activity than that of the previous biopsy, with only a minimal interstitial infiltrate of lymphocytes accompanied by a mild degree of interstitial fibrosis. Epithelial desquamation and necrosis were absent. P. carinii could not be demonstrated by special stains.*

Case 2

A 19-year-old white male was admitted to University of Nebraska Hospital with severe dyspnea, tachypnea, a low-grade fever, and night

---

*From Mak, H., Moser, R.L., Hallet, J.S., and Robotham, J.L.: Chest, *1*:124–126, 1982.[46]

sweats. Three years prior to this admission, the patient was found to have systemic lupus erythematosus and was treated with prednisone and azathioprine.

He complained of severe shortness of breath with pleuritis and some mid-epigastric distress. His medications on admission included prednisone 40 mg/d. The azathioprine had been discontinued the previous month. He was also taking propranolol 120 mg qid, furosemide 160 mg bid, and prazosin 1 mg q8h for hypertension.

Vital signs included T 99.5°F, BP 140/94 mm Hg, P 114, and R 50–60. Physical examination was consistent with chronic steroid usage. His examination revealed inspiratory and expiratory rhonchi without rales in the lungs, some evidence of peripheral cyanosis, and an ulcer in the pretibial area. Admission lab included a PO_2 of 49 with a PCO_2 of 29, pH 7.49.

The hospital course was complicated by a progressive anemia as documented by a decrease in hemoglobin from 12.3 to 7.2 g%. A continued leukocytosis from 11,200 to 16,100/mm³ with a marked left shift was observed. His blood urea nitrogen (BUN) and creatinine rose during this hospitalization from an admission BUN of 136 mg% and a creatinine of 3.3 mg% up to BUN 185 mg% and creatinine 7.2 mg%.

The day after admission, the patient underwent an open-lung biopsy, and a preliminary diagnosis of Pneumocystis carinii pneumonia was made. He was placed on a respirator with 50% FI_{O_2} to maintain his oxygenation. Following the open-lung biopsy, he was started on TMP 240 mg/SMX 1200 mg q6h by nasogastric tube. The following day, his dosage was increased to TMP 360 mg/SMX 1800 mg q6h. The absorption of the drug was questioned as the patient's condition deteriorated, and a decision was made to change to an intravenous solution of TMP/SMX (80 mg/400 mg per 5 ml); 1½ ampuls q8h were used initially, but increased to 2½ ampuls q8h after 1 day. Pentamidine 300 mg IM daily was added on hospital day 5.

Peritoneal dialysis was instituted on hospital day 3 and continued until the patient's demise. He was extremely hypoxic, requiring 50 to 100% oxygenation on the respirator with positive end expiratory pressure at 10 cm. No objective evidence of improvement wa seen throughout his hospital course. The patient expired on hospital day 7.

At autopsy, the findings of systemic lupus erythematosus and bilateral Pneumocystis carinii pneumonia were confirmed.*

---

*Reprinted with permission, Copyright 1981
Drug Intelligence & Clinical Pharmacy, Inc.
4906 Cooper Rd., P.O. Box 42435 Cincinnati, OH 45242[47]

Case 3

A 38-year-old homosexual man was in excellent health until July, 1980, 2 months before admission to the hospital, when recurrent sore throats, anorexia, and dyspnea began. These symptoms continued; 1 week before admission, fever, night sweats, headache, and a non-productive cough developed. Progressive fever to 39.4°C, substernal chest pain, and dyspnea on minimal exertion led to his admission. No coryza, myalgias, arthralgias, or mental changes were noted.

The patient appeared ill; respirations were 36/min; pulse rate, 88 beats per minute; and temperature, 40.3°C. Results of the physical examination were otherwise normal.

Laboratory evaluation disclosed a hematocrit reading of 37%; leukocyte count, 8400/cu mm, with 90 polymorphonuclear leukocytes, 15 lymphocytes, 4 band forms, and 1 monocyte; and sedimentation rate (Westergren), 120 mm/hour. Except for a nonfasting blood glucose level of 179 mg/dl, lactate dehydrogenase level of 252 units/L, and phosphorus level of 2.7 mg/dl, the laboratory findings were normal. Arterial blood gas analyses on room air were PO_2, 55 mm Hg and PCO_2, 24 mm Hg; pH was 7.50. Bilateral diffuse interstitial and alveolar infiltrates were present on chest roentgenogram.

Administration of erythromycin, 500 mg intravenously every 6 hours, and rifampin, 600 mg daily, were begun for therapy of possible Legionnaires' disease. One day later, open lung biopsy was performed because of worsening hypoxemia and pulmonary infiltration. Interstitial pneumonitis and alveolitis were found. Numerous P. carinii organisms were seen on Gram-Weigert and silver methenamine stains. No fungi, acid-fast bacilli, or Legionella pneumophila were noted on special stains. Further laboratory evaluation included levels of serum γ-globulin, 1.45 mg/dl; IgG, 15.2 mg/ml; IgA, 4.9 mg/ml; IgM, 1.0 mg/ml; and titers of antistreptolysin O, 333 Todd units; and cytomegalovirus, 1:16. A skin test for Candida showed 20 mm of induration at 48 hours, but a PPD skin test reaction was negative.

Oral trimethoprim, 20 mg/kg/day, and sulfamethoxazole, 100 mg/kg/day, were given and then changed to intravenous administration after 24 hours, due to further deterioration. Sulfamethoxazole levels were 110 μg/dl and 200 μg/dl after oral and intravenous therapy, respectively. Mechanical ventilation with positive end-expiratory pressure was required. After 4 days of intravenous administration of trimethoprim-sulfamethoxazole, pentamidine isethionate, 4 mg/kg/day, was added because of persistent fever and pulmonary infiltrates. Two days later, a chest tube was inserted for a right tension pneumothorax. Although the lung reexpanded, a large air leak persisted and failed to close despite a trial of high-frequency jet ventilation. Pulmonary infiltrates, hypercarbia, and hypotension progressed, and the patient died 14 days after trimethoprim-sulfamethoxazole therapy was begun.

At necropsy, lung consolidation, bilateral bronchopleural fistulae, and persistent Pneumocystis organisms were found throughout the lungs.*

SUMMARY

Human Pneumocystis infection has been recognized as a significant cause of morbidity and mortality in young infants for at least 4 decades. More recently, the etiologic agent, Pneumocystis carinii, has been isolated with increasing frequency from immunocompromised hosts with pneumonia. Clusters of cases of Pneumocystis carinii pneumonia (PCP), complicated by Kaposi's sarcoma in homosexual men living in large cities of the United States, have alerted public health officials to a new immunodeficiency syndrome. A human retrovirus is suspected as the possible etiologic agent of acquired immune deficiency syndrome (AIDS), but those individuals with the underlying immune deficiencies are susceptible to a number of opportunistic pathogens. The mode of transmission for P. carinii has been difficult to document. To date, the most valuable technique for establishing the presence of P. carinii has been microscopic examination, but the availability of an immunoassay technique may prove an effective tool for measuring P. carinii antigenemia in the future.

REFERENCES

1. Van der Meer, G., and Brug, S.L.: Infection par pneumocystis chez les animaux. Ann. Soc. Belg. Med. Trop., *22*:301, 1942.
2. Berdnikoff, G.: Fourteen personal cases of Pneumocystis carinii pneumonia. Can. Med. Assoc. J., *80*:1, 1959.
3. Post, C., Dutz, W., and Nasarian, I.: Endemic Pneumocystis carinii pneumonia in South Iran. Arch. Dis. Child., *39*:35, 1964.
4. Hyun, B.H., Varga, F., and Thalheimer, L.J.: Pneumocystis carinii pneumonitis occurring in an adopted Korean infant. JAMA, *195*:784, 1966.
5. Moragas, A., and Vidal, M.T.: Pneumocystis carinii pneumonia. First autopsy series in Spain. Helv. Paediatr. Acta, *26*:71, 1971.
6. Godell, B., Jacobs, J.B., and Powell, R.D.: Pneumocystis carinii: the spectrum of diffuse interstitial pneumonia in patients with neoplastic diseases. Ann. Intern. Med., *72*:337, 1970.
7. Wolff, J.J.: The causes of interstitial pneumonitis in immunocompromised children: an aggressive systematic approach to diagnosis. Pediatrics, *60*:41, 1977.
8. Singer, C.D., et al.: Diffuse pulmonary infiltrates in immunosuppressed patients: a prospective study of 80 cases. Am. J. Med., *66*:110, 1979.
9. Centers for Disease Control: Pneumocystis pneumonia—Los Angeles. Morbid. Mortal. Weekly Rept., *30*:250, 1981.
10. Waldhorn, R.E., Tsou, E., and Kerwin, D.M.: Pneumocystis carinii pneumonia in a previously healthy adult. JAMA, *247*:1860, 1982.
11. Centers for Disease Control: Unexplained immunodeficiency and opportunistic

---

*From Waldhorn, R.E., Tsou, E., and Kerwin, D.M.: JAMA, *247*:1860–1861, 1982. Copyright, 1982 American Medical Association.[10]

infection in infants—New York, New Jersey, California. Morbid. Mortal. Weekly Rept., *31*:665, 1982.

12. Centers for Disease Control. Kapsosi's sarcoma and Pneumocystis pneumonia among homosexual men—New York City and California. Morbid. Mortal. Weekly Rept., *30*:305, 1981.

13. Durack, D.T.: Opportunistic infections and Kaposi's sarcoma in homosexual men. N. Engl. J. Med., *305*:1465, 1981.

14. Gottlieb, M.S., et al.: Pneumocystis carinii pneumonia and mucosal candidiasis in previously healthy homosexual men—a report of eight cases: evidence of a new acquired cellular deficiency. N. Engl. J. Med., *305*:1425, 1981.

15. Masur, H., et al.: An outbreak of community-acquired Pneumocystis carinii pneumonia: initial manifestation of cellular immune dysfunction. N. Engl. J. Med., *305*:1431, 1981.

16. Frenkel, J.K.: Toxoplasmosis and pneumocystosis: clinical and laboratory aspects in immunocompetent and compromised hosts. *In* Opportunistic Infections. Edited by J.E. Prier and H. Friedman. Baltimore, University Park Press, 1974.

17. Ruskin, J. and Remington, J.S.: Pneumocystosis. *In* Infectious Diseases, 3rd Ed. Edited by P.D. Hoeprich. New York, Harper & Row, 1983.

18. Chagas, C.: Nova tripanzomiaze humane. Estudos sobre a morfolgia e o ciclo evolutivo do Schizotrypanum cruzi n. gen. n. sp., agente etiolojico de nova entidade morbida do homen. Mem. Inst., *1*:159, 1909.

19. Carini, A.: Formas de eschizogonia de Trypanosoma lewisii. Soc. Med. Cir. São Paulo, 16 Aout, 1910.

20. Campbell, W.G., Jr.: Ultrastructure of pneumocystis in human lung. Arch. Pathol., *93*:312, 1972.

21. Cohen, S.N.: Infection with Pneumocystis carinii. *In* Medical Microbiology and Infectious Diseases. Edited by A.I. Braude. Philadelphia, W.B. Saunders, 1981.

22. Frenkel, J.K., Good, J.T., and Schultz, J.A.: Latent Pneumocystis infection of rats, relapse, and chemotherapy. Lab. Invest., *15*:1559, 1966.

23. Lessiadro, R.J., Winkelstein, J.A., and Hughes, W.T.: Prevalence of Pneumocystis carinii pneumonitis. J. Pediatr., *99*:96, 1981.

24. Pedersen, F.K., et al.: Refractory Pneumocystis infection in chronic granulomatous disease: Successful treatment with granulocytes. Pediatrics, *64*:935, 1979.

25. Adinoff, A.D., et al.: Chronic granulomatous disease and Pneumocystis carinii pneumonia. Pediatrics, *69*:133, 1982.

26. Hamilton, J.R., Overall, J.C., Jr., and Glasgow, L.A.: Synergistic effect on mortality in mice with murine cytomegalovirus and Pseudomonas aeruginosa, Staphylococcus aureus, or Candida albicans infections. Infect. Immun., *14*:982, 1976.

27. Carney, D.P., et al.: Analysis of T lymphocyte subsets in cytomegalovirus mononucleosis. J. Immunol., *126*:2114, 1981.

28. Goode, E., and Troiden, R.R.: Amyl nitrite use among homosexual men. Am. J. Psychiatry, *136*:1067, 1979.

29. Centers for Disease Control: Pneumocystis carinii pneumonia among persons with hemophilia A. Morbid. Mortal. Weekly Rept., *31*:365, 1982.

30. Gentry, L.O., and Remington, J.S.: Pneumocystis carinii pneumonia in siblings. J. Pediatr., *76*:769, 1970.

31. Becroft, D.M., and Costello, J.M.: Pneumocystis carinii pneumonia in siblings: Diagnosis by lung aspiration. N.Z. Med. J., *64*:273, 1965.

32. Watanabe, J.M., Chinchinian, H., Weitz, D., and McIlvanie, S.K.: Pneumocystis carinii pneumonia in a family. JAMA, *193*:685, 1965.

33. Burke, B.A., and Good, R.A.: Pneumocystis carinii infection. Medicine, *52*:23, 1973.

34. Musto, L., Flanigan, M., and Elbadawi, A.: Ten-minute silver stain for Pneumocystis carinii and fungi in tissue sections. Arch. Pathol. Lab. Med., *106*:292, 1982.

35. Kagan, I.G., and Norman, L.: The laboratory diagnosis of Pneumocystis carinii pneumonia. Health Lab. Sci., *14*:155, 1977.

36. Deas, J.E.: Other tissue-swelling protozoa: Toxoplasma gondii and Pneumocystis carinii. *In* Manual of Clinical Microbiology, 3rd Ed. Edited by E.H. Lennette. Washington, D.C., American Society for Microbiology, 1980.

37. Hasleton, P.S., Curry, A., and Rankin, E.M.: Pneumocystis carinii pneumonia: a light microscopical and ultrastructural study. J. Clin. Pathol., *34*:1138, 1981.
38. Pifer, L.L., Hughes, W.T., and Murphy, M.J., Jr.: Propagation of Pneumocystis carinii in vitro. Pediatr. Res., *11*:305, 1977.
39. Latorre, C.R., Sulzer, A.J., and Norman, L.G.: Serial propagation of Pneumocystis carinii in cell line cultures. Appl. Environ. Microbiol., *33*:1204, 1977.
40. Bartlett, M.S., Verbanac, P.A., and Smith, J.W.: Cultivation of Pneumocystis carinii with WI-38 cells. J. Clin. Microbiol., *10*:796, 1979.
41. Meuwissen, J.H.E., et al.: Parasitologic and serologic observations of infection with Pneumocystis in humans. J. Infect. Dis., *136*:43, 1977.
42. Norman, L., and Kagan, I.G.: Some observations on the serology of Pneumocystis carinii infections in the United States. Infect. Immun., *8*:317, 1973.
43. Leggiadro, R.S., Yolken, R.H., Simkins, J.H., and Hughes, W.T.: Measurement of Pneumocystis carinii antigen by enzyme immunoassay. J. Infect. Dis., *144*:484, 1981.
44. Hughes, W.T.: Pneumocystis carinii pneumonia. N. Engl. J. Med., *297*:1381, 1977.
45. Sanyal, S.K., Mariencheck, W.C., and Mackert, P.W.: Course of pulmonary dysfunction in children surviving Pneumocystis carinii pneumonitis (PCP): a prospective study. Pediatr. Res., *15*:620, 1981.
46. Mak, H., Moser, R.L., Hallet, J.S., and Robotham, J.L.: Usual interstitial pneumonitis in infancy. Clinical and pathologic evaluation. Chest, *1*:124, 1982.
47. Johnson, J.F., Rehder, T.L., and Moore, G.F.: Pneumocystis carinii pneumonia: Review with a case study. Drug. Intell. Clin. Pharm., *15*:732, 1981.

CHAPTER 18 PSEUDALLESCHERIASIS

The fungus Pseudallescheria boydii (Allescheria boydii, Petriellidium boydii) and its asexual stage, Scedosporium apiospermum (Monosporium apiospermum), have long been associated with a mycetoma known as Madura foot.[1,2] Madura foot occurs in both temperate and tropical climates throughout the world. It is now recognized that the fungus can cause noninvasive or invasive disease in a variety of organs. The organism has been isolated from documented cases of sinusitis, necrotizing pneumonia, meningoencephalitis, endophthalmitis, keratitis, parotitis, otomycosis, chronic prostatitis, tenosynovitis, joint infections, osteomyelitis, soft-tissue infections, and disseminated disease.[3-12]

NONINVASIVE PSEUDALLESCHERIASIS

Noninvasive mycetomas of various organs have been described, but those associated with the eyes or lungs appear to be most common.[13,14] Noninvasive pulmonary pseudallescheriasis usually occurs in individuals with chronic cystic or cavitary lung disease caused by sarcoidosis, bronchiectasis, or tuberculosis. A fungus ball called a pseudallescherioma (formerly, petriellidioma) frequently can be observed in a cavity on a chest roentgenogram (Fig. 18–1). Cavities may erode into pulmonary blood vessels and cause hemoptysis. Sputum specimens are not consistently positive in the presence of fungus balls caused by P. boydii. Blood may or may not be present in the sputum. In the absence of a positive culture, surgical intervention is necessary.

INVASIVE PSEUDALLESCHERIASIS

Invasive pseudallescheriasis consists of progressive chronic infections in which the fungus invades cutaneous tissue, subcutaneous tissue, fascia, and bone.[15] Initial lesions frequently occur on the foot, but can be associated with the lung or eye. Relatively few cases of lung abscess or necrotizing pneumonia have been reported.[5,18,19] Most of these cases were in immunocompromised individuals, but at least one case of necrotizing pneumonia has been described in an apparently healthy host.[5] Lesions of the extremities are characterized by abscesses, granulomas, and sinus tracts, which drain granule-containing pus

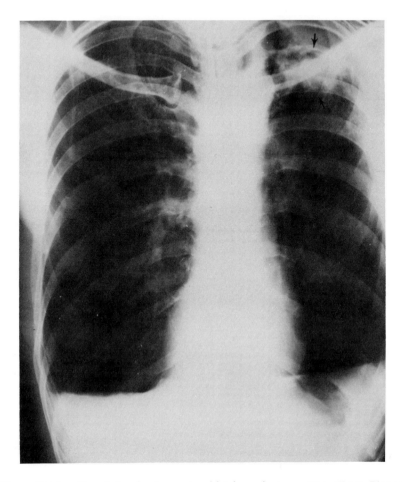

Figure 18–1. Pseudallescheriomas in old tuberculosis cavities. (From Rippon, J.W.: Medical Mycology—The Pathogenic Fungi and the Pathogenic Actinomycetes, 2nd Ed. Philadelphia, W.B. Saunders, 1982.)

(Fig. 18–2). Fever, chills, weight loss, and pain are either absent or minimal.

Increasing numbers of ocular infections following surgery or trauma have resulted from accidental exposure to P. boydii.[6,7] Impaired vision and inflammation are frequent complaints. If the fungi are resistant to local antimicrobial therapy, enucleation may be required to arrest or cure the infection.

Disseminated pseudallescheriasis was reported in an Italian military physician as early as 1938.[20] The physician had not been treated with any chemotherapeutic agents. More recently, disseminated pseudallescheriasis has been reported as a cause of morbidity or mortality in immunocompromised hosts with neoplastic disease, in a renal allo-

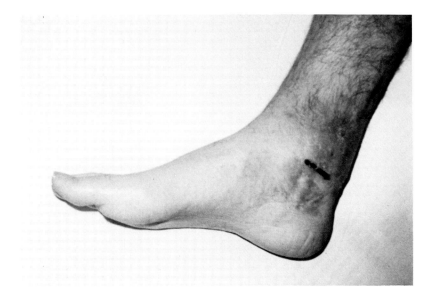

Figure 18–2. Mycetoma of the ankle caused by Pseudallescheria boydii. (Courtesy, J.P. Utz.)

graft recipient, and in Pancoast syndrome.[10,11] The brain, the meninges, and the thyroid have been frequent target sites in disseminated pseudallescheriasis, although no organ is invulnerable.[17–19]

ETIOLOGY

P. boydii and S. apiospermum appeared to be two distinct etiologic agents of Madura foot until 1944, when it was shown that S. apiospermum represents the imperfect state of P. boydii.[1] In invasive disease, the fungus produces brown, branching, septate hyphae in tissue. The hyphae are usually indistinguishable in histologic sections from the hyphae of Aspergillus species. Only rarely are conidia produced in vivo. The paucity or complete absence of hyphae in tissue in noninvasive disease has led to the hypothesis that tissue damage in pseudallescheriasis is related to a severe inflammatory response of the host.[4] Severe tissue damage may occur by a similar mechanism in other pulmonary mycoses, such as chronic histoplasmosis. It has been further postulated that dramatic host responses may be the result of the release and spread of fungal antigens from foci of infection.

PREDISPOSING FACTORS

Underlying disease, such as neoplastic disease and congenital immunodeficiencies, drug-related immunosuppression, and penetrating trauma, are important predisposing factors in pseudallescheriasis. The infection occurs infrequently in immunocompetent hosts.

It is often overlooked that the ubiquitous P. boydii can be introduced or disseminated by any invasive procedure, including surgery.[20] At least 1 case of chronic meningitis caused by the fungus followed administration of spinal anesthesia.[19] Meningitis developed 4 weeks after surgery, and the patient died after 8 months of severe illness. In another patient, a possibly airborne pulmonary infection is believed to have spread to the brain, thyroid, and heart by the bloodstream.[12]

EPIDEMIOLOGY

Pseudallescheria boydii is ubiquitous in nature. Since Ajello and Zeidberg first isolated it from the soil of Williamson County, Tennessee in 1951,[21] the organism has been isolated from soil, polluted water, sewage, sludge, and animal wastes in diverse geographical areas of the United States. Maduromycosis is associated with traumatic inoculation of P. boydii into a foot or hand. The infection occurs more frequently in men than in women and is more often seen in rural rather than urban areas.

It is assumed that initial pulmonary colonization with P. boydii is the result of inhaling ascospores.[22,23] It has been documented that transient colonization can occur secondary to underlying disease.[24] Aggressive searches for pulmonary colonization of P. boydii might yield more isolates of the fungus, but its mere presence may not be associated with disease. Although P. boydii has been incriminated in ocular infections, the organism does not appear to be a part of the indigenous flora of the outer eye.[25]

LABORATORY DIAGNOSIS

Pseudallescheria boydii is one of 17 common fungi known to cause eumycotic mycetomas. Several species of Actinomyces can cause actinomycotic mycetoma. Since pseudallescheriasis appears to be of increasing importance as a clinical entity, especially in severely immunocompromised patients, the alert laboratorian will want to review morphologic and cultural characteristics of P. boydii periodically.

Microscopic Examination

Pus or exudates from draining lesions and biopsy material in pseudallescheriasis are characterized by the presence of distinct white-to-yellow soft granules with diameters of approximately 2 mm. Granules of P. boydii can easily be mistaken for those of Aspergillus nidulans because they are similar in size and consistency. The granules consist of soft, compact masses of mycelia, which are carried along with serosanguineous fluid from infected sites. Granules of Actinomyces species are also white or yellow, but are hard in consistency and measure up to 5 mm in diameter.[26] Granules must be demonstrated for an infection to qualify as a mycetoma.

When crushed in 10% KOH preparations, granules of all eumycotic agents appear microscopically as broad, interwoven, septate hyphae measuring 2 to 5 μm in diameter.[27] Sometimes the hyphae contain swollen cells, which are at least 15 μm in diameter. Actinomycotic granules contain smaller interwoven fibers usually not greater than 1 μm in diameter. Coccoidal and bacillary forms are usually also present. The granules of P. boydii do not have the cement-like matrix found in the granules of other eumycotic agents. In an unusual case involving the parotid gland, granules of both Actinomyces israelii and P. boydii were observed.[5]

The morphologic units of crushed granules differ not only with etiologic agents, but also depending on the type of disease present. The mycelial units have large intercalary cysts or chlamydospores in the typical mycetoma-like lesion.

On Gram stains of pus or exudate, abundant septate branching hyphae can be observed in pseudallescheriasis (Fig. 18–3). The hyphae are not, however, morphologically distinct from the branching hyphae seen in aspergillosis. The periodic acid-Schiff (PAS) or the Gomori methenamine silver nitrate (GMSN) stain may be applied to a smear of crushed granules in physiologic saline or to tissue sections.

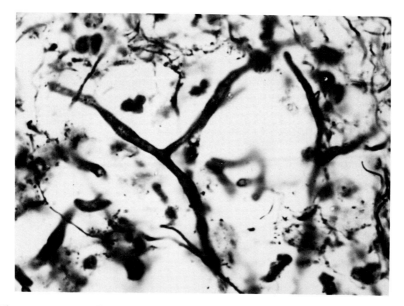

Figure 18–3. Hyphae of Pseudallescheria boydii in an area of edema and necrosis of a brain section. (From Walker, D.H., Adamec, T., and Krigman, M.: Disseminated petriellidosis (allescheriosis). Arch. Pathol. Lab. Med., *102*:158–160, 1978. Copyright 1978 American Medical Association.)

Cultural Techniques

Pseudallescheria boydii grows readily at 37°C on Sabouraud's dextrose agar containing chloramphenicol, but like Aspergillus species, the organism is inhibited by cycloheximide.[28] It is customary to set up duplicate plates and incubate one set at 25°C. Any granules should be washed several times with physiologic saline containing penicillin and streptomycin to free them from bacteria before setting up cultures.[26] All plates should be incubated for at least 6 weeks before they are discarded.

White to gray-green cottony, aerial mycelia are produced on the surface of agar. The reverse side takes on a gray-green appearance. On wet mounts made from cultures, the conidia measure 8 to 10 μm by 5 to 7 μm and are borne singly on short or elongated conidiophores arising from septate hyphae, which are 1 to 3 μm wide (Fig. 18–4). Coremia, consisting of clusters of connected conidiophores, may or may not be found. Typical thin-walled ascocarps (perithecia) containing asci and ascospores can be obtained by growing some isolates of P. boydii on potato dextrose or corn meal agar, but repeated transfers are sometimes required. The ascocarps measure 100 to 200 μm in size, and individual ascospores measure 4 to 5 μm by 7 to 8 μm (Fig. 18–5). The asexual phase (Scedosporium apiospermum) is usually cultured from clinical specimens. If the sexual phase (Pseudallescheria

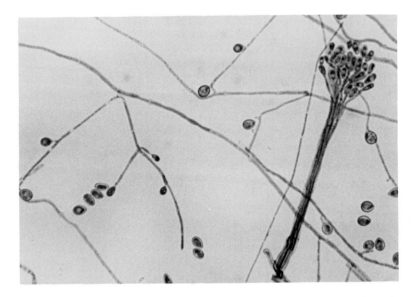

Figure 18–4. Microscopic appearance of asexual stage of Pseudallescheria boydii (Scedosporium apiospermum), showing single conidia borne on short or elongated conidiophores and a coremial phase in which a cluster of conidiophores are connected. (Courtesy of Janet Gallup, Garden Grove, California.)

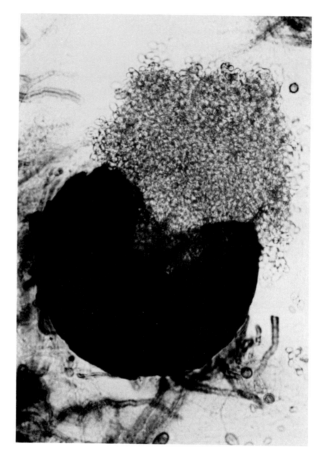

Figure 18–5. Ascocarp and ascospores of Pseudallescheria boydii. (Courtesy, Janet Gallup, Garden Grove, California.)

boydii) can be demonstrated, the name of the sexual phase is given to the isolate.[22] In pseudallescheriomas, as in aspergillomas, cultures may be unrewarding unless material can be obtained by needle aspiration.

Serologic Tests

Serologic tests as well as cultural studies may be necessary to differentiate pseudallescheriomas from aspergillomas. Direct fluorescent antibody (FA) staining may be applied to tissue sections to confirm the presence of Pseudallescheria boydii. An immunodiffusion (ID) test, using P. boydii antigen and the patient's serum, will usually demonstrate the presence of precipitating antibodies. As many as four to five precipitin bands on agar gel have been reported.[22] Repeated precipitin tests may have to be performed to demonstrate antibodies to P. boydii. A negative serologic test for precipitin bands does not necessarily rule out pseudallescheriasis, however, because a severely compromised host may be immunologically unresponsive.

PROGNOSIS

The lesions of mycetoma are almost invariably chronic and do not heal spontaneously. Dissemination does not usually occur in the absence of underlying disease or immunosuppression. Surgical intervention combined with miconazole treatment may improve the prognosis of individuals with mycetomas caused by P. boydii. Localized infections respond to miconazole, but not to amphotericin B.[29] The minimal inhibitory concentration (MIC) of 8 isolates of P. boydii has ben reported to be 0.25 µg/ml. Recovery following surgical excision of pseudallescheriomas has been documented in the absence of chronic debilitating disease.[8] The disseminated form of pseudallescheriasis in immunocompromised hosts is almost always fatal.

CASE REPORTS

Case 1

A 59-year-old woman had had a left groin lymph node dissection at Ochsner Foundation Hospital for possible recurrence of a melanoma of the thigh. The original lesion had been removed by local excision 5½ years previously. At the time of groin dissection, 2 of 10 nodes were positive for melanoma. Chest roentgenograms at this time showed a nodule in the upper lobe of the right lung. Planigrams disclosed a cystic lesion approximately 2½ cm in diameter, with an enclosed mass and a meniscus air sign. Because of the suspicion of tumor metastasis, a thoracotomy was performed and the lesion was removed by wedge resection.

Microscopic examination showed a benign cystic bronchial lesion measuring 2.1 cm in diameter. The epithelial lining was well preserved, consisting of ciliated respiratory epithelium. Within the cyst, soft necrotic material was present with solid clusters of fungi resembling Aspergillus species. The pathologist reported the lesion to be consistent with an aspergilloma; however, cultures showed the organism to be Monosporium apiospermum, and the pathologic diagnosis was therefore changed to allescheriasis.

The patient remained asymptomatic on follow-up visits to the clinic, and several chest roentgenograms taken at intervals to 3 years postoperatively did not show any major change.*

---

*From Arnett, J.C., Jr., and Hatch, H.B. Jr.: Arch. Intern. Med., *135*:1250–1253, 1975. Copyright 1975, American Medical Association.[22]

Case 2

A 76-year-old retired farmer had noted soft-tissue swelling, pain, and erythema of the fourth and fifth fingers of the right hand. Within a year, the symptoms gradually involved the entire hand, wrist, and distal forearm. There had been no history of preceding trauma to the hand. No antibiotic treatment had been attempted.

A small incision yielded small amounts of fibrous material. Subsequently, continuous drainage developed. His condition was treated with cephalosporins, without response for 1 week. He was then admitted to a local hospital.

On admission, the right arm, wrist, and hand were markedly swollen, indurated, erythematous, and warm. Yellow seropurulent drainage was evident from a small incision on the hypothenar eminence. Cultures of synovia and synovium taken at the time of surgical exploration of the wrist grew Petriellidium boydii. The identification was confirmed by the state laboratory. Routine and mycobacterial cultures of the material grew no other organisms. A synovial biopsy specimen showed chronic tenosynovitis with chronic inflammatory cells. Granules were not noted in the tissue; however, no fungal stains were performed. After 4 days of low doses of amphotericin B, the patient was transferred for further therapy.

On the patient's readmission, roentgenographic examination of the affected extremity showed marked demineralization consistent with disuse but no roentgenographic signs of osteomyelitis. A 30-day course of miconazole, 600 mg intravenously (IV) every 8 hours, was initiated. The minimal inhibitory concentration (MIC) of miconazole for the pathogen was 0.125 µg/ml. The method for susceptibility testing used in this report was that described by Lutwick, et al. The patient responded slowly but progressively, and at the time of discharge he had almost total resolution of the swelling, erythema, and tenderness.

Precipitins against a crude extract of P. boydii were detected by counterimmunoelectrophoresis with the patient's acute-phase serum. Follow-up visits showed complete resolution, and the patient regained complete use of his hand.

One year and 7 months after therapy, arthritis recurred at the wrist, and synovial fluid cultures again grew P. boydii. Serum precipitins were demonstrated in the same manner. Intravenous miconazole therapy was reinstituted, and 65.2 g was given for 52 days. Incision and drainage and local miconazole irrigation with 100 µg/ml of solution were also performed. There was progressive improvement with decreased swelling, drainage, and fluctuance, and aspirates of the wrist became sterile on culture. However, 6 weeks after completion of therapy, he relapsed a second time with wrist swelling and spontaneous purulent drainage. Miconazole therapy was reinstituted, with objective resolution a third time. A longer treatment course is planned.*

Case 3

A 33-year-old woman was admitted to the University of Texas Medical Branch, Galveston. Three months before admission, severe right frontoparietal headaches with occipital radiation developed. These persisted to the time of her admission. She had experienced recurrent rhinorrhea and nasal congestion for the 6 years before admission, but had otherwise enjoyed excellent health. There was no history of facial surgery or trauma, diabetes mellitus, recurrent infections, foreign travel, or use of immunosuppressive agents. Results of a physical examination disclosed no abnormalities. Complete blood cell counts, urinalysis, glucose tolerance test, serum protein electrophoresis, triiodothyronine test, thyroxine test, thyroid stimulating hormone, serum cortisol, and total hemolytic complement all showed normal values or results. Quantitative radioimmunodiffusion for IgG and IgA were also normal. The IgM levels were moderately increased at 332 mg/dl (normal, 70 to 210 mg/dl). Skin tests for mumps and Candida were positive. Chest roentgenographic studies showed a soft-tissue mass in the sphenoid sinus and destruction of the floor of the sella turcica. Her other sinuses were roentgenographically normal. Results of visual testing by the Department of Ophthalmology were normal.

A transseptal sphenoidotomy was performed, with curettage and drainage of 25 ml of purulent, non-foul-smelling material. Results of a histologic examination of the surgical specimen showed large masses of branching septate hyphae, with terminal conidiospores. There was focal superficial fungal invasion of the epithelium, with no involvement of the deeper mucosa or bone. Citrobacter freundii and P. boydii were cultured from the surgical specimen. Agar dilution fungal studies showed in vitro sensitivity to miconazole nitrate at 0.06 μg/ml, but resistance to amphotericin B and 5--fluorocytosine. She was treated with a 5-week course of miconazole nitrate (total dose, 41 g). Close follow-up during an 8-month period has shown no evidence of progression of the process. The patient is asymptomatic and roentgenographic study results are unchanged.†

SUMMARY

Pseudallescheriasis consists of a broad spectrum of noninvasive and invasive clinical diseases. The mycosis is being recognized with in-

---

*From Lutwick, L.I., et al.: JAMA, *241*:272–273, 1979. Copyright 1979, American Medical Association.[10]

†From Mader, J.T., Ream, R.S., and Heath, P.W.: JAMA, *239*:2368–2369, 1978. Copyright 1978, American Medical Association.[3]

creasing frequency as an opportunistic infection in debilitated or severely immunocompromised individuals. The etiologic agent, Pseudallescheria boydii, is a saprophytic fungus, which has been isolated from soil, polluted water, sludge, and animal wastes. The organism is believed to gain entrance by inhalation of ascospores or accidental inoculation during or following penetrating trauma. The manifestations of pseudallescheriasis often mimic those observable in aspergillosis. Rapid identification of P. boydii is essential because the organism does not respond to conventional antifungal agents.

REFERENCES

1. Emmons, C.W.: Allescheria boydii and Monosporium apiospermum. Mycologia, 36:188, 1944.
2. Mohr, J.A., and Muchmore, H.G.: Maduromycosis due to Allescheria boydii. JAMA, 204:335, 1968.
3. Mader, J.T., Ream, R.S., and Heath, P.W.: Petriellidium boydii (Allescheria boydii) sphenoidal sinusitis. JAMA, 239:2368, 1978.
4. Saadah, H.A., and Dixon, T.: Petriellidium boydii (Allescheria boydii) necrotizing pneumonia in a normal host. JAMA, 245:605, 1981.
5. Lutwick, L.I., Galgiana, J.N., Johnson, R.H., and Stevens, D.A.: Visceral fungal infections due to Petriellidium boydii. Am. J. Med., 61:632, 1976.
6. Glassman, M.I., Henkind, P., and Alture-Werber, E.: Monosporium apiospermum endophthalmitis. Am. J. Ophthalmol., 76:821, 1973.
7. Ernest, J.T., and Rippon, J.W.: Keratitis due to Allescheria boydii (Monosporium apiospermum). Am. J. Ophthalmol., 62:1202, 1966.
8. Rippon, J.W., and Carmichael, J.W.: Petriellidiosis (Allescheriosis): Four unusual cases and review of literature. Mycopathologia, 58:117, 1976.
9. Meyer, E., and Herrold, R.D.: Allescheria boydii isolated from a patient with chronic prostatitis. Am. J. Clin. Pathol., 35:155, 1961.
10. Lutwick, L.I., et al.: Deep infections from Petriellidium boydii treated with miconazole. JAMA, 241:272, 1979.
11. Winston, D.J., Jordan, M.C., and Rhodes, J.: Allescheria boydii infections in the immunosuppressed. Am. J. Med., 63:830, 1977.
12. Walker, D.H., Adamec, T., and Krigman, M.: Disseminated petriellidosis (allescheriosis). Arch. Pathol. Lab. Med., 102:158, 1978.
13. Paulter, E.R., Roberts, W., and Beamer, P.R.: Mycotic infection of the eye. Monosporium apiospermum associated with corneal ulcer. Arch. Ophthalmol., 53:385, 1955.
14. Travis, R.E., Urich, E.W., and Phillips, S.: Pulmonary allescheriasis. Ann. Intern. Med., 54:141, 1961.
15. Utz, J.P.: Mycetoma. In Infectious Diseases, 3rd Ed. Edited by P.D. Hoeprich. Hagerstown, Harper & Row, 1983.
16. Zaffiro, A.: Forma singulare di mycosi: cutanea de Monosporium apiospermum a sviluppo clinicamente setticemico: Considerazion diagnostiche deduzion. Medico-legal. Gior. Med. Mil., 86:636, 1938.
17. Forno, L.S., and Billingham, M.E.: Allescheria boydii infection of the brain. J. Pathol., 106:195, 1972.
18. Rosen, F., Deck, J.H., and Rewcastle, N.B.: Allescheria boydii—unique dissemination to thyroid and brain. Can. Med. Assoc. J., 93:1125, 1965.
19. Benham, R., and Georg, L.: Allescheria boydii, causative agent in a case of meningitis. J. Invest. Dermatol., 10:99, 1948.
20. Braude, A.I.: Miscellaneous fungi: The agents of mycetoma and Rhinosporidium. In Medical Microbiology and Infectious Diseases. Edited by A.I. Braude. Philadelphia, W.B. Saunders, 1981.
21. Ajello, L., and Zeidberg, L.D.: Isolation of Histoplasma capsulatum and Allescheria boydii from soil. Science, 113:662, 1951.

22. Arnett, J.C., Jr., and Hatch, H.B., Jr.: Pulmonary allescheriasis. Arch. Intern. Med., *135*:1250, 1975.
23. Spencer, H.: Pathology of the Lung, 2nd Ed. New York, Pergamon Press, 1968.
24. Shear, C.L.: Life history of an undescribed ascomyceta isolated from granular mycetoma of man. Mycetoma, *14*:239, 1922.
25. Wilson, L.A., Ahearn, D.G., Jones, D.B., and Sexton, R.R.: Fungi from the normal outer eye. Am. J. Ophthalmol., *67*:52, 1969.
26. Padhye, A.A., and Ajello, L.: Fungi causing eumycotic mycetomas. *In* Manual of Clinical Microbiology, 3rd Ed. Edited by E.H. Lennette. Washington, D.C., American Society for Microbiology, 1980.
27. Georg, L.K.: Diagnostic procedures for the isolation and identification of the etiological agents of actinomycosis. Pan. Am. Health Organ. Sci. Publ., *205*:71, 1970.
28. Campbell, M.C., and Stewart, J.L.: The Medical Mycology Handbook. New York, John Wiley & Sons, 1980.
29. Mohr, J.A. and Muchmore, H.G.: Susceptibility of Allescheria boydii to amphotericin B. *In* Antimicrobial Agents and Chemotherapy. Edited by G.L. Hobby. Washington, D.C., American Society for Microbiology, 1968.

CHAPTER 19 REYE SYNDROME

Reye syndrome was first described in Australia in 1963 as an acute encephalopathy of children.[1] Since that time, it has become apparent that the syndrome is actually a multi-organ system disease associated with diffuse fatty infiltration of the viscera and that it can occur in nonpediatric patients. The illness usually occurs following an upper respiratory viral infection and is frequently life-threatening. Interest in Reye syndrome has heightened with the recognition that use of salicylates has been associated with the sometimes rapidly fulminating course of the disorder.[2]

The clinical features of Reye syndrome include fever, vomiting, altered respiratory rhythm, abnormal reflexes and muscle tone, rapidly progressive encephalopathy, and fatty degeneration of the viscera. The criteria of Lovejoy and his colleagues are widely applied in staging of the syndrome (Table 19–1).[3] In infants under 6 months of age, vomiting may be minimal and delayed, but hyperventilation occurs early. The Moro and tonic neck reflexes are often not demonstrable, and the course is more rapidly fulminant.[4] Although recurrent Reye syndrome has been reported, the recurrent nature of the illness has not been established to the satisfaction of all pediatricians.[5]

Table 19–1. Clinical stages of Reye syndrome.

Stage	Clinical Criteria
Stage 1	Vomiting and lethargy
Stage 2	Disorientation, delirium, combativeness, hyperactive deep tendon reflexes, hyperventilation, inappropriate responses to noxious stimuli
Stage 3	Coma, hyperventilation, decorticate rigidity, preservation of pupillary reflexes
Stage 4	Deepening coma, decerebrate rigidity, loss of oculocephalic reflexes, dilated pupils unresponsive to light, dysconjugate eye movements in response to caloric stimulation
Stage 5	Seizures, loss of deep tendon reflexes, respiratory arrest, flaccidity

From Lovejoy, F.H., et al.: Clinical staging in Reye's syndrome. Am. J. Dis. Child., 128:36–41, 1974. Copyright 1974, American Medical Association.

The most outstanding pathologic feature in Reye syndrome is the accumulation of panlobular neutral lipid microdroplets in the liver.[1] The mechanisms that cause fatty generation of the liver are not known, but evidence is consistent with a metabolic or a toxic reaction. It is generally assumed that excessive lipolysis of adipose tissue and subsequent free fatty acidemia play a role in the accumulation of the hepatic triglycerides.[6]

The cause of the progressive encephalopathy is less well understood. Studies of brain tissue from autopsy material do not reveal increased lipid concentrations. The coma of Reye syndrome has been attributed to ammonia intoxication, free fatty acidemia, accumulation of biogenic amines, and lactic acidemia.[7–10]

The magnitude of protein breakdown in patients with Reye syndrome is well documented.[11] As a consequence of the catabolic state, large quantities of ammonia are produced. The toxic metabolite normally does not accumulate in more than trace amounts in individuals in nitrogen balance. Ammonia is recycled to form a variety of essential nitrogen-containing compounds. It is likely that only excess ammonia is used for the synthesis of urea.

Synthesis of urea is defective in Reye syndrome. The impairment is associated with a decrease in the activity of the enzymes carbamylphosphate synthetase (CPS) and ornithine transcarbamylase (OTC).[12–14] A descriptive analogy contained in a recent review on encephalopathy of Reye syndrome compares the metabolic disorder to flooding conditions. The origin of the systemic hyperammonia flood is a catabolic outburst of urea coupled with a metabolic downstream dam blocking synthesis of urea.[14] One could extend that analogy to include a rate-limiting disposal system that works adequately when precipitation is normal, but that is overburdened by flash floods.

Urea is synthesized mainly in the liver. The initial reaction involves the formation of carbamylphosphate (Fig. 19–1). It occurs when ammonia and carbon dioxide are activated by adenosine triphosphate (ATP) in the presence of N-acetylglutamic acid and CPS.[15] In a second step, carbamylphosphate combines with ornithine in the presence of OTC to produce citrulline. In the absence of sufficient quantities of CPS and OTC, activities of the urea cycle are blocked, and ammonia accumulates in the blood. The ammonia burden in the cerebral blood supply markedly impairs brain function. A correlation between hyperammonemia and increases in intracranial pressure has been documented.[16]

Free fatty acidemia is a consistent finding in Reye syndrome.[6,8,17] Proprionate, butyrate, isobutyrate, isovalerate, and valerate levels are reported to be as much as twice those of normal values early in the syndrome. The free fatty acidemia disappears in patients after glucose and insulin infusion but is not necessarily correlated with clinical im-

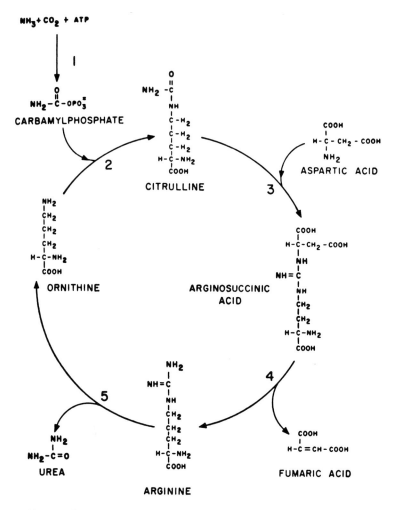

Figure 19–1.   The urea cycle. (From Searcy, R.L.: Diagnostic Biochemistry. New York, McGraw-Hill, 1969. Copyright 1969 McGraw-Hill. By permission of the publisher.)

provement. Since the rise in free fatty-acid levels seen in fasting does not promote brain dysfunction, it is unlikely that the encephalopathy of Reye syndrome is related to free fatty acidemia.[18]

There is growing evidence that the accumulation of certain biogenic amines may contribute to the encephalopathy of Reye syndrome.[9] Normally, the aromatic amino acids, tyrosine and phenylalanine, are converted into the keto acids by hepatic enzymes. In Reye syndrome, marked elevations of tyrosine and its intermediate decarboxylated metabolite, tyramine, occur in the plasma. Hypertyraminemia could be caused by an increased rate of synthesis or a decreased rate of degradation of tyramine.

Lactic acidemia appears to be a metabolic component of Reye syndrome, but correlation with the clinical state has not been clearly established.[10,19–21] Since patients often receive hypertonic glucose infusions of 10 to 20%, it has been difficult to ascertain whether elevations in lactate levels are associated with a metabolic disturbance or with a management regimen. If, however, blood glucose levels are maintained at a constant level throughout the course of Reye syndrome, glucose cannot be correlated with severity of illness.[21] In one study, lactic acidemia appeared to be a reflection of lactate production associated with anoxia or hypoperfusion. The most plausible explanation for lactic acidemia is that damage to the mitochondria of the liver causes a decrease in the activity of pyruvate decarboxylase and pyruvate dehydrogenase.[22,23]

Since beta oxidation of fatty acids occurs chiefly in the matrix of mitochondria, damage to those organelles could be expected to cause an increase in serum fatty acids.[24] Conversely, accumulation of fatty acids could injure mitochondria.[25] The complexity of the metabolic disturbances in Reye syndrome may be explained by an insult that is potentiated in a complex cause-effect relationship involving hyperammonemia, an accumulation of fatty acids, an interference in tyramine catabolism, and lactic acidemia. It is generally accepted that the ammonia burden in the brain is directly associated with the encephalopathy that characterizes Reye syndrome.[14]

ETIOLOGY

The factors that trigger the metabolic derangement of Reye syndrome are unknown. Prodromal illnesses of viral origin are universal in patients with Reye syndrome. There is growing evidence that other factors may either cause identical symptoms or act in a synergistic manner to promote the severe metabolic disturbances. In 1 study of 379 cases of Reye syndrome, 89% had an antecedent upper respiratory infection, 7% had varicella determined by clinical evidence, and 4% had gastroenteritis.[26]

The role of aspirin in promoting the metabolic disorder has been the subject of continuing controversy. It has been difficult to obtain reliable data to substantiate salicylate intoxication because of the lack of control cases. Carefully controlled studies in Arizona, Michigan, and Ohio, completed in 1982, suggest that aspirin is a risk factor for Reye syndrome.[27–29] Those epidemiologic investigations prompted a Surgeon General's advisory on the use of salicylates and Reye syndrome in the United States.[2,29] Independent groups of the American Academy of Pediatrics on Infectious Diseases and the Food and Drug Administration have found a relationship between ingestion of aspirin and Reye syndrome.[30] After an extensive review process, the Surgeon General determined that salicylate and salicylate-containing medications should not be given to children with influenza or chickenpox.

Acetaminophen (paracetamol), which is widely available in the United States and Great Britain, is sometimes used as an alternative analgesic for children as well as for adults during epidemics of influenza or influenza-like illnesses. Approximately 300 prescription and nonprescription drugs containing acetaminophen are sold in the United States.[31,32] In the Ohio study, use of acetaminophen showed a reverse relationship when cases of Reye syndrome were compared with a control group not using the medication.[28] Nevertheless, if recommended doses of acetaminophen are exceeded, acetaminophen may be more toxic than aspirin.[33] It has been suggested that young children may metabolize acetaminophen differently than do adults.[34]

It may be also that salicylates are degraded more slowly in young children than in adults. Conversely, aspirin could modify a host's response to particular viruses. More study is required before the exact role of aspirin in the production of Reye syndrome can be determined. Of special interest is the fact that Reye syndrome has been reported in the absence of salicylate ingestion.[35]

Various environmental factors, including insecticides, aflatoxins, and other chemicals have long been suspected of having a synergistic role in the etiology of Reye syndrome.[36-38] Whereas definitive relationships are difficult to establish, it appears possible that clearance of toxic agents may be slower in some children. The half-life of salicylate in two pediatric patients was found to be as much as four or more times that of normal.[39] The relationship between the increased half-life of salicylate and the hepatic derangement in Reye syndrome is not known, but the deficit in hepatic function may be the common factor in more than one type of chemical intoxication. No one disagrees that the severity of the illness in pediatric or nonpediatric patients requires prompt diagnosis and immediate institution of therapy designed to minimize or correct the effects of the metabolic derangements.

PREDISPOSING FACTORS

Although Reye syndrome has been reported in nonpediatric patients, children up to 16 years of age seem to be at higher risk. In an epidemic associated with influenza B virus in 1973 to 1974, only 4% of the individuals with Reye syndrome were more than 16 years of age.[39,40] The presence of an antecedent prodromal viral infection is a consistent finding. The consequences of the disorder, however, appear to be more serious in children under 12 months of age. The use of aspirin as an analgesic-antipyretic constitutes an additional risk factor that cannot be overlooked.

EPIDEMIOLOGY

Reye syndrome appears to be worldwide in distribution and to occur with equal frequency in both sexes.[41] Most cases of Reye syndrome occur during times of increased influenza activity, but sporadic and family outbreaks are common.[42] Limited information is available regarding racial differences in susceptibility, but the syndrome has been reported most frequently in Caucasians.[29] Infants with Reye syndrome tend to come from urban lower socioeconomic groups.[43] It has been suggested that earlier introduction of babies to table food in economically depressed families may expose infants to enteroviruses or aflatoxins.[44]

LABORATORY DIAGNOSIS

Attempts to culture viruses from patients with Reye syndrome have not produced consistent results.[45–47] No single biochemical alteration in serum or urine components is pathognomonic for Reye syndrome. Hyperammonemia, fatty acidemia, accumulation of biogenic amines, and lactic acidemia are commonly found, but may also be evident in other types of liver dysfunction.

Biochemical Parameters

Most body fluids contain substantive amounts of ammonia (Table 19–2). Accurate measurements of ammonia are difficult to obtain because ammonia is generated during analysis. Marked hyperammonemia occurs in Reye syndrome. Blood ammonia levels ranging from 91 mg to 760 mg/dl have been reported in patients with the metabolic dysfunction characterizing the syndrome.

Elevated levels of serum glutamic oxaloacetic transaminase (SGOT), serum glutamic pyruvic transaminase (SGPT), decreased prothrombin activity, and hypoglycemia are consistent biochemical features of Reye syndrome. Increase in creatine phosphokinase (CPK) reflects muscle and central nervous system disorders. Isoenzyme CPK studies on a limited number of patients suggest that the CPK is of muscle

Table 19–2. Ammonia content of some body fluids.

Body Fluid	Ammonia Concentration (μg/dl)
Breast milk	28.1–33.6*
Cerebrospinal fluid	96.0–97.0
Gastric juice	500.0–4000.0
Pancreatic juice	12.2–18.2*
Urine	30.0–70.0†
Whole blood	120.0–365.0

*Values expressed in terms of mg/dl
†Values expressed in terms of mEq/day

Adapted from Searcy, R.L.: Diagnostic Biochemistry. New York, McGraw-Hill, 1969.

rather than brain origin in Reye syndrome.[47] The myopathy involving skeletal or cardiac muscle has been largely overshadowed by the dramatic symptoms associated with dysfunction of the central nervous system.

At least 1 study has attempted to relate serum carnitine levels with Reye syndrome.[24] Carnitine is known to aid in the transport of fatty acid esters across the inner membranes of mitochondria. Since serum carnitine is not altered in some hepatic diseases, measurements of serum carnitine may have diagnostic value in a differential diagnosis. In 9 patients diagnosed clinically as Stage II or Stage III of Reye syndrome, a mean serum carnitine level of 27.2 μmol/dl was found. A group matched for age and presence of viral infections had a mean of only 6.6 μmol/dl. More studies are needed to document the value of serum carnitine levels in establishing a definitive diagnosis of Reye syndrome.

Microscopic Examination

Unequivocal diagnosis of Reye syndrome has depended on microscopic studies of liver tissue obtained on autopsy or on material obtained from a biopsy. Diffuse microvesicular, fatty infiltration of hepatocytes without necrosis or with minimal or no evidence of inflammation is characteristic of Reye syndrome (Fig. 19–2). The disturbance in coagulation, which often occurs in hepatic dysfunction, makes a liver biopsy an undesirable procedure because of the risk of hemorrhage.

Needle biopsy of muscle may be a reliable and safer alternative to a liver biopsy. Infiltration of muscle fibers with fat microdroplets can be observed on muscle sections stained with oil red O and examined by electron microscopy. A study limited to three children with Reye syndrome admitted to Hadassah University Hospital in Israel showed pronounced infiltration of fat microdroplets in muscle fibers.[48] These findings support the hypothesis that the lipid deposition is caused by injury to the mitochondria and inability to oxidize lipids. More studies will be required to confirm the value of muscle biopsies in Reye syndrome.

PROGNOSIS

Although Reye reported a mortality rate of 80% in his case studies in 1963, early diagnosis and aggressive treatment have reduced the mortality rate for Reye syndrome to approximately 20 to 40%.[2,4,48] Because the major cause of death is cerebral edema, control of intracranial pressure is crucial to the recovery of patients.[49]

Blood ammonia and α-amino acid nitrogen levels have been used in the prognosis of cases of Reye syndrome. Patients with blood ammonia concentrations in excess of 270 μg/dl and α-amino acid nitrogen

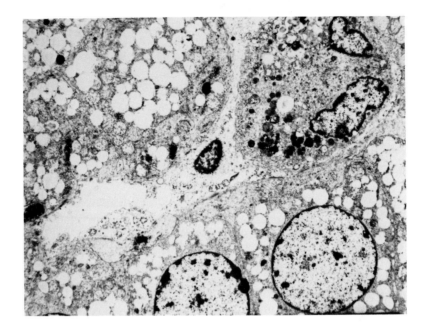

Figure 19–2. Electron micrograph of hepatocytes with noncoalescing lipid droplets in Reye syndrome. (From Shapira, Y., et al.: Reye's syndrome: Diagnosis by muscle biopsy? Arch. Dis. Child., 56:287, 1981.)

levels above 14 μg/dl almost inevitably deteriorate rapidly and lapse into comas.[50] One advantage of α-amino acid determinations over total amino acid measurements is that less time is required to perform tests. It is important that appropriate therapy be instituted promptly. Despite aggressive and supportive therapeutic regimens, some survivors of Reye syndrome sustain permanent neurologic damage as evidenced by mental retardation, spasticity, or epileptic-type seizures.[4]

CASE REPORTS

Case 1

A 14-year-old female of Yemenite origin was hospitalized because of fever, abdominal pains and vomiting. Until 3 weeks prior to the hospitalization she was healthy. At that time, she developed an upper respiratory tract infection with low grade fever, rhinorrhea, and cough, which subsided after a few weeks. Three days before the admission she started to complain of upper abdominal pains, repeated vomiting, and fever up to 39°C without chills.

The physical examination revealed an alert patient with some jaundice and a temperature of 37.4°C. The edge of the liver and spleen were palpated below the respective costal margins. No lymphadenopathy or abnormal neurologic findings were noted.

Laboratory work showed: hemoglobin 12.5 g/dl, hematocrit 40%, WBC 6100/cmm with 43% segmented and 10% band form neutrophils, 44% lymphocytes, 1% monocytes and 2% plasmacytoid cells. Platelet count was 150,000/cmm. Total bilirubin was 2.6 mg%, direct— 2.0 mg%, SGOT 212 U, SGPT 92 U, 5′-nucleotidase 108 U (normal, up to 20 U). Serum alkaline phosphatase 300 U (normal, up to 80 U). Kidney function tests were normal. Serologic tests for typhoid fever, infectious mononucleosis, brucellosis and hepatitis B antigen, mumps, herpes virus, and adenovirus were negative.

On the following day, the patient became confused, disoriented, and developed diffuse clonic convulsions. Gradually she became comatose. A lumbar puncture showed 65 mg% protein, 62 mg% glucose, a few lymphocytes, and a pressure of 19 mm H_2O. A needle biopsy of the liver showed massive fatty infiltration with only mild infiltration by lymphocytes. After 1 additional day, she regained consciousness and her condition gradually improved. Two weeks later, all the liver function tests returned to normal values. The patient refused to undergo another liver biopsy.*

Case 2

A 6-year-old Arab girl was admitted to this hospital with a history of vomiting and progressive loss of consciousness of 2 days' duration. There was no history of pre-existing infection, headaches, or intoxication. The day before admission she had been treated at another hospital with intravenous glucose for hypoglycaemia and this had temporarily improved her level of consciousness. On admission, she was in semicoma and had sluggish responses to painful stimuli. Her blood pressure was 150/80 mm Hg, pulse rate 80/min, respiratory rate 40/min. Pupils were equal and reacted to light, funduscopic examination showed no papilloedema. The oculocephalic reflex was normal. Muscle tone was generally decreased. Deep tendon and abdominal reflexes were decreased. Babinski's sign was negative. The liver was palpable 4 cm below the costal margin. Treatment consisted of dexamethasone, arginine, glutamate, ampicillin, vitamin K, mannitol, dopamine, and later, mechanical respiratory support. Her condition quickly deteriorated, and she went into deep coma with Cheyne-Stokes respiration. The oculocephalic reflexes ceased and the pupils became dilated and no longer responded to light; she died in cardiorespiratory arrest. Necropsy was not performed but liver tissue was obtained by needle biopsy immediately after she died.

---

*From Lewinski, H., and Djaldetti, M.: J. Submicrosc. Cytol., *13*:697–701, 1981.[51]

Laboratory findings: Hb 9.4 g/dl, haematocrit 34%, and platelets 240 × 10^9/L, plasma urea 32.1 mg/ml (11.3 mmol/L), glucose 160 mg/100 ml (8.88 mmol/L), bilirubin 1.4 mg/100 ml (23.9 μmol/L), calcium 9.8 mg/100 ml (2.45 mmol/L), phosphate 5.0 mg/100 ml (1.6 mmol/L), uric acid 10 mg/100 ml (0.59 mmol/L), cholesterol 110 mg/100 ml (2.85 mmol/L), sodium 139 mmol/L, potassium 4.9 mmol/L, diastase 120 IU, aspartate transaminase (AST) 2000 IU, alkaline phosphatase 255 IU, prothrombin time 22%, partial thromboplastin time 16 seconds, arterial blood ammonia 532 μg/100 ml (312.3 μmol/L), total protein 5.6 g/100 ml (56 g/L), albumin 3.8 g/100 ml (38 g/L), Australia antigen negative.

The cerebrospinal fluid (CSF) was clear with no cells. Pressure was 300 mm H$_2$O, protein 29 mg/100 ml (0.29 g/L), glucose 65 μg/100 ml (3.6 mmol/L). Electroencephalogram (EEG) showed pronounced diffuse slowing, which later became isoelectric.

Special biochemical studies. Plasma alanine 336 (normal <30) μmol/100 ml, plasma glutamine 392 (normal <50) μmol/100 ml, urinary lactic acid 325 (control 5–15) mg/100 ml, g lactic acid/g creatinine = 18 (control 0.24).

The activity of the liver ornithine-transcarbamylase was 757 μmol/g per hour (20% of normal activity). Enzymatic activity of the liver carbamylphosphatase-synthetase was 57 μmol/g per hour (half that of normal).*

Case 3

A 19-year-old woman noted a sore throat 7 days before admission. Two days later, a typical varicelliform rash appeared on her face and trunk. Thirty-six hours before admission, she experienced nausea and vomiting. She was examined in the emergency room of another hospital and was treated with trimethobenzamide hydrochloride suppositories, antacids, and anticholinergics. Deteriorating mental status prompted her to return to the emergency room later that evening. She was irritable, combative, with alternating episodes of agitation and somnolence. She was admitted.

Several family members had symptoms suggestive of upper respiratory tract infection but without mental changes. Findings of a lumbar puncture were normal except for an opening pressure of 30 cm of water, which was attributed to the patient's agitated behavior. The blood ammonia level was 261 μ/L (normal, 50 to 70 μ/L), and the SGOT value was 271 IU/L. The next morning the patient was transferred to Milwaukee County General Hospital.

The pulse rate was 120 beats per minute; axillary temperature,

*From Shapira, Y., et al.: Arch. Dis. Child., 56:287–291, 1981.[48]

37°C; respirations, 24/min; and BP, 110/60 mm Hg. There was no icterus. A dark-red, crusting, papular rash was visible over her trunk and face. The patient was intermittently combative and somnolent. The extremities moved equally, and no decerebrate or decorticate activity was noted. The neck was supple. The pupils were dilated but reacted briskly to light. The corneal and oculocephalic reflexes were intact. The optic margins were sharp. The plantar response was extensor bilaterally. The deep-tendon reflexes were symmetrical and hyperactive. Palmomental and snout reflexes were present. The liver was palpable 3 cm below the right costal margin. Except for a mild respiratory alkalosis, the electrolyte levels were normal. The glucose value was 129 mg/dl; BUN, 13 mg/dl; creatinine, 1.1 mg/dl; hematocrit, 42.9%; and WBCs, 12,200/cu mm. The prothrombin time was 15.0 s (control, 12.0 s). The total bilirubin value was 0.7 mg/dl, and the SGOT value was 270 IU/L.

The patient was treated with mannitol and furosemide for incipient cerebral edema. Three and a half hours after admission, spontaneous movements ceased, and decerebrate posturing occurred in response to pain. An EEG showed continuous high voltage synchronous delta activity. At periodic intervals, suppression of activity was also noted in a generalized fashion. These findings were consistent with a metabolic encephalopathy and compatible with Reye's syndrome.

Since the patient's condition was clinically deteriorating, an exchange transfusion with fresh-frozen plasma and saline-washed RBCs was performed. The patient remained somnolent, but decerebrate posturing was no longer noted, and the deep-tendon reflexes were less hyperactive. A second exchange transfusion was performed on the second hospital day. A percutaneous liver biopsy was performed without complications. Specimens were submitted for light and electron microscopy, viral culture, and enzyme assays. Early on the third hospital day, she dramatically became oriented and alert. The deep-tendon reflexes became normoactive, and the plantar responses became flexor. On the seventh hospital day, she was discharged.

The liver biopsy specimen was grossly yellow. Light microscopy of the liver biopsy specimen disclosed panlobular fatty infiltration consistent with findings of Reye's syndrome. By electron microscopy, the hepatocyte cytoplasm contained various-sized lipid vacuoles. Large numbers of residual bodies and microbodies were noted. The mitochondria demonstrated degenerative changes characterized by loss of cristae. No viral particles were found. Carbamyl phosphate synthetase, ornithine transcarbamylase, and arginase levels in liver tissue were measured and were 0.6 mg (normal, 1.3 ± 0.3 SD), 19.5 μmole/mg protein (normal, 37.2 ± 8.7 μmole/mg protein), and 253.0 μmole/

mg protein (177.0 ± 63.0 μmole/mg protein), respectively. Acute and convalescent sera disclosed a fourfold increase in titers to Varicella.*

SUMMARY

Reye syndrome is an acute encephalopathy with hepatic dysfunction, uually seen in children. Whereas it can still be considered a rare clinical entity, it has occurred with greater frequency in many countries since it was first described in 1963 in Australia. The increasing frequency, the recent discovery of the syndrome in nonpediatric patients, the high fatality rate, and neurologic sequelae challenge pediatricians, family practitioners, emergency room attendants, internists, pathologists, and neurologists in a unique manner. An antecedent viral infection followed by 2 to 5 days of vomiting before onset of neurologic symptoms is characteristic in Reye syndrome. The deepening coma occurring in Stages III, IV, and V of the derangement has been attributed to specific metabolic disturbances.

Although the cause of Reye syndrome remains an enigma, an association between salicylate ingestion and the syndrome has been established. Recently described myopathy in patients with Reye syndrome may provide an alternative to liver biopsy in establishing a definitive diagnosis for Reye syndrome. Specific biochemical tests may be valuable in monitoring treatment and as an aid in establishing the prognosis in individual cases.

REFERENCES

1. Reye, R.D., Morgan, G., and Baral, J.: Encephalopathy and fatty degeneration of the viscera: A disease entity in childhood. Lancet, 2:749, 1963.
2. Centers for Disease Control.: Surgeon general's advisory on the use of salicylates and Reye syndrome. Morbid. Mortal. Weekly Rept., 31:389, 1982.
3. Lovejoy, F.H., et al.: Clinical staging in Reye's syndrome. Am. J. Dis. Child., 128:36, 1974.
4. Trauner, D.A.: Reye's syndrome. In Medical Microbiology and Infectious Disease. Edited by I.A. Braude. Philadelphia, W.B. Saunders, 1981.
5. Newman, S.L.: Recurrent Reye's syndrome. Am. J. Dis. Child., 133:657, 1979.
6. Pollack, J.D., et al.: Serum and tissue lipids in Reye's syndrome. In Reye's Syndrome. Edited by J.D. Pollack. New York, Grune & Stratton, 1975.
7. Huttenlocher, P.R., Schwarts, A.D., and Klatskin, G.: Reye's syndrome: Ammonia intoxication as a possible factor in encephalopathy. Pediatrics, 43:443, 1969.
8. Mamunes, P., et al.: Fatty acid quantitation in Reye's syndrome. In Reye's Syndrome. Edited by J.D. Pollack. New York, Grune & Stratton, 1975.
9. Faraj, B.A., et al.: Evidence for hypertyraminemia in Reye's syndrome. Pediatrics, 64:76, 1979.
10. Moore, T.A.: Association of hyperammonemia and lactic acidosis in Reye's syndrome. J. Pediatr., 84:440, 1974.
11. Snodgrass, P.J., and De Long, G.R.: Urea cycle enzyme deficiencies and an in-

*From Varma, R.R., et al.: JAMA, 242:1373–1375, 1979. Copyright 1979, American Medical Association.[52]

creased nitrogen load producing hyperammonemia in Reye's syndrome. N. Engl. J. Med., *294*:855, 1976.

12. Sinatra, F., et al.: Abnormalities of carbamyl phosphate synthetase and ornithine transcarbamylase in liver of patients with Reye's syndrome. Pediatr. Res., *9*:829, 1975.

13. Brown, T., et al.: Transiently reduced activity of carbamylphosphate synthetase and ornithine transcarbamylase in liver of children with Reye's syndrome. N. Engl. J. Med., *294*:861, 1976.

14. Delong, G.R., and Glick, T.H.: Encephalopathy of Reye's syndrome: A review of pathogenetic hypotheses. Pediatrics, *69*:53, 1982.

15. Searcy, R.L.: Diagnostic Biochemistry. New York, McGraw-Hill, 1969, p. 537.

16. Ware, A.J., D'Agostino, A.N., and Combes, B.: Cerebral edema: A major complication of massive hepatic necrosis. Gastroenterol., *61*:877, 1971.

17. Trauner, D., et al.: Biochemical correlates of illness and recovery in Reye's syndrome. Ann. Neurol., *2*:238, 1977.

18. Corvilain, J., et al.: Effect of fasting on levels of plasma nonesterified fatty acids in normal children, normal adults, and obese adults. Lancet, *1*:534, 1961.

19. Haymond, M., et al.: Metabolic response to hypertonic glucose administration in Reye syndrome. Ann. Neurol., *3*:207, 1978.

20. Shannon, D.C., et al.: Studies on the pathophysiology of encephalopathy in Reye's syndrome. Hyperammonemia in Reye's syndrome. Pediatrics, *56*:999, 1975.

21. Tonsgard, J.H., Huttenlocher, P.R., and Thisted, R.A.: Lactic acidemia in Reye's syndrome. Pediatrics, *69*:64, 1982.

22. Robinon, B.H., Gall, D.G., and Cutz, E.: Deficient activity of hepatic pyruvate carboxylase and pyruvate dehydrogenase in Reye's syndrome. Pediatr. Res., *11*:279, 1977.

23. De Vivo, D.C.: Reye syndrome: A metabolic response to an acute mitochondrial insult. Neurology, *28*:165, 1978.

24. Hinshaw, W.B., Glenn, J.L., and Hatch, K.M.: Serum carnitine in Reye's syndrome. N. Engl. J. Med., *302*:1423, 1980.

25. Zborowski, J., and Wojtczak, L.: Induction of swelling of liver mitochondria by fatty acids of various chain lengths. Biochem. Biophys. Acta, *70*:596, 1963.

26. Corey, L., et al.: Diagnostic criteria for influenza B-associated Reye's syndrome: Clinical vs. pathologic criteria. Pediatrics, *60*:702, 1977.

27. Waldman, R.J., Hall, W.N., McGee, H., and van Amburg, G.: Aspirin as a risk factor in Reye's syndrome. JAMA, *247*:3080, 1982.

28. Halpin, T.J., et al.: Reye's syndrome and medication use. JAMA, *248*:687, 1982.

29. Centers for Disease Control: National surveillance for Reye syndrome, 1981: Update, Reye syndrome and salicylate usage. Morbid. Mortal. Weekly Rept., *31*:53, 1982.

30. Committee on Infectious Dieases, American Academy of Pediatrics: Special report: Aspirin and Reye syndrome. Pediatrics, *69*:810, 1982.

31. Prescott, L.F., et al.: Successful treatment of severe paracetamol overdosage with cysteamine. Lancet, *1*:588, 1974.

32. Crome, P., et al.: The use of methionine for acute paracetamol poisoning. J. Int. Med. Research, *4* (Suppl.):105, 1976.

33. American Academy of Pediatrics Committee on Drugs: Commentary on acetaminophen. Pediatrics, *61*:108, 1978.

34. Miller, R.C., Roberts, R.J., and Fischer, L.J.: Acetaminophen elimination kinetics in neonates, children, and adults. Clin. Pharmacol. Ther., *19*:284, 1976.

35. Partin, J.S., et al.: Serum salicylate concentrations in Reye's disease: A study of 130 biopsy-proven cases. Lancet, *1*:191, 1982.

36. Crocker, J.F.S., et al.: Insecticides and viral interaction as a cause of fatty visceral changes and encephalopathy in the mouse. Lancet, *2*:22, 1974.

37. Pollack, J.D., et al.: The interaction of chemicals and viruses and their role in Reye's syndrome. Chemosphere, *7*:55, 1978.

38. Nelson, et al.: Aflatoxin and Reye's syndrome: A case control study. Pediatrics, *66*:865, 1980.

39. Rodgers, G.C., et al.: Salicylate and Reye's syndrome. Lancet, *1*:616, 1982.

40. Corey, L., et al.: A nationwide outbreak of Reye's syndrome: Its epidemiological relationship to influenza B. Am. J. Med., *61*:615, 1976.
41. Bellman, M.H., et al.: Epidemiological association with Reye's syndrome. Arch. Dis. Child., *55*:820, 1980.
42. Glick, T.H., et al.: Reye's syndrome: An epidemiologic approach. Pediatrics, *46*:371, 1970.
43. Hottenlocher, P.R., and Trauner, D.A.: Reye's syndome in infancy. Pediatrics, *62*:84, 1978.
44. Ryan, N.J., et al.: Aflatoxin B_1: Its role in the etiology of Reye's syndrome. Pediatrics, *64*:71, 1979.
45. Golden, G.S., and Duffell, D.: Encephalopathy and fatty change in the liver and kidney. Pediatrics, *36*:67, 1965.
46. Dvorackova, I., Vortel, V., and Hroch, M.: Encephalitis syndrome with fatty degeneration of viscera. Arch. Pathol., *81*:240, 1966.
47. Roe, C.R., et al.: Enzymatic alterations in Reye's syndrome: Prognostic implications. Pediatrics, *55*:119, 1975.
48. Shapira, Y., et al.: Reye's syndrome: Diagnosis by muscle biopsy? Arch. Dis. Child., *56*:287, 1981.
49. Ansevin, C.F.: Reye syndrome: Serum-induced alterations in brain mitochondrial function are blocked by fatty-acid-free albumin. Neurology, *30*:160, 1980.
50. McArthur, B.S., Arcinue, E.L., and Schultz, G.E.: Total-α-amino acid nitrogen quantification as prognosticator in Reye's syndrome. Am. J. Dis. Child., *135*:765, 1981.
51. Lewinski, H., and Djaldetti, M.: Ultrastructural alterations of the lymphocytes from a patient with Reye's syndrome. J. Submicrosc. Cytol., *13*:697, 1981.
52. Varma, R.R., et al.: Reye's syndrome in nonpediatric age groups. JAMA, *242*:1373, 1979.

CHAPTER **20** TOXIC-SHOCK SYNDROME

Toxic-shock syndrome (TSS) is a severe multisystem disease, which was first observed in 1978 in children with staphylococcal infections.[1] Since that time, most cases of TSS have occurred in young menstruating women who use tampons and in whom Staphylococcus aureus was a part of the indigenous flora of the cervix or vagina.[2] TSS has been reported also in males and in nonmenstruating women with staphylococcal infections.[3] Symptoms of TSS include a fever greater than 39.9°C (102°F), hypotension, vomiting, diarrhea, development of an erythematous rash, which is followed by desquamation, and multiple-organ-system dysfunction (Table 20–1). Women in whom TSS has been diagnosed have become ill usually between the second

Table 20–1. Toxic-shock syndrome case definition.

1. Fever (temperature ≥ 38.9°C 102°F).
2. Rash (diffuse macular erythroderma).
3. Desquamation, 1–2 weeks after onset of illness, particularly of palms and soles.
4. Hypotension (systolic blood pressure ≤ 90 mm Hg for adults or < 5th percentile by age for children < 16 years of age, or orthostatic dizziness).
5. Involvement of 3 or more of the following organ systems:
   A. Gastrointestinal (vomiting or diarrhea at onset of illness).
   B. Muscular (severe myalgia or creatinine phosphokinase level ≥ 2 × ULN*).
   C. Mucous membrane (vaginal, oropharyngeal, or conjunctival hyperemia).
   D. Renal (BUN† or Cr‡ ≥ 2 × ULN or ≥ 5 white blood cells per high-power field— in the absence of a urinary tract infection).
   E. Hepatic (total bilirubin, SGOT,§ or SGPT# 2 ≥ × ULN).
   F. Hematologic (platelets ≤ 100,000/mm³).
   G. Central nervous system (disorientation or alterations in consciousness without focal neurologic signs when fever and hypotension are absent).
6. Negative results on the following tests, if obtained:
   A. Blood, throat, or cerebrospinal fluid cultures.
   B. Serologic tests for Rocky Mountain spotted fever, leptospirosis, or measles.
7. Positive or negative results on blood cultures.

---

*Twice upper limits of normal for laboratory
†Blood urea nitrogen level
‡Creatinine level
§Serum glutamic oxaloacetic transaminase level
#Serum glutamic pyruvic transaminase level

From Center for Disease Control: Morbid. Mortal. Weekly Rept., 29:442, 1980, and Centers for Disease Control: Morbid. Mortal. Weekly Rept., 31:201, 1982.

and fifth day of their menstrual periods. In some instances, complications of acute renal failure, adult respiratory distress syndrome (ARDS), disseminated intravascular coagulation (DIC), or ischemic necrosis of the extremities have followed the staphylococcal toxemia.[2-4]

ETIOLOGY

The etiologic agents of toxic-shock syndrome are toxigenic strains of the gram-positive coccus Staphylococcus aureus. The symptoms appear to be mediated by a toxin rather than an invasive process.[5] Two staphylococcal exotoxins have been implicated in TSS. In 1 study, staphylococcal enterotoxin F was isolated from over 90% of staphylococci from TSS patients.[6] In another study, 100% of the TSS case-strains produced exotoxin C.[7] The toxins are pyrogenic, stimulate lymphocyte mitogenicity, appear to enhance susceptibility to shock by endotoxin and may represent a single entity.[9-12]

Presumably, trauma to the vaginal mucosa during insertion of tampons provides the opportunity for toxin to be absorbed.[8] Alternatively, it has been proposed that contaminated blood may flow in a retrograde manner up the Fallopian tubes into the peritoneal cavity, where absorption of toxin into the general circulation can occur with ease. It has been suggested that full expression of TSS may require unique host susceptibility or another toxin in a synergistic role.[7]

PREDISPOSING FACTORS

Young, white non-Hispanic menstruating women in their early twenties who use tampons or vaginal contraceptive sponges constitute a high-risk group for TSS. In over 90% of cases, the onset has been during a menstrual period. Some women who have survived an attack of TSS have an increased risk of getting it again. Recurrence rates up to 30% have been reported in the United States.[7] Staphylococcal infection at a variety of sites may represent a predisposing factor. As with other newly described microbial illnesses, however, as yet unrecognized predisposing factors may exist.

EPIDEMIOLOGY

Toxigenic strains of S. aureus frequently colonize the vaginal tract of healthy women as transient residents, but the use of tampons appears to provide favorable conditions for the growth of these organisms in some individuals.[13] TSS has been reported in all 50 states of the United States and in the District of Columbia, with more than one third of the cases occurring in the states of California, Minnesota, and Wisconsin. More than 90% of the cases of TSS have occurred in menstruating women.[14]

No person-to-person transmission of TSS has been documented, and TSS has not been reported in other countries.[15] This may be associated with the more frequent use of tampons by menstruating women in the United States, where it is estimated that 70% of menstruating women use the product. Although 11 postpartum cases have been reported, a case of mother-to-neonate transmission in which the infant died suggests that surveillance studies of maternal vaginal colonization and even of mild erythroderma in infants might be indicated.[16] The fatality rate based on cases reported to the Centers for Disease Control (CDC) for 1980 and 1981 is 5.6%.[17]

LABORATORY DIAGNOSIS

The first step in the laboratory diagnosis or confirmation of TSS is to recognize a staphylococcus; however, some micrococci appear morphologically similar to staphylococci. On cervical or vaginal smears, cocci may occur singly, in pairs, in short chains, in small clusters, or in tetrads. Although staphylococci can be recovered with regularity from vaginal secretions, the microbial flora of the vagina varies with age and even during the menstrual cycle.

Microscopic Examination

Gram stains of smears prepared from the vagina, cervix, or cultures reveal gram-positive cocci, which are approximately 1 μm in diameter, frequently occurring in clusters (Fig. 20–1). A variety of microorganisms colonize the vagina. The cervix may contain a few bacteria, but it is often sterile. Any bacteria present reflect to a large degree the microbiota of the vagina. Demonstration of gram-positive cocci on vaginal or cervical smears is predictable even in the absence of disease.

Cultural Techniques

Staphylococci grow readily on sheep blood agar after 18 to 24 hours of incubation at 37°C. The colonies are white to yellow, convex, opaque, moist, and measure approximately 1 to 2 mm in diameter. Some strains of Staphylococcus aureus produce beta hemolysis on sheep blood agar. Most strains of S. epidermidis are nonhemolytic.

Biochemical Characterization

The coagulase test is used in hospital laboratories for the presumptive identification of S. aureus.[18–21] S. aureus clots normal rabbit plasma after incubation for 4 to 24 hours at 37°C. It is not always recognized, however, that coagulase-positive and coagulase-negative strains of staphylococci coexist in many infectious states. A high percentage of staphylococcal colonies isolated in a major county teaching hospital were heterogeneous with respect to coagulase activity.[22] Colony selection, therefore, can constitute a significant variable. Although

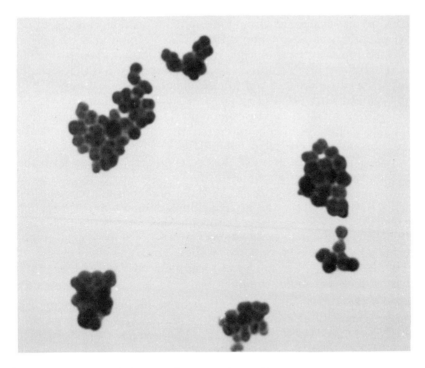

Figure 20–1. Typical clusters of cocci as formed by S. aureus and revealed by the Gram stain. (Courtesy Carolina Biological Supply Company, Burlington, North Carolina.)

multiple colony selection can be time-consuming, it can be expected to increase the probability of recovering coagulase-positive organisms. Most hospital laboratories report coagulase-negative staphylococci as S. epidermidis, but at least 14 species of Staphylococcus are coagulase-negative, and others are currently under investigation.[23]

The recommended test for coagulase activity, which is performed in a test tube, detects the presence of free coagulase. Because the test requires isolated staphylococcal colonies, identification of S. aureus could take up to 48 hours. Although a slide test for bound coagulase or clumping factor is not as definitive, it can be used as a screening procedure. The method employs a heavy suspension of the colony in distilled water and a drop of rabbit plasma. Observable clumping occurs within 10 minutes if bound coagulase is present. If this test is negative, the slide tube test should be performed.

A recently developed screening test that differentiates S. aureus from S. epidermidis and other micrococci appears to be both rapid and reliable.[24] The method employs an extracellular mixture of proteins produced by S. staphylolyticus.[25] The mixture, called lysostaphin, contains a lytic peptidase that acts on the bridging pentapeptides of staphylococcal cell walls.[26,27] S. aureus and S. epidermidis differ in the quantities of serine and glycine in the pentapeptide moieties of cell-wall peptidoglycans.[28–31] The differences in amino acid content are reflected in differences in sensitivity to lysostaphin. When small aliquots of diluted broth cultures of S. aureus are mixed with lysostaphin (final concentration of 2 μg/ml) and incubated for 30 min at 37°C, the organisms are lysed (Fig. 20–2). As with any characteristic of a microorganism, there can be exceptions. Lysostaphin-resistant strains of S. aureus have been encountered in the clinical laboratory.[24,32] The test tube test for coagulase should be performed on lysostaphin-resistant strains of S. aureus. Most screening procedures have their limitations, but their use can be justified in life-threatening situations.

Strains of S. aureus grow in 7.5% sodium chloride, ferment mannitol, produce catalase, and usually exhibit deoxyribonuclease activity. A typical micrococcus differs in several ways from a staphylococcus, but most notably, it lacks the ability to ferment glucose anaerobically (Table 20–2).

Phage Typing and Antibiograms

Phage typing and antibiograms have been valuable in epidemiologic studies of infectious disease caused by staphylococci; however, many different phage types are represented by toxigenic strains of S. aureus.[16] The isolation of staphylococcal exotoxin could be a useful marker for identifying strains of S. aureus capable of causing TSS.[8]

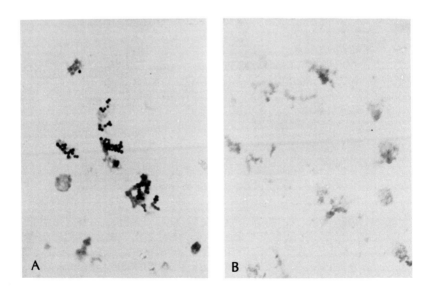

Figure 20–2.   A. Gram stain of a culture of S. aureus. **B.** Gram stain of the same culture after exposure to lysostaphin at 2 μg/ml. (From Severance, P.J., Kauffman, C.A., and Sheagren, J.N.: Rapid identification of Staphylococcus aureus by using lysostaphin sensitivity. J. Clin. Microbiol., *11*:724, 1980.)

Table 20–2. Characteristics for differentiating Staphylococci from Micrococci.

Genus and/or Species	Resistance to*		Acid (aerobically) from glycerol-erythromycin medium (0.4 µg erythromycin/ml)*	Growth on selective medium of Schleifer and Kramer†	Modified oxidase and benzidine tests‡
	Lysozyme (25 µg/ml)	Lysostaphin (200 µg/ml)			
Staphylococcus	+	−	+/− (rare)	+	−
S. sciuri	+	−/±	+/− (rare)	+	+
Micrococcus	−/+	+/±	−	−	+
M. kristinae	+	+	+/−	±	+

*Methods described by Schleifer and Kloos. Lysozyme and lysostaphin susceptibilities could be alternatively tested by using impregnated discs.
†Composition and preparation of medium described by Schleifer and Kramer. Selective agents included sodium azide, potassium thiocyanate, lithium chloride, and glycine.
‡Methods described by Faller and Schleifer.

The availability of a test for toxigenicity that can be applied to suspected strains of S. aureus in the hospital laboratory awaits additional study, however.

Negative cultures, chemical analyses that detect abnormalities in organ systems, or specific serologic tests can be significant in the differential diagnosis of TSS. Elevated levels of BUN or creatinine with sterile pyuria are seen frequently in TSS. Elevated levels of serum bilirubin, serum glutamic oxalic transaminase (SGOT), and/or serum glutamic pyruvic transaminase (SGPT) occur when there is hepatic involvement. Thrombocytopenia, leukocytosis with a shift to the left, and normochromic, normocytic anemia are sometimes present. Rocky mountain spotted fever, leptospirosis, measles, Kawasaki syndrome, and Reye syndrome need to be ruled out in a diagnosis of TTS. The causes of Kawasaki and Reye syndromes are unknown. In Kawasaki syndrome, multiple organs are involved, but findings do not include azotemia or hypovolemic shock.[33] A viral infection precedes Reye syndrome. Although multiple organs may be affected in Reye syndrome, it is most frequently described as an acute encephalopathy of children. Only rarely is significant azotemia found.[34]

PROGNOSIS

The prognosis of TSS is largely dependent on the time elapsing between first symptoms and the time medical aid is sought. With institution of aggressive therapy, including administration of intravenous fluids to maintain blood pressure, most patients respond favorably in 4 or 5 days.[34] Desquamation of the skin occurs 1 or 2 weeks after onset of symptoms (Fig. 20–3). The risk of a primary or secondary attack can be significantly reduced if tampons are not used or are used intermittently during menses.

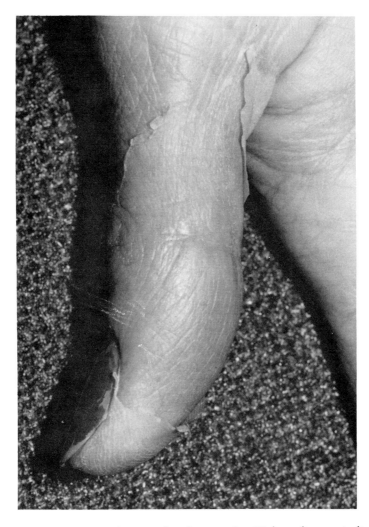

Figure 20–3. Desquamation on a thumb, occurring 12 days after onset of toxic-shock syndrome. (From Thomas, S.W., Baird, I.M., and Frazier, R.D.: Toxic shock syndrome following submucous resection and rhinoplasty. JAMA, 247:2402, 1982. Copyright 1982, American Medical Association.)

CASE REPORTS

Case 1

A 40-year-old woman was seen in October, 1979, because of fever and low blood pressure. The patient had had a sore throat and fever during 2 previous menstrual cycles, beginning in May, 1979. She was treated with penicillin during one of these episodes. She became ill again in October, 1 day following the onset of her menstrual period. Dysuria, chills, fever, myalgia, vomiting, and diarrhea developed. She was admitted to a local hospital 2 days after becoming ill. On admission, she was febrile, her skin was flushed and she was hypotensive, with orthostatic light-headedness. She had pyuria and was treated for a urinary tract infection with co-trimoxazole and cefazolin. Over the next 12 hours her blood pressure remained 60/40 mm of mercury, her fever persisted, and the diffuse redness increased.

The patient was referred to a regional hospital. On admission there, blood pressure was 80/40 mm of mercury, temperature was 38.9°C (102°F), and her respiratory rate was 22 per minute. The most striking aspects of her appearance were a generalized erythema and edema of the face. The patient was irritable, uncooperative, and in considerable discomfort from diffuse pain. However, she was mentally alert and her recent memory appeared intact. Also noted were a diffuse redness of the throat without edema, supple neck, clear chest, bilateral costovertebral angle tenderness and unremarkable heart sounds. There was bilateral lower quadrant tenderness of the abdomen with questionable rebound in the left lower quadrant, but there was no distention. No circumoral pallor was noted, nor were the conjunctiva noted to be injected. A foul-smelling tampon was removed. Findings of a pelvic examination included a mucopurulent vaginal discharge and a uterus that was very tender on manipulation.

Laboratory findings on admission were serum creatinine 4.1 mg/ dl, BUN 57.9 mg/dl, direct bilirubin 1.0 mg/dl, indirect bilirubin 0.3 mg/dl, alkaline phosphatase 258 IU/L (normal, 546 IU/L), SGPT within normal limits, CPK within normal limits, hemoglobin 9.4 g/dl, leukocyte count 10,400 per cu mm with 26% segmented neutrophils and 70% bands, triglycerides 298 mg/dl (normal, 155 mg/dl), albumin 3.5 g/dl (normal, 2.9 g/dl), calcium 6.6 mg/dl, phosphorus 4.1 mg/dl, hilar infiltrates especially on left on x-ray of the chest, prothrombin time 12.5 seconds (control 16 seconds), partial prothrombin time <40 seconds (normal, 44 seconds), fibrinogen/fibrin split products 275/ negative, and platelet count 93,000 per cu mm.

Analysis of urine showed a pH of 5, 5 to 8 leukocytes per high-power field, and proteinuria (1 +). Electrolyte values included sodium 124, potassium 3.9, chloride 92, and carbon dioxide content 18 mEq per liter. Antistreptolysin (ASO) titer was negative. Vaginal cultures were positive for Staphylococcus aureus and Klebsiella pneumoniae. Blood, urine, and pharynx cultures were negative. An x-ray study of the chest and intravenous pyelogram (IVP) done on admission showed no abnormalities. The electrocardiogram indicated sinus tachycardia and nonspecific ST-T changes.

During her first 24 hours in the regional hospital she was treated with ampicillin and gentamicin and was given supportive care. The patient's irritability and uncooperativeness improved, and she became afebrile. On the day after admission the following occurred: a spontaneous diuresis of 4 liters with the patient's weight dropping from 57 to 54 kg, resolution of the generalized edema, the appearance of a macular rash and the development of mild dyspnea associated with perihilar infiltrates on x-ray studies of the chest. By discharge, these signs had resolved and renal function had returned to normal. Abdominal tenderness persisted 2 days into the hospital stay. The patient reported peeling of the skin of her hands following discharge from the hospital.*

Case 2

A 17-year-old woman was admitted to the Wilmington Medical Center on November 2, 1980, with the chief complaints of fever and malaise of 5 days' duration. She had been well until October 27, 1980, when she developed a dry cough and sore throat. On October 29, she felt flushed; during the day she vomited twice. She felt intermittently better and worse during the next day, and sought the attention of her family physician. A throat culture was taken, and amoxicillin and Actifed (Burroughs Wellcome) were started.

On November 1, she awakened feeling "stiff and sore all over," with fever during the day between 104 and 105°F (40 and 40.5°C). In addition, she noticed that her hands were swollen and her palms bright red. Her feet and perineum were also red; the skin in these areas began peeling that day. Her eyes were red and burned. She remained in bed throughout the day, with little appetite and taking only a small quantity of liquids. Her fever and malaise continued. She was admitted to the hospital on the night of November 2.

In addition to fever, malaise, and rash, she described a yellow, stringy, vaginal discharge which had been present for 3 days, beginning October 29 and ending November 1. She denied any diarrhea. She was sexually active, using foam and condoms for birth control. During her menstrual periods, she used Playtex tampons (International Playtex Incorporated), changing them every 4 to 6 hours. She

---

*From Tanner, M.H., Pierce, B.J., and Hale, D.C.: West. J. Med., *134*:477–484, 1981.[36]

had used these tampons throughout her most recent menstrual period. She had never had a pelvic examination.

A similar illness, albeit less severe, had occurred 1 month prior to admission. This illness, which also was during her menstrual period, was also associated with a red, peeling rash, and, in addition, with diarrhea. It resolved spontaneously within a week of its onset.

Her past medical history was significant in that she had developed a draining pilonidal cyst in the presacral area during June of 1980, which was removed surgically in August, 1980.

Physical examination on admission revealed a weak and pallid 17-year-old female whose temperature was 38.8°C. Her pulse was 150; her respiratory rate, 24; and her blood pressure, 100/60. A rash resembling sunburn was present on her palms and a desquamating rash on her toes. Her bulbar and palpebral conjunctiva were moderately injected. Her tongue seemed enlarged and slightly injected, and was tender to palpation. Examination of her perineum revealed a 10 × 10 cm area of erythema with peripheral desquamation. The vaginal mucosa and cervix appeared normal, but there was a copious mucopurulent discharge emanating from the cervical os. Her uterus was normal in size and nontender as was the right adnexal area; the left adnexal area was moderately tender.

Total WBC was 14,300/cmm with 60% polymorphonuclear leukocytes and 26% bands. Hemoglobin was 10.4 gm/dl. Urinalysis revealed 100 to 200 WBCs per high-power field. The serum SGOT was 43 IU/L. LDH was 136 IU/L and alkaline phosphatase was 175 IU/L. Throat culture taken on October 30 was negative for pathogens. Gram stain of the endocervical discharge showed only numerous pus cells and no bacteria. The patient was treated with cephalothin and gentamicin as well as intravenous fluids after cultures of the urine and endocervix were performed. She responded well; a day later she was afebrile and felt much stronger. Three days after admission she was eating and walking without difficulty. At that time, her palms began to peel.

When the endocervical and urine cultures were both reported to have grown Staphylococcus aureus, the gentamicin and cephalothin were discontinued, and the patient continued on oral cloxacillin to complete a 10-day course of antibiotics. The staphylococcal organisms were sent to the Centers for Disease Control in Atlanta for phage-group typing.*

Case 3

A 31-year-old woman underwent bilateral breast augmentation in September, 1980. Subsequently, a superficial wound infection devel-

---

*From Abrahamsen, C.E.: Del. Med. J., 53:9–10, 1981.[37]

oped in the left breast, which was treated initially with local care and oral antibiotics. However, at the end of 4 weeks, the incision had failed to heal satisfactorily, and a second operation to remove granulation tissue was done. Within 24 hours of this procedure, the patient noted the sudden onset of profuse watery diarrhea, vomiting, severe myalgias, and generalized weakness.

When the patient was examined in the emergency room she was found to be cyanotic and obtunded, with a rectal temperature of 38.9°C and an unobtainable blood pressure. Minimal purulent drainage was noted from the left breast incision, and a culture of the fluid yielded S. aureus that was resistant to ampicillin and penicillin. During the next 24 hours, a fiery-red pharyngitis, bilateral conjunctival hyperemia, and a macular erythroderma over the patient's chest, neck, and arms developed. Laboratory studies disclosed a WBC count of 22,000/cm mm, with 40% segmented neutrophils and 52% band-form cells; a platelet count of 12,500/cm mm; urine containing 20 to 30 WBCs per high-power field; and proteinuria (4+). Additional laboratory results included a BUN level of 30 mg/dl; serum creatinine level of 7.3 mg/dl; SGOT level of 207 units/ml; total bilirubin level of 12.8 mg/dl; creatine phosphokinase level of 3100 IU/L; and serum calcium level of 5.7 mg/dl. Blood cultures yielded no organisms, and cultures of the throat, anterior nares, and vagina were negative for S. aureus. The patient was treated initially with cefamandole nafate and gentamicin sulfate. Despite vasopressors and massive volumes of intravenous fluids, the patient's urinary output remained low, and she required peritoneal dialysis. The left breast incision was reopened, the prosthesis removed, and the wound irrigated thoroughly. Subsequently, adult respiratory distress syndrome developed and she required ventilatory assistance with positive end-expiratory pressure to maintain adequate oxygenation. The patient's medical condition was improving by the sixth hospital day, when desquamation over the neck, face, and chest began. Ten days after the onset of her illness, while making good progress toward recovery, bilateral pneumonia with Pseudomonas aeruginosa developed. The patient died 4 days later; no autopsy was performed.*

SUMMARY

The disease entity known as toxic-shock syndrome (TSS) is caused by toxigenic strains of Staphylococcus aureus, which often colonize the vaginal tract of women. Most TSS patients have been young, white, menstruating women who use tampons, but TSS also occurs in a variety of clinical situations. Although two exotoxins have been iso-

---

*From Bartlett, P., et al.: JAMA, *247*:1448–1450, 1982. Copyright 1982, American Medical Association.[38]

lated from cultures taken from TSS patients, recent evidence has shown them to be immunologically identical. A specific role for the toxins in the pathogenesis of TSS has not been demonstrated. Clinically recognizable disease may depend on host susceptibility or another toxin in a synergistic role. The risk of TSS can be reduced by discouraging or limiting the use of tampons. Recovery from TSS is dependent on prompt medical attention after onset of symptoms.

REFERENCES

1. Todd, J., Fishaut, M., Kapral, F., and Welch, T.: Toxic-shock syndrome associated with phage-group I staphylococci. Lancet, *2*:1116, 1978.
2. Shands, K.N., et al.: Toxic-shock syndrome in menstruating women: its association with tampon use and Staphylococcus aureus and the clinical features in 52 cases. N. Engl. J. Med., *303*:1436, 1980.
3. Tofte, R., and Williams, D.: Toxic-shock syndrome: clinical and laboratory features in 15 patients. Ann. Intern. Med., *94*:149, 1981.
4. Tofte, R., and Crossley, K.: Clinical experience with toxic shock syndrome. N. Engl. J. Med., *303*:1417, 1980.
5. Lentino, J.R., Rytel, M.W., and Davis, J.P.: Serologic evidence of noninvasive nature of S. aureus infection in toxic-shock syndrome. N. Engl. J. Med., *305*:641, 1981.
6. Bergdoll, M.S., Crass, B.A., Reiser, R.F., and Davis, J.P.: A new staphylococcal enterotoxin, enterotoxin F, associated with toxic-shock syndrome S. aureus isolates. Lancet, *1*:1017, 1981.
7. Centers for Disease Control: Follow-up on toxic-shock syndrome—United States. Morbid. Mortal. Weekly Rept., *29*:297, 1980.
8. Schlievert, P.M., Shands, K.N., Dan, B.B., and Nishimura, R.D.: Identification and characterization of an exotoxin from Staphylococcus aureus associated with toxic-shock syndrome. J. Infect. Dis., *143*:509, 1981.
9. Brunson, K.W., and Watson, D.W.: Pyrogenic specificity of streptococcal exotoxins, staphylococcal enterotoxin, and gram-negative endotoxin. Infect. Immun., *10*:347, 1974.
10. Sugiyama, H., McKissic, E.M., Jr., Bergdoll, M.S., and Heller, B.: Enhancement of bacterial endotoxin lethality by staphylococcal enterotoxin. J. Infect. Dis., *114*:111, 1964.
11. Peavy, D.L., Adler, W.H., and Smith, R.T.: The mitogenic effects of endotoxin and staphylococcal enterotoxin B on mouse spleen cells and human peripheral lymphocytes. J. Immunol., *115*:49, 1975.
12. Bonventre, P.F., et al.: Production of staphylococcal enterotoxins F and pyrogenic exotoxin C by Staphylococcus aureus isolates from toxic shock syndrome-associated sources. Infect. Immun., *40*:1023, 1983.
13. Centers for Disease Control: Follow-up on toxic-shock syndrome. Morbid. Mortal. Weekly Rept., *29*:441, 1980.
14. Centers for Disease Control: Toxic-shock syndrome, United States, 1970–1980. Morbid. Mortal. Weekly Rept., *30*:25, 1981.
15. Rotheram, E.B.: Nonvenereal infections of the female genitalia. *In* Medical Microbiology and Infectious Disease. Edited by A.I. Braude. Philadelphia, W.B. Saunders, 1981.
16. Green, S.L., and La Peter, K.S.: Evidence for postpartum toxic-shock syndrome in a mother-infant pair. Am. J. Med., *72*:169, 1982.
17. Centers for Disease Control: Toxic-shock syndrome, United States, 1970–1982. Morbid. Mortal. Weekly Rept., *31*:201, 1982.
18. Chapman, G.H., Berens, C., Peters, A., and Curcio, L.: Coagulase and hemolysin tests as measures of the pathogenicity of staphylococci. J. Bacteriol., *28*:343, 1934.
19. Cruickshank, R.: Staphylocoagulase. J. Pathol. Bacteriol., *45*:295, 1937.
20. Baird-Parker, A.C.: The basis of the present classification of staphylococci and micrococci. Ann. N.Y. Acad. Sci., *236*:7, 1974.
21. Smith, W.J., Hale, H., and Smith, M.M.: The role of coagulase in staphylococcal infections. Br. J. Exp. Pathol., *28*:57, 1947.
22. Gross, T.D., Bergquist, L.M., and Searcy, R.L.: Clinical trial of a new capillary-tube technique for rapid detection of coagulase activity. *In* Antimicrobial Agents

and Chemotherapy. Edited by J.C. Sylvester. Washington, D.C., American Society for Microbiology, 1965.

23. Kloos, W.E.: Coagulase-negative staphylococci. Clin. Microbiol. Newsl., *4*:75, 1982.
24. Severance, P.J., Kauffman, C.A., and Sheagren, J.N.: Rapid identification of Staphylococcus aureus by using lysostaphin sensitivity. J. Clin. Microbiol., *11*:724, 1980.
25. Schindler, C.A., and Schubardt, V.T.: Lysostaphin: a new bacteriolytic agent for the staphylococcus. Proc. Natl. Acad. Sci. U.S.A., *51*:414, 1964.
26. Browder, H.P., Zygmunt, W.A., Young, J.R., and Tavormina, P.A.: Lysostaphin: enzymatic mode of action. Biochem. Biophys. Res. Commun., *19*:383, 1965.
27. Iversen, O.J., and Grov, A.: Studies on lysostaphin: Separation and characterization of three enzymes. Eur. J. Biochem., *38*:293, 1973.
28. Ghuysen, J.M.: Use of bacteriolytic enzymes in determination of wall structure and their role in cell metabolism. Bacteriol. Rev., *32*:425, 1968.
29. Ghuysen, J.M., Tipper, D.J., Birge, C.H., and Strominger, J.L.: Structure of the cell wall of Staphylococcus aureus strain Copenhagen. VI. The soluble glycopeptide and its sequential degradation by peptidases. Biochemistry, *4*:2245, 1965.
30. Tipper, D.J.: Structure of the cell wall peptidoglycan of Staphylococcus epidermidis Texas 26 and Staphylococcus aureus Copenhagen. II. Structure of neutral and basic peptides from hydrolysis with Myxobacter A1-1 peptidase. Biochemistry, *8*:2192, 1969.
31. Zygmunt, W.A., and Tavormina, P.A.: Lysostaphin: model for a specific enzymatic approach to infectious disease. Prog. Drug Res., *16*:309, 1972.
32. Zygmunt, W.A., Browder, H.P., and Tavormina, P.A.: Lytic action of lysostaphin on susceptible and resistant strains of Staphylococcus aureus. Can. J. Microbiol., *13*:845, 1967.
33. Melish, M.E.: Kawasaki syndrome: A new infectious disease? J. Infect. Dis., *143*:317, 1981.
34. Trauner, D.A.: Reye's syndrome. *In* Medical Microbiology and Infectious Diseases. Edited by A.I. Braude. Philadelphia, W.B. Saunders, 1981.
35. DeHertogh, D.: Toxic-shock syndrome. Clin. Microbiol. Newsl., *4*:61, 1982.
36. Tanner, M.H., Pierce, B.J., and Hale, D.C.: Toxic shock syndrome. West. J. Med., *134*:477, 1981.
37. Abrahamsen, C.E.: Toxic-shock syndrome: A case report. Del. Med. J., *53*:9, 1981.
38. Bartlett, P., et al.: Toxic shock syndrome associated with surgical wound infections. JAMA *247*:1448, 1982.

CHAPTER 21 PERSPECTIVES FOR THE FUTURE OF INFECTIOUS DISEASE

Two significant scientific advances during the last decade could have a profound effect on the future of infectious disease. One development, which generates recombinant DNA molecules, has been used by taxonomists for years in determining relatedness of microorganisms.[1] The other, more recent, discovery is a method for fusing plasma cells with mutants of mouse myeloma cells.[2] The products of the fusion, known as hybridomas, can provide readily available sources of antibodies of predefined specificity. The monoclonal antibodies, produced by hybridomas, have been used to elucidate some of the enigmatic intricacies of immune responses.

The development of recombinant DNA and hybridoma techniques has led to the rapidly growing expansion of technologies that can be applied to the diagnosis and control of infectious disease. The two technologies can be expected to have a sizable impact on the incidence of infectious disease in the not too distant future.

RECOMBINANT DNA MOLECULES

Natural mechanisms for the transfer and recombination of genetic material have been recognized for over 40 years. The methods for gene transfer, which include transformation, transduction, and conjugation, occur in nature as random and rare events and only between closely related species of certain microorganisms. In the 1970s, a series of discoveries made it possible to join segments of DNA in vitro to create biologically active recombinant DNA in the form of units known as plasmids.

The construction of recombinant DNA molecules is dependent on enzymes called restriction endonucleases. The endonucleases act on the phosphodiester bonds of specific base sequences. The fragments of DNA can be cloned or mixed with DNA molecules which are self-replicating in a host cell. When pieces of donor and host DNA are mixed, some circular recombinant molecules are formed. Other enzymes, known as DNA ligases, are needed to successfully join the molecules. The recombinant DNA molecules can be introduced into host cells by transformation or transduction. The transplanted genes may function immediately or may require additional engineering.

Eucaryotic donor genes have been successfully incorporated and cloned in both eucaryotic and procaryotic host cells. The bacterium Escherichia coli can host DNA extracted from insulin- or growth-hormone-producing human cells. Insulin and growth hormone, produced in E. coli, are currently undergoing clinical trials in human subjects. The successful transplantation of three types of interferon-producing genes into E. coli and the yeast Saccharomyces cerevisiae was announced in 1980. Interferons are species-specific antiviral proteins normally produced by virus-infected cells. The interferons appear to inhibit synthesis of virus-specific proteins. Interferons are currently being investigated for use in the treatment of some types of cancer and of acquired immune deficiency syndrome (AIDS).

The potential for the insertion of various kinds of recombinant DNA into host microorganisms for use in limiting the spread of infectious disease and controlling neoplastic disease staggers the imagination. It offers an opportunity for the most brilliant scientists to alter the course of evolution by genetic engineering. Already, genetically-modified microorganisms are being used in the development of vaccines. The new technology offers many advantages over conventional methods. Purified antigen can be produced without the time-consuming, and often ineffective, techniques designed to free the antigen from extraneous material. Moreover, it is possible to produce toxins that are antigenic, but not toxic, by gene modification and cloning.

The use of cloned genes can be extended as a definitive technique for the diagnosis of infectious disease. A specific gene can be cloned, cut out, labeled with radioactive material, such as $^{32}PO_4$, and used to detect the same gene in lysed bacterial colonies or in clinical specimens. Radioactive-labeled probes have been employed for the identification of enterotoxigenic strains of Escherichia coli, for the detection of Epstein-Barr virus in lymphoid cell lines, for the demonstration of hepatitis B virus (HBV) in serum, and for screening urine for the presence of human cytomegalovirus (HCV).[3-6] Although such exacting techniques are still expensive and not available to clinical laboratories, there is no doubt that radioactive probes will be a part of the future of diagnostic microbiology. Alternative systems using enzyme reactions also hold promise as DNA probes and are currently under investigation.

MONOCLONAL ANTIBODIES

Until 1975, inoculation of laboratory animals was the only way to produce large quantities of antisera. The in vivo technique has many serious limitations. Not only do individual animals vary in response to the immunogenic material, but polyclonal antibodies are synthesized in the presence of a single species of bacterium.[7] In order to obtain antibody of a single type, it has been necessary to treat antisera produced in animals with time-consuming adsorption techniques. Although antisera of animal origin have been valuable in diagnostic testing, their application in the prevention of infectious disease to date has been limited. Many individuals either react unfavorably to the presence of extraneous material or develop sensitivities to animal proteins.

In hybridoma technology, selected antigens are used to immunize mice or rats. The plasma cells are isolated from the spleens of the immunized animals and fused with mutant mouse myeloma cells. The mutant cells no longer have the ability to produce immunoglobulins so the hybridomas synthesize only the specific antibodies the plasma cells have been programmed to produce. Individual hybridoma cells are cloned and the clones tested for the desired antibody. Hybridoma cells may be frozen and recovered as needed, thereby providing a permanent reservoir for monoclonal antibodies. After cloning and subcloning, yields up to 100 μg/ml of specific antibody can be obtained. Before use, antibodies are separated from hybridomas by centrifugation.

Monoclonal and polyclonal antibody-based reagents have been used to identify a variety of microbial pathogens and particular populations of monocytes and lymphocytes.[8–18] In the future, it is anticipated that such reagents will permit the rapid identification of an increasing number of infectious agents directly from clinical specimens within a few minutes or a few hours. Optimism exists among oncologists that monoclonal antibodies could be the "magic bullets" for treatment of cancer. Investigations are under way at many major cancer centers, and the remissions obtained through the use of cancer-cell-specific monoclonal antibodies are encouraging.

A LOOK AHEAD

Despite the remarkable progress envisioned for the application of recombinant DNA and hybridoma technologies, new infectious microorganisms will evolve, additional antibiotic-resistant strains of microorganisms will emerge, life styles will afford opportunistic modes of transmission, and the pool of susceptible individuals will increase as medical breakthroughs permit people to live longer. Microorganisms will remain formidable enemies of humankind. No end is in sight for the ongoing battle between human hosts and their microbial parasites.

The challenges of infectious disease for health-care personnel and for scientific investigators are clear. The continuum of alterations in parasites and their human hosts is so awesome that the contribution of any single individual to such complex problems appears at times to be minor. It will take the collective diligence and surveillance of all microbial sleuths to minimize the human suffering and economic loss caused by the ever changing patterns of infectious disease.

REFERENCES

1. Wetzel, R.: Applications of recombinant DNA technology. Am. Sci., *68*:664, 1980.
2. Köhler, G., and Milstein, C.: Continuous cultures of fused cells secreting antibody of predefined specificity. Nature, *256*:495, 1975.
3. Moseley, S.L., et al.: Identification of enterotoxigenic Escherichia coli by colony hybridization using three enterotoxin gene probes. J. Infect. Dis., *145*:863, 1982.
4. Brandsma, J., and Miller, G.: Nucleic acid spot hybridization: rapid quantitative screening of lymphoid cell lines for Epstein-Barr viral DNA. Proc. Natl. Acad. Sci. U.S.A., *77*:6851, 1980.
5. Berninger, M., Hammer, M., Hoyer, B., and Gerin, J.L.: An assay for the detection of the DNA genome of hepatitis B virus in serum. J. Med. Virol., *9*:57, 1982.
6. Chou, S., and Merigan, T.C.: Rapid detection and quantitation of human cytomegalovirus in urine through DNA hybridization. N. Engl. J. Med., *308*:921, 1983.
7. McCarthy, L.R.: The impact of new technology on clinical microbiology. Clin. Microbiol. Newsl., *5*:68, 1983.
8. Alves, M.J., Aikawa, M., and Nussenzweig, R.S.: Monoclonal antibodies to Trypanosoma cruzi inhibit motility and nucleic acid synthesis of culture forms. Infect. Immun., *39*:377, 1983.
9. Greenblatt, C.L., Slutky, G.M., de Ibarra, A.A., and Snary, D.: Monoclonal antibodies for serotyping Leishmania strains. J. Clin. Microbiol., *18*:191, 1983.
10. Polin, R.A., and Kennett, R.: Use of monoclonal antibodies in an enzyme immunoassay for rapid identification of group B Streptococcus types II and III. J. Clin. Microbiol., *11*:332, 1980.
11. Nachamkin, I., Cannon, J.G., and Mittler, R.S.: Monoclonal antibodies against Neisseria gonorrhoeae: production of antibodies directed against a strain-specific cell surface antigen. Infect. Immun., *32*:641, 1981.
12. Robertson, S.M., et al.: Monoclonal antibodies directed against a cell-surface exposed outer membrane protein of Haemophilus influenzae, type b. Infect. Immun., *36*:80, 1982.
13. Robertson, S.M., Kettman, J.R., Miller, J.N., and Norgard, M.V.: Murine monoclonal antibodies specific for virulent Treponema pallidum (Nichols). Infect. Immun., *36*:1076, 1982.
14. Goldstein, L.C., et al.: Monoclonal antibodies to cytomegalovirus: rapid identification of clinical isolates and preliminary use in diagnosis of cytomegalovirus pneumonia. Infect. Immun., *38*:273, 1982.
15. Stamm, W.E., Tam, M., Koester, M., and Cles, L.: Detection of Chlamydia trachomatis inclusions in McCoy cell cultures with fluorescein-conjugated monoclonal antibodies. J. Clin. Microbiol., *17*:666, 1983.
16. Cukor, G., Perron, D.M., Hudson, R., and Blacklow, N.R.: Detection of rotavirus in human stools by using monoclonal antibody. J. Clin. Microbiol., *19*:888, 1984.
17. Maruyama, S., et al.: Preparation of a monoclonal antibody against human monocyte lineage. J. Clin. Immunol., *3*:57, 1983.
18. Kung, P.C., Goldstein, G., Reinherz, E.L., and Schlossman, S.F.: Monoclonal antibodies defining distinctive human T cell surface antigens. Science, *206*:347, 1979.

INDEX

Page numbers in *italics* indicate figures; page numbers followed by t indicate tables.